T0262077

以史為鑒

為《中國心胸外科·歷史與現狀》題

韓啟德 二〇〇七年元旦

# *"History is our mirror."*

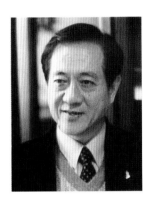

**Professor Qi-De Han**
Vice-chairman, Standing Committee of the National People's Congress of China
Chairman, Chinese Association for Science and Technology
President, Peking University Health Science Center
Director, Peking University Institute of Cardiovascular Sciences
Member, Chinese Academy of Science

**韓啟德教授**
全國人民代表大會常務委員會副委員長
中國科技協會主席
北京大學醫學部主任
北京大學心血管研究所所長
生理學教授
中國科學院院士

# CARDIOTHORACIC SURGERY IN CHINA

## Past, Present and Future

*Edited by*

Song Wan
Anthony P. C. Yim

## The Chinese University Press

*Cardiothoracic Surgery in China: Past, Present and Future*
Edited by Song Wan and Anthony P. C. Yim

© **The Chinese University of Hong Kong**, 2007

ISBN-10: 962–996–321–3
ISBN-13: 978–962–996–321–7

**THE CHINESE UNIVERSITY PRESS**
The Chinese University of Hong Kong
SHA TIN, N.T., HONG KONG
Fax: +852 2603 6692
    +852 2603 7355
E-mail: cup@cuhk.edu.hk
Web-site: www.chineseupress.com

Printed in Hong Kong

# Contents

Foreword (*Michael E. DeBakey*) . . . . . . . . . . . . . . . . . . . . . . . . . .   viii

Foreword (*Arthur K C Li*) . . . . . . . . . . . . . . . . . . . . . . . . . . . . .   x

Preface . . . . . . . . . . . . . . . . . . . . . . . . . . . . . . . . . . . . . . . .   xiii

The Editors . . . . . . . . . . . . . . . . . . . . . . . . . . . . . . . . . . . . .   xvi

List of Contributors . . . . . . . . . . . . . . . . . . . . . . . . . . . . . . .   xvii

### Prologue   The Legacy of Three Thoracic Surgeons

"A Surgeon and Something More"—Dr. Jia-Si Huang . . . . . .   1
   *Song Wan, Anthony P. C. Yim*

Ying-Kai Wu and His Two Decisions . . . . . . . . . . . . . . . . . . . . .   27
   *Song Wan, Anthony P. C. Yim*

Dr. Norman Bethune in China: 1938–1939 . . . . . . . . . . . . . . . .   47
   *Larry Hannant*, with *Editorial Comments*

### Section 1   The Development of Cardiothoracic Surgery in China

The Evolution of Cardiovascular Surgery in China . . . . . . . . .   80
   *Song Wan, Anthony P. C. Yim*

The Historical Perspective of Surgery for Congenital
Heart Disease . . . . . . . . . . . . . . . . . . . . . . . . . . . . . . . . . . . .   113
   *Wen-Xiang Ding*

The History, Current Status and Future of Coronary
Heart Disease . . . . . . . . . . . . . . . . . . . . . . . . . . . . . . . . . . . .   134
   *Qing-Yu Wu, Ming-Kui Zhang*

The Made-in-China Mechanical Valve Prostheses . . . . . . . . . . 143
  *Bao-Ren Zhang, Zhi-Yun Xu, Jian-Zhou Xing*

The History of Cardiothoracic Surgery at the Shanghai
Chest Hospital . . . . . . . . . . . . . . . . . . . . . . . . . . . . . . . . . . . 154
  *Ying-Ze Li*

The Development of Thoracic Surgery at Peking Union
Medical College . . . . . . . . . . . . . . . . . . . . . . . . . . . . . . . . . . 167
  *Le-Tian Xu, Qi Miao*

The Development of Esophageal Surgery in China . . . . . . . . . 174
  *Guo-Jun Huang*

The Surgical Treatment of Pulmonary Tuberculosis in
China . . . . . . . . . . . . . . . . . . . . . . . . . . . . . . . . . . . . . . . . . . . 192
  *Yu-Ling Xin, Xiao-Jia Chen*

Open Heart Operation under Acupuncture Anesthesia . . . . . 198
  *Yi-Shan Wang*

The Evolution of Cardiology in China . . . . . . . . . . . . . . . . . . 204
  *Tsung O. Cheng*

### Section 2   Current Status

Minimally Invasive Thoracic Surgery—A Personal
Perspective . . . . . . . . . . . . . . . . . . . . . . . . . . . . . . . . . . . . . . . 306
  *Anthony P. C. Yim*

Heart Transplantation in China . . . . . . . . . . . . . . . . . . . . . . . 311
  *Wang-Fu Zang*

Lung Transplantation in China . . . . . . . . . . . . . . . . . . . . . . . . 314
  *Song-Lei Ou, Song Wan*

Cellular Therapy for Heart Failure . . . . . . . . . . . . . . . . . . . . . 322
  *Ren-Ke Li, Chung-Dann Kan*

The Evolution of Mitral Valve Surgery: 1902–2002 . . . . . . . . . . 354
  *Lawrence H. Cohn, Edward G. Soltesz*

Mitral Valve Surgery in China: Where Are We Now? . . . . . . . 371
  *Xu Meng, Song Wan*

Cardiology in China: Current Status and New Trends . . . . . . 380
  *Shu Zhang, Ming-Zhe Chen*

## Section 3    Forging Global Links

Forging a Link  . . . . . . . . . . . . . . . . . . . . . . . . . . . . . . . . . . . .    396
  *Thomas B. Ferguson*

Pediatric Cardiovascular Surgery: Project Hope and the
Shanghai Children's Medical Center  . . . . . . . . . . . . . . . . . . .    408
  *Richard A. Jonas*

My Relationship with China's Cardiac Surgery  . . . . . . . . . . .    431
  *Albert Starr*

China: Personal Reminiscences  . . . . . . . . . . . . . . . . . . . . . . .    440
  *W. Gerald Rainer*

Leo Eloesser: An American Cardiothoracic Surgeon in
China  . . . . . . . . . . . . . . . . . . . . . . . . . . . . . . . . . . . . . . . . . . . .    449
  *Yi-Shan Wang, Tsung O. Cheng*

Forging Global Links: Asian Perspectives  . . . . . . . . . . . . . . .    455
  *Chuen-Neng Lee*

Forging Global Links: European Perspectives  . . . . . . . . . . . .    464
  *Carlos-A. Mestres*

English for Chinese Cardiothoracic Surgeons  . . . . . . . . . . . .    507
  *John R. Benfield*

The Interaction between Chinese and Western Cardiac
Surgery Communities—Reflections on the Personal
Career of a Cardiac Surgeon  . . . . . . . . . . . . . . . . . . . . . . . . .    520
  *Guo-Wei He*

Research Perspectives in Chinese Cardiothoracic Surgery:
Towards the International Standard  . . . . . . . . . . . . . . . . . . . .    556
  *Y. John Gu*

The Development of Cardiothoracic Surgery in China:
A Historical Perspective  . . . . . . . . . . . . . . . . . . . . . . . . . . . . .    565
  *Ray Chu-Jeng Chiu*

A Selective Glossary  . . . . . . . . . . . . . . . . . . . . . . . . . . . . . . . . .    577

# Foreword

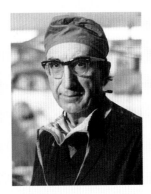

**Michael E. DeBakey, MD**
Chancellor Emeritus
Olga Keith Wiess and Distinguished Service Professor
Michael E. DeBakey Department of Surgery
Director, DeBakey Heart Center, Baylor College of Medicine
Houston, TX, USA
*Past President, American Association for Thoracic Surgery (1958–1959)*

*Cardiothoracic Surgery in China* provides a comprehensive review of this field in China. The book is divided into three sections, the first of which reviews the historical development and current status of surgery in the major centers in China. In addition to the editors' special insight, chapters by a number of Chinese surgical leaders present the development of surgery in specialized areas such as valvular disease, coronary disease, congenital lesions, esophageal and pulmonary diseases. An interesting chapter by one of the authors, Dr. Tsung O. Cheng, relates the evolution of cardiology in China.

The second section, "Current Status," emphasizes trends in cardiology and cardiovascular surgery, such as transplantation, cellular therapy and minimally invasive valve surgery. This section also includes a chapter on minimally invasive thoracic surgery.

In the final section, entitled "Forging Global Links," a chapter describes a visit by Dr. Leo Eloesser to China. Another chapter concerns the experiences of Dr. Norman Bethune [editors' note: this chapter has been moved to the *Prologue* section] and other well-recognized authors regarding specialized areas in cardiovascular surgery in relation to China.

This is a fascinating textual resource that has been compiled by the editors, who have assembled Chinese expertise in cardiovascular surgery. The editors deserve high commendation for their efforts to demonstrate that no real borders exist in medicine.

*Michael E. DeBakey*, MD

# *Foreword*

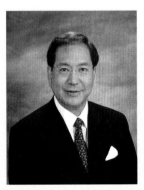

**Professor the Honourable Arthur K C Li**
**Emeritus Professor of Surgery, The Chinese University of Hong Kong**
**Secretary for Education and Manpower, Hong Kong SAR**
GBS; BA(Cantab); MA(Cantab); MB BChir(Cantab); MD(Cantab); HonDSc(Hull);
HonDLitt(HKUST); HonDoc(Soka); HonLLD(CUHK); HonDSc(Med)(UCL);
HonLLD(UWE); FRCS; FRCSEd; FRACS; FCSHK; FHKAM(Surgery); HonFPCS;
HonFRCSGlas; HonFRSM; HonFRCS(I); HonFACS; HonFRCP(Lon); HonFCSHK; JP

There is an old Chinese saying: "When one drinks the water, one should think of its source." In other words, to understand the present development, one should consider its history. The editors and contributors of *Cardiothoracic Surgery in China* has reviewed the history, present development and charted the course of cardiothoracic surgery in China. They have given us invaluable insight into the status and potential of cardiothoracic surgery in China.

Without doubt, this is an important resource for surgeons who wish to have a global perspective and who wish to understand specialized healthcare for a quarter of the people living on this planet.

The editors are to be congratulated for the work well done.

*Arthur K C Li*

# *Preface*

"以古為鏡，可以知興替；以人為鏡，可以明得失。"

*"We can use history as a mirror to reflect the vicissitude of society; we can use people as a mirror to judge the good from the bad."*

The above quotation is from the Tang Dynasty (618–907 AD), which represents one of the most glorious periods in ancient Chinese history. Professor Han's calligraphy on the first page of this book is an adaptation from this quote which emphasizes the importance of history. Harry S. Truman, the 33rd American president, once pointed out, "There is nothing new in the world, except the history you don't know." His sentiment in fact echoed nicely the Chinese saying.

The history of the development of cardiothoracic surgery in China is not widely known to the West, as there have been few publications on this subject in the English language. Moreover, very often we might not even realize how little we actually know about the true history of a given period in a given region, especially in developing countries. One of the editors (S. W.) got this feeling during a long conversation in 1998 with the late Professor Ying-Kai Wu at Anzhen Hospital, Beijing.

Deeply moved by Dr. Wu's personal account, we both felt this story should be shared with colleagues worldwide. This was the beginning of a small series of *Surgical Heritage articles*, which subsequently appeared in *The Annals of Thoracic Surgery*. To our delighted surprise, the response to these articles from our peers around the world was very positive and the response from our Chinese colleagues was overwhelming. The feedback from our readership was a powerful impetus encouraging us to move forward, and the idea of editing a book on this subject was born. However, true history may sometimes be difficult to ascertain. We started to appreciate the importance of making an accurate and complete record of this piece of medical history. We believed it essential to obtain the information first hand from those individuals who made history.

This book is a tribute to the crusading spirit of many people, Chinese and non-Chinese alike, who struggled to establish cardiothoracic surgery in China as we know it today. Editing this book has been an enriching experience, a labor of love, and a journey of discovery. It would not have been possible without the help and support of many dedicated colleagues. We are deeply grateful to our contributors—all of them are acknowledged experts and leaders in our specialty. By accepting our invitation, they took time from their busy work schedules to share with us their experiences.

We also wish to express our heartfelt gratitude to many Chinese cardiothoracic pioneers, whose names are not listed as contributors but whose expertise and guidance have been invaluable. They include Professors Jia-Qiang Guo (郭加強), Mei-Hsin Shih (石美鑫), Hong-Xi Su (蘇鴻熙), Yan-Qing Sun (孫衍慶), Wei-Yong Liu (劉維永), and Xiao-Dong Zhu (朱曉東). We are also grateful to the many colleagues and friends who helped us with this project, including Professors Sheng-Shou Hu (胡盛壽), Zhao-Su Wu (吳兆蘇), Ming-Di Xiao (肖明第), Chang-Qing Gao (高長青), Cun Long (龍村), Yi-Fei Yu (余翼飛), Feng Wan (萬峰), and Qiang Zhao (趙強). Our sincerely thanks are extended to the Chinese Society for Thoracic and Cardiovascular Surgery for their support.

A special thanks must go to the following visiting professors of the Chinese University of Hong Kong for their encouragement and suggestions over the past few years: Denton A. Cooley, MD, Andrew S. Wechsler, MD, Marco I. Turina, MD, and L. Henry Edmunds, Jr, MD.

Last but not least we are indebted to our publisher, the Chinese University Press, and in particular to Mr. Wai-Keung Tse and Mr. Kingsley Ma for their diligence and meticulous editorial assistance.

We recognize there will be unavoidable omissions and oversights in this volume. We earnestly invite readers to give us their comments and advice so that we may be able to improve on the contents for the planned Chinese edition.

Song Wan, Anthony P. C. Yim

# *The Editors*

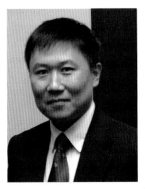

**Song Wan, MD, PhD, FRCS (萬松)**
Associate Professor, Division of Cardiothoracic Surgery
The Chinese University of Hong Kong
Prince of Wales Hospital
Hong Kong, China

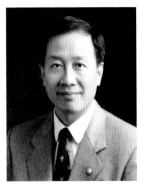

**Anthony P. C. Yim, MD, FRCS, FACS (嚴秉泉)**
Professor of Surgery
The Chinese University of Hong Kong
Hong Kong, China

# *List of Contributors*

**John R. Benfield, MD, FACS**
Professor of Surgery Emeritus
David Geffen School of Medicine at UCLA
Los Angeles, USA
*Past President, Society of Thoracic Surgeons (1996)*

**Ming-Zhe Chen, MD (陳明哲)**
Professor of Medicine (Cardiology)
Tsinghua University School of Medicine
Beijing, China

**Xiao-Jia Chen, MD (陳肖嘉)**
Department of Thoracic Surgery
Beijing Institute for Treatment of Tuberculosis and Thoracic Tumor
Beijing, China

**Tsung O. Cheng, MD (鄭宗鍔)**
Professor of Medicine
George Washington University Medical Center
Washington, D.C., USA

**Ray C. J. Chiu, MD, PhD**
Professor and Chair Emeritus, Department of Cardiothoracic Surgery
Montreal General Hospital, McGill University Health Center
Montreal, Canada

**Lawrence H. Cohn, MD**
Virginia and James Hubbard Professor of Cardiac Surgery
Harvard Medical School
Division of Cardiac Surgery, Brigham and Women's Hospital
Boston, USA
*Past President, American Association for Thoracic Surgery (1998–1999)*

**Wen-Xiang Ding, MD** (丁文祥)
Professor and Surgeon-in-Chief, Department of Cardiovascular Surgery
Shanghai Children's Medical Center
Shanghai, China

**Thomas B. Ferguson, MD**
Professor Emeritus
Washington University School of Medicine
St. Louis, MO, USA
*Past President, Society of Thoracic Surgeons (1977)*
*Past President, American Association for Thoracic Surgery (1981–1982)*

**Y. John Gu, MD, PhD** (顧嚴己)
Cardiopulmonary Surgery Research Division
University Hospital Groningen
The Netherlands

**Larry Hannant, PhD**
Adjunct Associate Professor of History, University of Victoria
Instructor, History, Camosun College, Victoria
British Columbia, Canada

**Guo-Wei He, MD, PhD, DSc** (何國偉)
Clinical Professor of Surgery, Division of Cardiothoracic Surgery
Oregon Health and Science University, Portland, OR, USA
Co-Director, Cardiovascular Research Lab, Department of Surgery
The Chinese University of Hong Kong
Hong Kong, China

**Guo-Jun Huang, MD** (黃國俊)
Professor Emeritus, Department of Thoracic Surgery
Cancer Center of the Chinese Academy of Medical Science
Beijing, China

**Richard A. Jonas, MD**
Cohen Funger Chair of Cardiac Surgery, Children's National Medical
    Center
Co-Director, Children's National Heart Institute
Professor of Surgery, George Washington University Medical School
Washington D.C., USA
*Past President, American Association for Thoracic Surgery (2005–2006)*

**Chung-Dann Kan, MD** (甘宗旦)
Division of Cardiothoracic Surgery, University of Toronto
Toronto General Research Institute
Canada

**Chuen Neng Lee, MD, FRCS, FACC** (李俊能)
Professor & Head, Department of Surgery, National University of Singapore
Director, The Heart Institute, National Healthcare Group
Chief, Department of Surgery and Department of Cardiac, Thoracic & Vascular Surgery
National University Hospital, Singapore

**Ren-Ke Li, MD, PhD** (李仁科)
Professor of Cardiovascular Surgery, University of Toronto
Senior Scientist, Toronto General Research Institute
Canadian Chair of Cardiac Regenerative Medicine
Career Investigator, Heart and Stroke Foundation of Canada
Canada

**Ying-Ze Li, MD** (李穎則)
Professor, Department of Cardiovascular Surgery
Shanghai Chest Hospital
Shanghai, China

**Xu Meng, MD** (孟旭)
Professor, Capital Medical University
Department of Cardiac Surgery, Anzhen Hospital
Beijing, China

**Carlos-A. Mestres, MD, PhD**
Department of Cardiovascular Surgery
Hospital Clinic
Barcelona, Spain

**Qi Miao, MD** (苗齊)
Chief, Department of Cardiovascular Surgery
Beijing Union Hospital (PUMC)
Beijing, China

**Song-Lei Ou, MD** (區頌雷)
Department of Thoracic Surgery
Capital Medical University, Anzhen Hospital
Beijing, China

**W. Gerald Rainer, MD, MS, FACS**
Distinguished Clinical Professor of Surgery, UCHSC
St. Joseph Hospital
Denver, USA
*Past President, Society of Thoracic Surgeons (1990, 1991)*
*Historian, Society of Thoracic Surgeons*

**Albert Starr, MD**
Starr-Wood Cardiac Group of Portland
Professor of Cardiac Surgery, Oregon Health and Science University
Portland, OR, USA
*Past President, Society of Thoracic Surgeons (1986)*

**Edward G. Soltesz, MD**
Harvard Medical School
Division of Cardiac Surgery, Brigham and Women's Hospital
Boston, USA

**Song Wan, MD, PhD, FRCS (萬松)**
Associate Professor, Division of Cardiothoracic Surgery
The Chinese University of Hong Kong
Prince of Wales Hospital
Hong Kong, China

**Yi-Shan Wang, MD (王一山)**
Professor Emeritus, Department of Cardiothoracic Surgery
Renji Hospital, Shanghai Second Medical University
Shanghai, China

**Qing-Yu Wu, MD (吳清玉)**
Professor and Chairman, Department of Cardiovascular Surgery
Tsinghua University School of Medicine
Beijing, China

**Yu-Ling Xin, MD (辛育齡)**
Professor and Director Emeritus
Department of Thoracic Surgery, Sino-Japan Friendship Hospital
Beijing, China

**Jian-Zhou Xing, MD (邢建州)**
Department of Cardiovascular Surgery
Changhai Hospital, Second Military Medical University
Shanghai, China

**Le-Tian Xu, MD** (徐樂天)
Professor and Director Emeritus, Department of Cardiothoracic Surgery
Beijing Union Hospital (PUMC)
Beijing, China

**Zhi-Yun Xu, MD** (徐志雲)
Professor and Chief, Department of Cardiovascular Surgery
Changhai Hospital, Second Military Medical University
Shanghai, China

**Anthony P. C. Yim, MD, FRCS, FACS** (嚴秉泉)
Professor of Surgery
The Chinese University of Hong Kong
Hong Kong, China

**Wang-Fu Zang, MD** (臧旺福)
Professor and Chief, Department of Cardiothoracic Surgery
Shanghai Jiao-Tong University Medical School
Ruijin Hospital, Shanghai, China

**Bao-Ren Zhang, MD** (張寶仁)
Professor and Chairman Emeritus, Department of Cardiovascular Surgery
Changhai Hospital, Second Military Medical University
Shanghai, China

**Ming-Kui Zhang, MD** (張明奎)
Department of Cardiovascular Surgery
Tsinghua University School of Medicine
Beijing, China

**Shu Zhang, MD** (張澍)
Professor and Director, Electrophysiology Unit
Department of Cardiology
The Cardiovascular Institute of Chinese Academy of Medical Sciences
Fuwai Hospital, Beijing, China

# "A Surgeon and Something More" — Dr. Jia-Si Huang

Song Wan, Anthony P. C. Yim

*The growth of thoracic surgery in China was much more difficult than in many industrialized countries over the first five decades because of the ever-changing political and harsh socioeconomic conditions. The struggle to establish this specialty in a developing country with more than one fifth of the world population was certainly one of the most crucial challenges in the last century. The unique story of a pioneering Chinese thoracic surgeon—Dr. Jia-Si Huang (1906–1984)—is a glorious example of heroic leadership and self sacrifice. His fundamental role in developing cardiothoracic surgery in China is clearly reflected not only by some first-in-China operations he personally performed, but also by his continued contributions in educating younger generations of Chinese surgeons.*

Two decades ago, if some senior North American thoracic surgeons were asked to name two of their colleagues in China, the answer might simply have been Huang in the South and Wu in the North. Interestingly, there were many similarities between Doctors Jia-Si Huang (previously spelled as Chia-Ssu Huang) and Ying-Kai Wu. Both of them obtained their general surgical training at Peking Union Medical College (PUMC) and were subsequently trained under two American thoracic surgical leaders in the 1940s (Huang trained with John Alexander and Wu with Evarts A. Graham).

Both of them returned to China at the end of World War II and, during the next four to five decades, they both made fundamental contributions to the development of cardiothoracic surgery in their motherland. Eventually both of them played a leading role in Chinese surgical societies and became highly respected figures, representing thoracic surgeons in China. In fact Jia-Si Huang was the only Chinese surgeon elected to be one of the 229 founder members of the American Board of Thoracic Surgery, whereas Ying-Kai Wu was the only Chinese honorary member of the American Association for Thoracic Surgery (AATS) to date.

In May 1985, exactly one year after the death of Huang, an American thoracic surgical delegation led by Dr. Herbert Sloan (who had just retired as the editor of *The Annals of Thoracic Surgery*) visited Beijing, China. On behalf of the Lyman A. Brewer III International Surgical Society, Dr. Sloan presented two oil paintings to the PUMC and the Chinese Academy of Medical Sciences—portraits of Drs. Huang and Wu (Figs. 1A, 1B), which symbolized the long-term friendship among colleagues of the two countries.

This chapter will highlight the life of Dr. Huang who was not only a great surgeon but also an inspiring mentor and leader for the younger generations of surgeons in China.

## The Man

Jia-Si Huang was born on July 14, 1906 (which was May 23 according to the Chinese lunar calendar) to an intellectual family in Yushan County, Jiangxi Province, China. Both his grandfather and his father were officials of the regional Qing government. He was the fourth son among eight children of the family (five were boys, one younger brother of Huang died at the age of 2 and another elder brother at age 8. Eventually only three of the boys survived beyond childhood). Unfortunately, his father died of massive hemoptysis at the age of 36 when Huang was only 5 years old. Huang's well-educated mother, then 35 years old, brought up her five sons alone and she herself never married again. It's understandable that, being the favorite son (Fig. 2), Huang was deeply influenced by his mother. When Huang

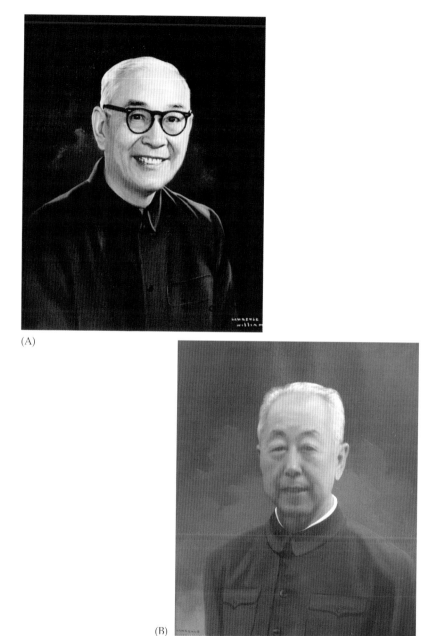

(A)

(B)

*Fig. 1. Gift to PUMC from the Lyman A. Brewer III International Surgical Society in 1985: portraits in oils of [A] Dr. Jia-Si Huang and [B] Dr. Ying-Kai Wu.*

approached 18 years of age, his marriage was pre-arranged (which was then a well accepted tradition in China) by his mother and grandfather. Although reluctant at first, Huang eventually accepted such an arrangement due to his high respect for his mother. His mother died in 1925 when Huang just entered PUMC for pre-medical study. He never met his bride until the wedding day in April 1926 (Fig. 3). Interestingly, the young couple fell in love with each other soon after the wedding and stayed happily together ever after. In fact, apart from Huang's 4-year stay in the US, they were never separated over the following 58 years [1].

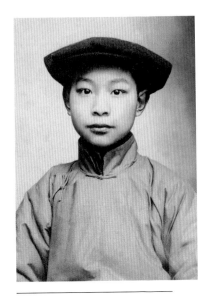

*Fig. 2. Jia-Si Huang in his childhood.*

The decision to pursue medical studies was again not initially made by Huang himself. He showed talent in mathematics and physics early in his primary school days. When he spent his 1-week spring vacation in 1924 with his elder brother in Beijing, Huang was only a first-year high school student. One day when they walked by the beautiful PUMC Chinese-palace-style campus in downtown Beijing (Fig. 4), Huang was casually asked by his brother whether he would like to study there in the future. "Sure," Huang answered without thinking. Six months later, his brother applied to PUMC on behalf of Huang. "Your English is good," Huang was strongly encouraged by the brother. "Why not just try, so that 2 years later you could be better prepared for the real examination?" his brother added. Huang did and was accepted by PUMC (Fig. 5)!

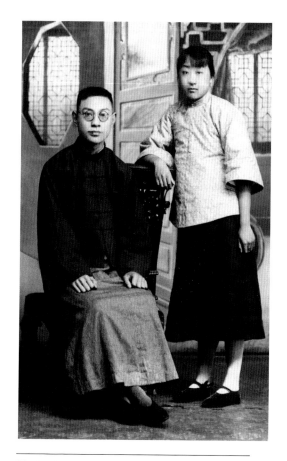

Fig. 3. The wedding of Jia-Si Huang and Chun-Li Xu in April 1926.

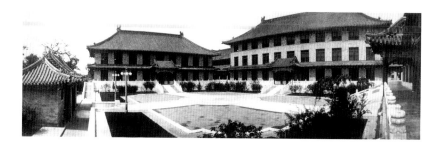

Fig. 4. PUMC in 1924.

**[Historical note]**

*Aimed high from the very beginning, PUMC was established by the China Medical Board of the Rockefeller Foundation to be the "Johns Hopkins in China." At the Dedication Ceremony of PUMC on September 19, 1921, John D. Rockefeller Jr. opened his address by reading a cable from his father:*

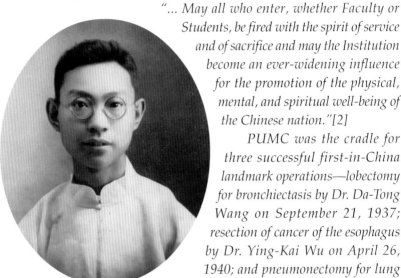

*"... May all who enter, whether Faculty or Students, be fired with the spirit of service and of sacrifice and may the Institution become an ever-widening influence for the promotion of the physical, mental, and spiritual well-being of the Chinese nation."[2]*

*PUMC was the cradle for three successful first-in-China landmark operations—lobectomy for bronchiectasis by Dr. Da-Tong Wang on September 21, 1937; resection of cancer of the esophagus by Dr. Ying-Kai Wu on April 26, 1940; and pneumonectomy for lung cancer by Dr. Ji-Zheng Zhang on March 14, 1941 [3].*

*Fig. 5. Jia-Si Huang at PUMC in 1924.*

Huang graduated from PUMC in 1933. After his 2-year basic surgical training at the same institution, he moved to the National Shanghai Medical College and subsequently became Lecturer in Surgery in 1939—at the same time as Shanghai was invaded by the Japanese troops. The college and its teaching hospital were relocated in 1940 to Kunming and then to Chongqing—two major cities in South China where Huang had a chance to participate in Tsinghua University's selection examination for advanced study in the USA.

**[Historical note]**

*In 1908 the American government rebated the excess amount of the Boxer*

*Indemnity for funding Chinese students to go to the US. Apart from setting up the Office for Selection of Students for America, the Qing government also founded a preparatory school in Beijing. Located in the western suburb of Tsinghua Gardens, the school was thus named Tsinghua School. From 1909 to 1929, some 1,800 Chinese went to the US to study on Boxer Indemnity funds. After the outbreak of the War of Resistance against Japan in 1937, the Nationalist government adopted stringent measures regulating students going abroad for education, and this policy was only relaxed when the Pacific War broke out in 1941. It standardized the qualification for studying abroad through examination. In 1940 a total of 20 students were sent to the US, only one of them for medical training (on a monthly scholarship of US$100).*

Huang successfully passed the exam and became the only candidate selected for medical specialty training. A family picture (Fig. 6) was taken in 1941, just prior to his departure.

On October 23, 1941, he arrived at the University of Michigan in Ann Arbor, Michigan, where the first surgical residency program in thoracic surgery in the US had been established by Dr. John Alexander (Fig. 7, the 17th president of AATS) [4]. It was natural that under Dr. Alexander's guidance (Fig. 8), Jia-Si Huang's study interest was focused on the collapse therapy for pulmonary tuberculosis. He was extremely active not only in the operating rooms but also in the laboratory [5]. In 1943, he received his Master of Science degree (Fig. 9A) and also passed the American Board of Surgery examination (Fig. 9B).

At that juncture, he could have chosen to stay in the US. The easiest path for him was to join the army (a green card could usually be obtained just months after joining the army during wartime). As Huang was already a board-certified thoracic surgeon, the military hospital offered him a job with a monthly salary of US$3,000. However, he decided to return to China to establish thoracic surgery as a specialty there (Fig. 10).

His trip was unfortunately delayed by a disease with which he was only too familiar, namely pulmonary tuberculosis, for which he was hospitalized for several weeks. Then Huang got on the first army

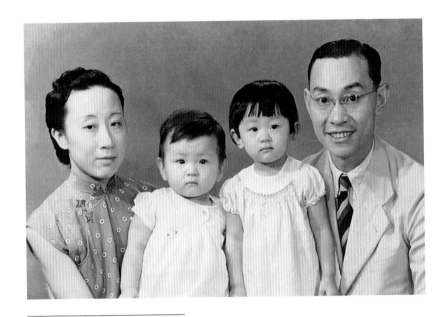

*Fig. 6. Huang's family photo in 1941.*

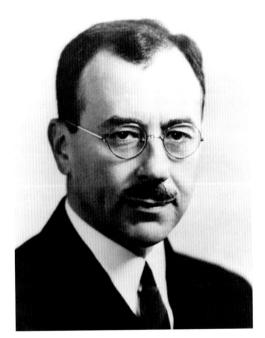

*Fig. 7. John Alexander, MD*

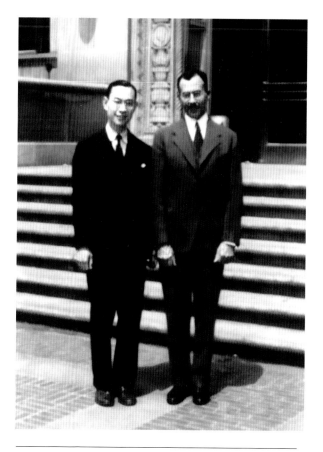

Fig. 8. Drs. Huang and Alexander at the University of Michigan in Ann Arbor, Michigan.

plane across the Pacific Ocean from New York to Chongqing, China on October 23, 1945. Unluckily again, he lost his luggage while stopping in India; his two suitcases were eventually located four months later, and they were empty except for a few papers (i.e., the graduate certificate from PUMC, the Master's degree certificate from the University of Michigan, and the American Board of Surgery certificate). Nevertheless, his hand luggage containing a full set of thoracic surgical instruments was safely brought back home [1].

Between 1945 and 1951 Huang was a professor of surgery at

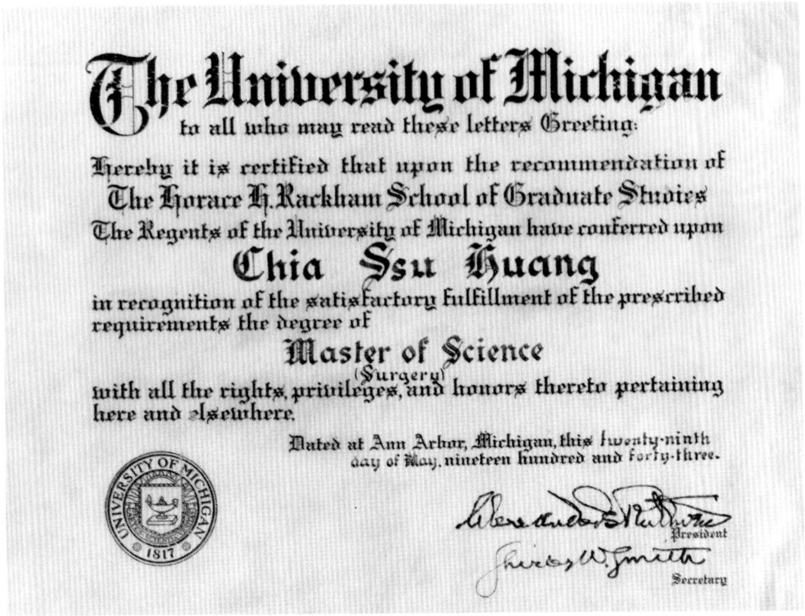

The University of Michigan
to all who may read these letters Greeting:
Hereby it is certified that upon the recommendation of
The Horace H. Rackham School of Graduate Studies
The Regents of the University of Michigan have conferred upon
Chia Ssu Huang
in recognition of the satisfactory fulfillment of the prescribed requirements the degree of
Master of Science
(Surgery)
with all the rights, privileges, and honors thereto pertaining here and elsewhere.
Dated at Ann Arbor, Michigan, this twenty-ninth day of May, nineteen hundred and forty-three.
University of Michigan 1817
President
Secretary

(A)

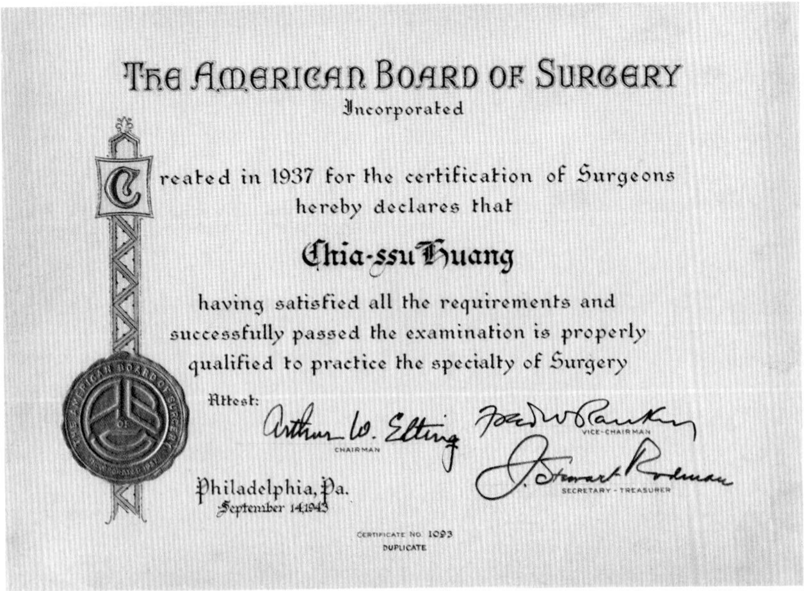

The American Board of Surgery
Incorporated
Created in 1937 for the certification of Surgeons
hereby declares that
Chia-ssu Huang
having satisfied all the requirements and successfully passed the examination is properly qualified to practice the specialty of Surgery
Attest:
Arthur W. Elting
Chairman
Vice-Chairman
Secretary-Treasurer
Philadelphia, Pa.
September 14, 1943
Certificate No. 1093
Duplicate

(B)

Fig. 9. Huang's certificates: [A] Master of Science from the University of Michigan; [B] American Board of Surgery certificate.

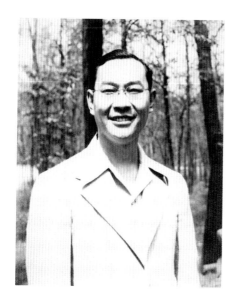

*Fig. 10. Jia-Si Huang in Ann Arbor, Michigan in 1945.*

Shanghai Medical College and the surgeon-in-chief at two hospitals (China Red Cross Hospital and Shanghai Zhongshan Hospital). He was elected the second President of the Chinese Surgical Association in 1947.

The Korean War broke out in the winter of 1950. Huang served at the army hospital and was appointed as the chief of the Shanghai medical team (Fig. 11), oversee more than 300 healthcare workers. During the next six months he and his associates performed 942 operations (including 204 major procedures) at the Second Military Hospital in Northeast China, with an overall surgical mortality rate of 0.6%. Huang was invited to report on his experiences, at a national congress in November 1951 in Beijing. He was seated to sit next to Chairman Ze-Dong Mao during the congress dinner (Fig. 12).

## [Historical note]

*In 1951 Huang was elected to be one of the 229 members of the Founder's Group of the American Board of Thoracic Surgery (Fig. 13). However "this honor was withdrawn by the Board when it was thought that he supported*

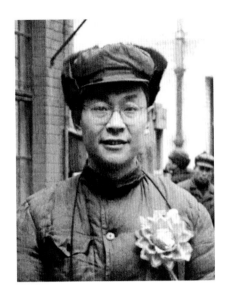

*Fig. 11. Huang as chief of the Shanghai medical team in January 1951.*

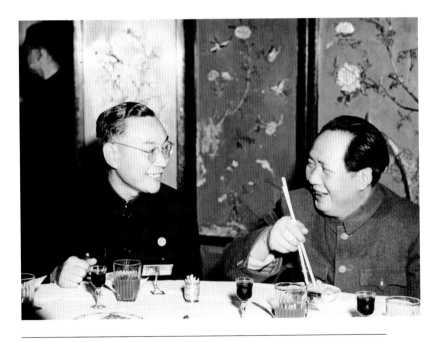

*Fig. 12. Dr. Jia-Si Huang and Chairman Ze-Dong Mao at a national congress dinner in November 1951, Beijing, China.*

*China during the Korean War." Twenty-eight years later, Dr. Huang visited the United States again as the President of the Chinese Academy of Medical Sciences. "Shortly after that his original certificate was found in the Board office, and it was felt to be appropriate to award it to him. It was delivered to him in China, with appropriate ceremony, by Dr. Myron Wegman, Dean of the University of Michigan School of Public Health, who was visiting China at that time."*

— *From "A 50 Year Perspective,"* American Board of Thoracic Surgery, *1998; pp 40–42.*

## The Leader

Over the next few years, Huang played an important leadership role in developing thoracic surgery in Shanghai. As Vice Dean of the

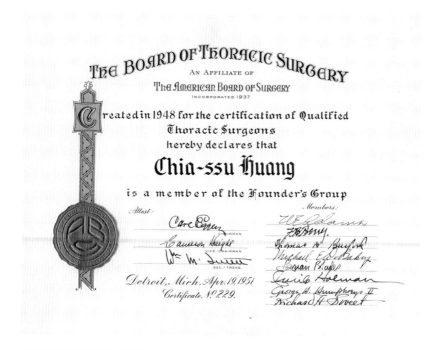

*Fig. 13. Huang's certificate as a member of the Founder's Group of the American Board of Thoracic Surgery.*

Shanghai Medical College and President of Zhongshan Hospital, he had to deal with heavy administrative duties. However he continued to operate and to train young surgeons (Figs. 14A, 14B). The number of beds in his department increased from less than 30 to 96. In 1956 Huang became the Founding President of the Shanghai Chest Hospital, a newly established specialty center for thoracic surgery. He reported their large series of pulmonary resections for tuberculosis, which totaled 1,376 cases [6, 7]. Their experience in surgical treatment for bronchiectasis was also one of the largest in China [8]. In addition, the first Chinese-made heart-lung machine was first used at Shanghai Chest Hospital in July 1958 [9].

During the same period, Huang also dedicated much of his energy to edit the first surgical textbook in the Chinese language (Fig. 15), which was distributed for evaluation at medical schools nationwide in 1958. Based on the feedback, it was re-edited and published in May 1960. Subsequently, a much-improved 2nd edition of this surgical textbook was published in 1964 (Fig. 16).

In late 1958 Huang was appointed the President of the Chinese Academy of Medical Sciences (Fig. 17). One of his major tasks then was to build a top-notch medical university similar to PUMC. It was a daunting task for Huang and his associates as they had to overcome not only various technical obstacles, but also many political and socioeconomic burdens. Initially called "China Medical University" it was then the only medical school in China providing an 8-year education and training program. This university was officially opened in September 1959 and Huang was assigned to be its first President. He remained in that position for the next 25 years, including the 10-year shut-down period (1968–1978) during the "Cultural Revolution" disaster. From 1959 through 1968, 506 students studied at this university and many of them eventually became national leaders in their own fields. In the late 1970s the university was renamed "China Union Medical University." Medical education, research, and clinical services were redeveloped under the leadership of Jia-Si Huang. Part of the funding for the university was raised by Dr. Huang from the China Medical Board of the Rockefeller Foundation and the total amount exceeded US$ 1 million in the early 1980s. He re-established

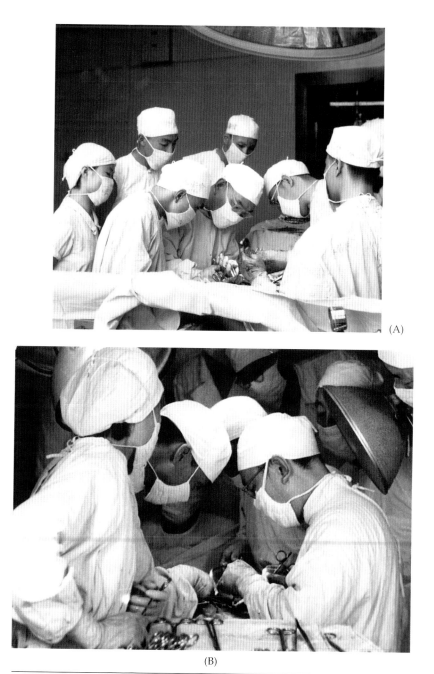

(A)

(B)

Fig. 14. [A, B] Dr. Huang performing thoracic surgical operation in Shanghai.

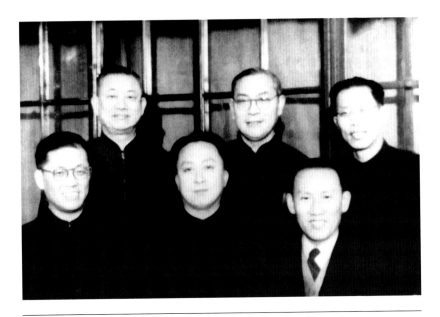

Fig. 15. Editors of the 1st edition of Textbook of Surgery in 1957 (from left to right): Drs. Xian-Jiu Ceng, Xi-Chun Lan, Jie-Ping Wu, Jia-Si Huang, Xian-Zhi Fang, Fa-Zu Qiu.

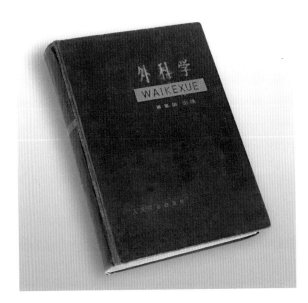

Fig. 16. 2nd edition of Textbook of Surgery (1964).

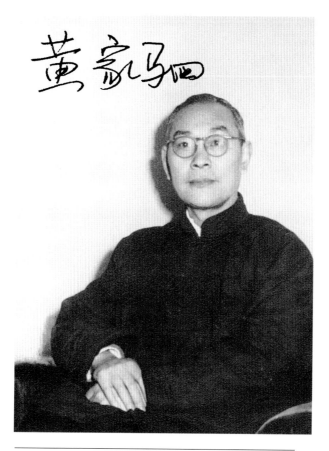

Fig. 17. *Dr. Huang in 1958 as President of the Chinese Academy of Medical Sciences and his signature.*

the regular scientific exchanges and collaborations with the Johns Hopkins University (Fig. 18) and the National Institutes of Health in the USA. As a result, this university has been repeatedly ranked as one of the top two medical schools in China in the past two decades.

In 1975 Drs. Jia-Si Huang and Jie-Ping Wu (a pioneering urologist in China) and their colleagues started to work on a new edition of the *Textbook of Surgery*. When this updated two-volume 3rd edition was published in April 1979, it was immediately used by all medical schools across the country.

In 1980 Dr. Lyman A. Brewer III (the 54th president of AATS) and his wife visited Beijing where they met Drs. Jia-Si Huang, Ying-Kai Wu, and Ji-Zheng Zhang (Fig. 19). All of them except Dr. Wu had previous working experience at the University of Michigan in Ann Arbor. Dr. Brewer trained under Dr. Evarts Graham at Barnes Hospital in St. Louis earlier than Dr. Wu. Following his visit, Dr. Brewer generously gave a supporting hand to some Chinese thoracic

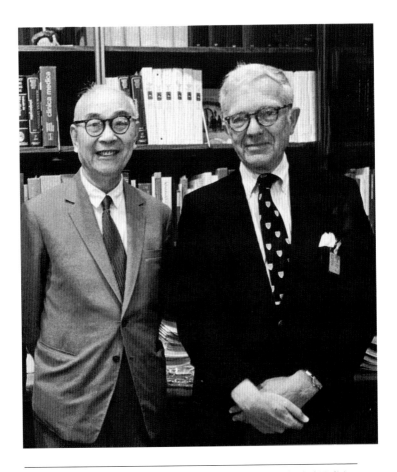

*Fig. 18. Dr. Huang in 1979 with Dr. Richard Ross, Dean of School of Medicine, Johns Hopkins University.*

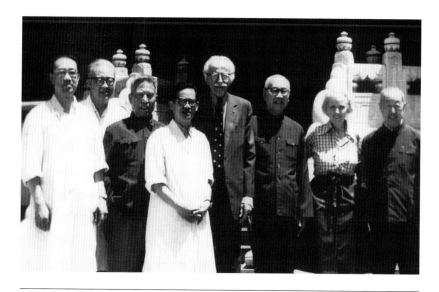

*Fig. 19. Drs. Jia-Si Huang (third from right), Ying-Kai Wu (first from right), Ji-Zheng Zhang (third from left), with Dr Lyman A. Brewer III (fourth from right) and his wife in Beijing in 1980. Courtesy of Dr. Le-Tian Xu (first from left).*

surgeons by granting them advanced training opportunities in the USA (Fig. 20). His visit also resulted in a symposium jointly organized in October 1981 by the Chinese Medical Association and the Lyman A. Brewer III International Surgical Society. Focusing on the latest advances in cardiothoracic surgery, this 4-day "East-meet-West" symposium was the first of its type ever held in China (Fig. 21). The invited foreign speakers included many world-renowned experts of the time from North America, Europe, South America, and Asia. With more than 150 Chinese surgeons attending the meeting, the impact of this symposium on the future development of cardiothoracic surgery in China was tremendous.

### The Mentor

If the success of a surgeon can be gauged at good outcome for his/her patients, the accomplishments of a mentor are best reflected by

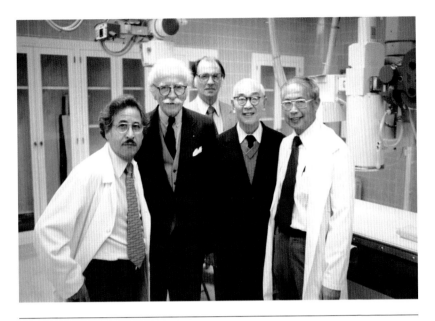

*Fig. 20. Huang was awarded the outstanding member of the Lyman A. Brewer III International Surgical Society on January 11, 1980 in Los Angeles, California. He also visited Dr. Brewer's institution.*

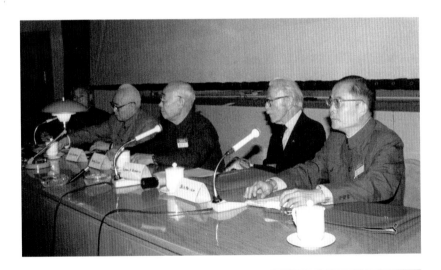

*Fig. 21. At the International Symposium on Cardiothoracic Surgery in October 1981 in Beijing (from right to left): Drs. Mei-Hsin Shih, Lyman A. Brewer III, and Jia-Si Huang.*

the achievements of his/her students. Jia-Si Huang's legacy unquestionably is the surgeons he trained, as many of his residents became leaders in cardiothoracic surgery at major medical centers across the country. Among them, a well-known example is Dr. Mei-Hsin Shih—a pioneer cardiac surgeon in Shanghai [9], who can still recall those early days they spent together in the operating room as well as in the laboratory. Dr. Huang personally guided Shih in almost every aspect of a surgical career, even back to Shih's days at medical school.

The very first time Mei-Hsin Shih, then a year-four medical student, personally benefited from Dr. Huang's care was somewhat dramatic. One day he was absent from the morning class and missed Dr. Huang's surgical lecture. Knowing that the reason for the absence was a sudden onset of abdominal pain, Dr. Huang visited his student in the afternoon. Acute appendicitis was diagnosed and Huang performed an appendectomy on Shih. In 1948, Mei-Hsin Shih contracted pulmonary tuberculosis at the end of his chief residency in surgery. After more than three months of medical treatment, Shih underwent a phrenic nerve division operation. The surgeon was again Huang, then Professor of Surgery and Chairman of the Department. Huang also persuaded Shih to stay at Zhongshan Hospital in Shanghai as a Faculty staff member. It did not take long to prove this was important to the development of cardiac surgery in China [9].

On May 9, 1979, Huang was invited to deliver a lecture at the American Medical Association's 75th Congress on Medical Education in Washington D.C. [10–12]. At that meeting, he received the "World Outstanding Medical Educator" award along with nine peers (Fig. 22). Several similar talks were given at subsequent international meetings [13–16] which enabled Western colleagues to understand the medical system in China after the "Cultural Revolution." Scientific collaborations with several North American institutions were re-established.

On June 22, 1983, Huang underwent surgical repair of his abdominal aortic aneurysm which was unfortunately complicated by postoperative myocardial infarction. He rested for only two months before returning to work. Although officially retired, he was

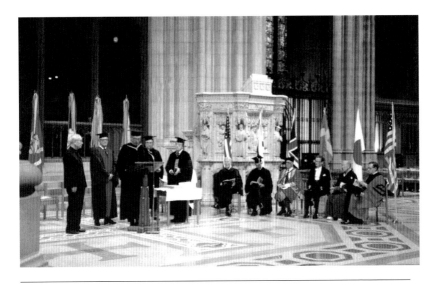

*Fig. 22. At the 75th AMA Congress on Medical Education in Washington D.C. in May 1979.*

still very active in many academic activities in China. One of his top priorities was the 4th edition of the *Textbook of Surgery*.

Huang's frequent visit to western universities in the early 1980s strengthened his thoughts on the importance of surgical training. Therefore the guidelines for the new edition of the textbook changed fundamentally. It was decided that the book should reflect the most updated knowledge and techniques in the field. Accordingly, the targeted readers are surgeons rather than medical students. Dr. Huang personally re-wrote a chapter entitled "Trauma to the Chest." On May 11 and 12, 1984, Dr. Huang chaired the editorial meeting for the 4th edition of the *Textbook of Surgery* (Fig. 23). His chapter was used as a sample representing the new format of the book. Two days later, he died from a cardiac arrest while attending out-patient clinic at PUMC.

The 4th edition of the *Textbook of Surgery* was published in December 1986. In Huang's honor, the book was named "Huang Jia-Si's Textbook of Surgery." Within the next two years, it underwent five reprints with over 136,000 copies sold. In mainland China to date, the only medical textbook which is named after an editor and has been serially published over half a century is "Huang Jia-Si's Textbook of Surgery." Its three volume sixth edition appeared in 1999 (Fig. 24) and the 7th edition is currently in press.

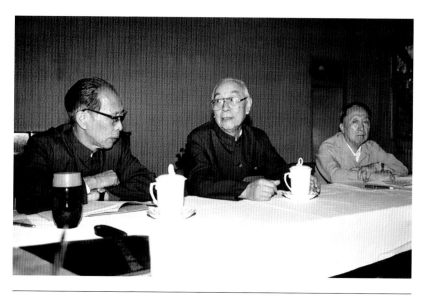

*Fig. 23. At the editorial meeting on May 12, 1984 (from left to right): Drs. Fa-Zu Qiu, Jia-Si Huang, Jie-Ping Wu.*

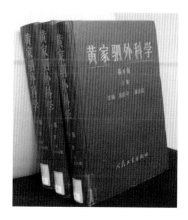

*Fig. 24.* Huang Jia-Si's Textbook of Surgery (*6th edition, 1999*).

## *"The Spirit of Service and of Sacrifice"*

A plate was mounted on the right lower corner of the oil portrait of Huang (Fig. 25) with the following remarks:

**Huang Jia-Si**
May 23, 1906 – May 14, 1984
This portrait is presented to the
**Peking Union Medical College**
To assure that new generations of physicians remain recognized of Huang Jiasi's leadership in the development of a medical care system for the people of China and his inspiration to worldwide community of medical care providers.

Lyman A. Brewer III, MD
and Richard M. Peters, MD, President
Lyman A. Brewer III International Surgical Society

A pioneering cardiac surgeon once made the following remarks, "the *good* surgeon has the ability to apply proper standard techniques skillfully; the *very good* surgeon reduces those standard techniques to their simplest terms, improves them, and applies them with scholarly flexibility; the *great* surgeon has all the qualities of the very good surgeon; in addition, he is innovative and creative, and he passes the improved standard and new techniques on to others. Thus, the *great* surgeon serves many more than one at a time, one at a time."[17] Undoubtedly Jia-Si Huang was one of the *great* surgeons who worked for something even greater than themselves, something which lies in the future and which would be effected by their successors (Fig. 26).

## *Acknowledgements*

The generous support of Mr. Wen-Kun Huang and Ms. Wen-Mei Huang (son and daughter of Dr. Jia-Si Huang) in providing the photographs used in this chapter is deeply appreciated.

A major part of this chapter is reproduced from: Wan S, Yim APC (2006) Jia-Si Huang: "a surgeon and something more." Ann Thorac Surg 82:1147–1151, with permission from the Society of Thoracic Surgeons and Elsevier Inc.

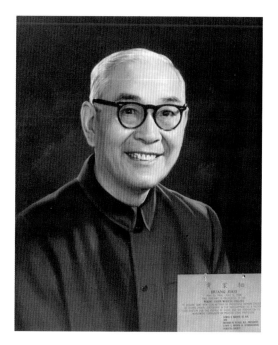

*Fig. 25. Portrait in oils of Jia-Si Huang from the Lyman A. Brewer III International Surgical Society.*

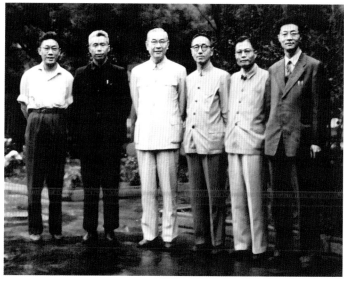

*Fig. 26. Huang and his students at a national symposium on cardiovascular surgery in May 1963 in Tianjin (from left to right): Drs. De-Xing Wan, Ying-Heng Su, Jia-Si Huang, Shou-Qi Tao, Mei-Hsin Shih, Zhong-Xi Qian.*

# References

1.  Literature and History Research Committee of Jiang-Xi Province (1990) Selected review on literature and history of Jiang-Xi (Volume 33rd): Huang Jia-Si. First edition. Beijing: China Literature and History Press (in Chinese).
2.  Bowers JZ (1972) Western medicine in a Chinese palace: Peking Union Medical College, 1917–1951. The Josiah Macy Jr. Foundation, Philadelphia, 1972.
3.  Xu LT (2004) The development of cardiothoracic surgery in China. Proceedings of 2004 national symposium on advance in thoracic surgery. Urumqi, Xinjiang, August 21–24, pp 14–16 (in Chinese).
4.  Sloan H. (2005) Historical perspective of the American Association for Thoracic Surgery: John Alexander (1891–1954). J Thorac Cardiovasc Surg 129:435–436.
5.  Huang CS (1943) Tuberculos Tracheobronchitis: a pathological study. Am Rev Tubercul 47:500–508.
6.  Huang CS, Liang QC, Shi MH, Gu KS (1956) Lung resection for 1376 patients with pulmonary tuberculosis: Shanghai experience. Chin J Surg 4:781–785 (in Chinese).
7.  Huang CS, Liang QC, Shi MH, Gu KS (1957) Pulmonary resection for tuberculosis: analysis of 1376 cases. Chin Med J 75:171–180.
8.  Huang CS, Shi MH, Wan TH, Jen CY (1958) Surgical treatment for bronchiectasis. Chin Med J 77:587–595.
9.  Wan S, Yim APC (2003) The evolution of cardiovascular surgery in China. Ann Thorac Surg 76:2147–2155.
10. Huang JS (1979) Medical education in China. Invited lecture at American Medical Association's 75th Congress on Medical Education (May 9, Washington DC).
11. Huang JS (1979) Medical education in China. Am Med News (October 26).
12. Huang JS (1979) Medicine in the People's Republic of China. Maryland State Med J 28:35–39.
13. Huang JS (1979) Medical and health work in new China. Invited lecture at McGill University's 50th anniversary ceremonial meeting, Canada.
14. Huang JS (1981) Medical education in China. Invited lecture at "Medical education in Asia: a Symposium" (June 1981, New York, USA), pp 79–86.
15. Huang JS (1982) Medical education in China: its historical background, present status, and further development. Invited lecture at Cumberland College of Health Science, Australia.
16. Huang JS (1983) Health service for one billion people including care of the aged. Hospital Association Magazine, Australia.
17. Harken DE (1984) Foreword. In: Cooley DA (ed) Techniques in cardiac surgery. 2nd ed. Philadelphia: W. B. Saunders.

# Ying-Kai Wu and His Two Decisions

*Song Wan, Anthony P. C. Yim*

**D**r. Ying-Kai Wu (1910–2003) is known to many in the thoracic surgical academia worldwide. This chapter focuses on the two decisions he made at the age of 34 and 70 that profoundly influenced the development of thoracic and cardiovascular medicine in China. His successful career was gauged not so much by the position he has achieved, but by the obstacles he had to overcome to get there.

## 1933–1941: Initial Steps

Ying-Kai Wu was born on May 8, 1910, in the last years of the Qing Dynasty. His family originated in Xinmin County, Liaoning Province. Wu's father was a teacher and the family was not well off. Wu had three brothers and a sister. Eventually all of them (Fig. 1) received university education, which was indeed unusual and remarkable in that particular days of age in China. His elder brother, Zhi-Zhong Wu (old style spelled as Chi-Chong Wu, 1906–1980), was trained in the UK and qualified as a Fellow of Royal College of Physicians and Surgeons of Glasgow in 1935. Wu's younger sister, Zhen-Zhong Wu, was a professor of ophthalmology. Wu's other two younger brothers were Wei-Zhong Wu who studied agricultural chemistry in Japan, and Xian-Zhong Wu who became a Professor of Surgery in 1949 and later the Dean of Tianjin Medical College.

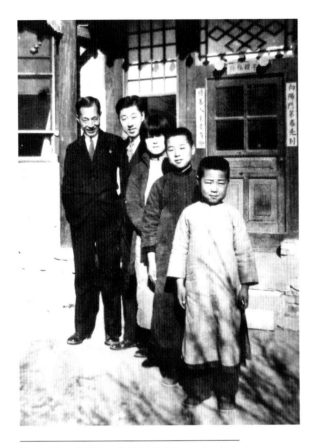

*Fig. 1. Ying-Kai Wu with his 3 brothers and a sister.*

Ying-Kai Wu's long surgical career started in 1933 with setback right from the beginning. He was diagnosed to have tuberculosis three months into his surgical internship at Peking Union Medical College (PUMC), after having just completed his medical education at Moukden Medical College in northeast China. Streptomycin was not available then and the young Dr. Wu was sent to a sanatorium to recuperate. Under such circumstances, one may be persuaded to give up medicine or at least choose a career less physically demanding than surgery, but Wu decided to repeat his one-year surgical internship after spending nine months in the sanatorium (Fig. 2).

PUMC was established by the Rockefeller Foundation in 1917 and was designed to promote research in addition to clinical excellence. Wu was chosen to be the research fellow immediately after his internship. Only the most promising intern out of a dozen could obtain such an honor each year. He was referred as "Y. K.," instead of "Dr. Wu," and was invited to join the afternoon tea everyday with the professors. During his one-year fellowship, Wu had two articles published in English [1, 2]. The first one, interestingly, happened to be related to tuberculosis. He went on to become the Chief Resident in Surgery in June 1938 and, one year later, instructor in surgery at PUMC (Fig. 3).

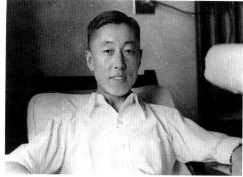

*Fig. 2. Y. K. Wu in 1933: Internship at PUMC.*

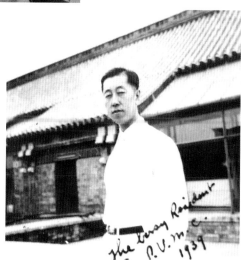

*Fig. 3. Dr. Wu in 1939: Chief Resident at PUMC.*

On April 26, 1940 (12 days before his 30th birthday), Wu performed the first successful resection of cancer of the esophagus with intrathoracic esophagogastrostomy in China [3]. There were earlier attempts at esophagectomy by the former chief of surgery at PUMC, but there were no survivors. The next chief, Dr. Harold H. Loucks (Fig. 4), together with a group of investigators including oncologists, pathologists, radiologists, and ENT surgeons, continued the task. As Loucks assistant, Wu joined this team of investigators as soon as he completed his residency. At that time, they were encouraged by isolated case reports of Samuel Marshall from Boston [4] and William Adams from Chicago [5]. Loucks and Wu were impressed by the Adams approach and decided to carry it out in China.

A male patient in his fifties with known carcinoma of the lower thoracic esophagus was soon scheduled for surgery. Unfortunately, Loucks got a severe cold the day before the operation and had to stay at home. Wu called Loucks and proposed postponing the operation. Much to his surprise, the answer came: "Go on, Ying-Kai, since the patient is ready. I am sure you can do the job. I wish you all the best." Loucks was correct. Although lasted for more than seven hours, the operation was uneventful. Through a left thoracotomy, Wu excised an "apple-sized" tumor and did a two-layer end-to-side esophagogastric anastomosis below the aortic arch. The patient, Mr. Feng, was discharged home 3 weeks after surgery. Every team member was invited to dinner to celebrate. Wu was glad to pay the bill, which came to one third of his monthly salary.

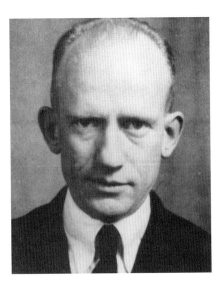

*Fig. 4. Harold H. Loucks, MD*

Within the following year, Drs. Wu and Loucks performed 10 more cases with only 3 early deaths. It was certainly not just a "beginner's luck." In August 1941, PUMC decided to send a few promising staff members, including one surgeon, to the United States for further training. Logically, the choice of surgeon was Wu. The initial arrangement for him, however, was to study plastic surgery at Barnes Hospital in St. Louis, Missouri.

## *1943: The First Decision*

Ying-Kai Wu would have become a plastic surgeon if Dr. Evarts A. Graham (Fig. 5), then chairman of the Department of Surgery at Washington University in St. Louis, had not called on him during the third month after this young Chinese surgeon joined the plastic surgery unit at Barnes Hospital. One day, Graham showed Wu a letter from Dr. Loucks, saying that the chief thoracic surgeon at PUMC had just resigned and so it would be better for Wu to learn thoracic surgery abroad. To this young surgeon, it was like a dream come true to learn a

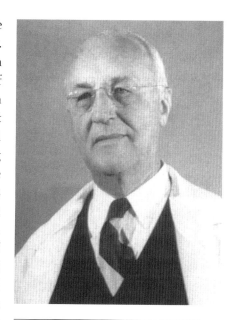

Fig. 5. *Evarts A. Graham, MD (1883–1957)*

trade he was interested in, under a world-renowned expert [6]. Dr. Wu then started to work in the chest service at Barnes Hospital (Fig. 6).

Two weeks later, two cases of carcinoma of the esophagus were presented at the weekly surgical pathology meeting. The operations, just done by Graham, were believed to be among the first few in the USA. Dr. Lischer recalled the following incidence:

Towards the end of the conference, in a very modest and quiet manner, Dr. Wu said, "I just happen to have a couple of slides." So, he got up and discussed his own personal experience with some ten patients. From then on Dr. Graham had the highest admiration for Dr. Wu, who always went about his work in a quiet, modest way [7].

Wu was then invited to a St. Louis Surgical Society meeting to give a more detailed account of his work on esophagectomy [8]. That report was subsequently published in *The Journal of Thoracic Surgery* [9], of which Graham was the founding editor.

After 10-month training at the chest service of Barnes Hospital, Wu went on to be the chief resident of thoracic surgery at Robert Koch Hospital, a 700-bed municipal tuberculosis hospital in St. Louis, where the previous chief resident Thomas Burford left for war (Fig. 7). Wu and his colleague Dr. Mario Pianetto, a surgical fellow from Argentina, were soon sharing almost all the cases (Fig. 8). This

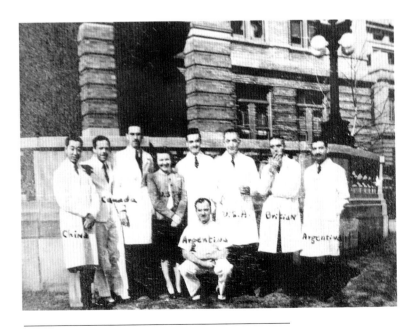

*Fig. 6. Wu with colleagues at Barnes Hospital, St. Louis (1941).*

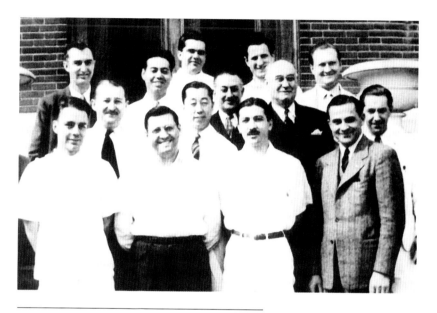

*Fig. 7. Wu with colleagues at Robert Koch Hospital (1942).*

proved to be a great opportunity for them. They set a record for not having a single wound infection in 150 consecutive stages of thoracoplasty [8, 10], which was an outstanding improvement comparing to an infection rate of 12% only ten months earlier [10].

In March 1943, Dr. Wu decided to return to China to fight in the war against Japanese invasion. This was certainly not an easy decision. Many may have chosen to stay in the United States where the standard of living was much higher and research facility far superior than in China. However, as a patriot, Wu had no hesitation of returning home. This decision, in fact, had a major impact on the development of thoracic and cardiovascular surgery in China for the next 50 years.

> One day I went to Dr. Graham and told him about my wish to return to China soon. At first he said, "Wu, you better stay here. We are allies and fighting the same war. You can make your contribution here just as well as in China." I said, "Thank you, Dr. Graham, but I feel I should be in China while my country is at war. Dr. Graham

understood and promptly said, "Yes, that is true. I am sorry we cannot keep you longer. Then what can I do for you before you go?" I asked for his advice concerning a study tour through some surgical clinics before I left the United States for home. About 1 week later, Miss Hanvey, Dr. Graham's capable secretary, gave me more than 30 letters of introduction.... Armed with these letters, I visited many famous surgical clinics during the next 4 months [11].

More than 100 patients at Robert Koch Hospital presented to Dr. Wu a wristwatch as a farewell souvenir (Fig. 9). Dr. Wu has been wearing that watch since [8].

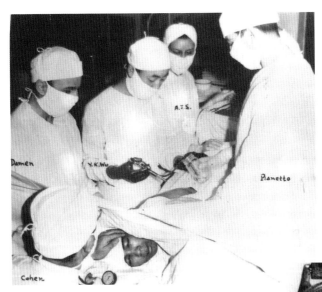

*Fig. 8. Performing thoracic operation at Robert Koch Hospital.*

*Fig. 9. Wristwatch presented to Wu by the patients of Robert Koch Hospital on March 23, 1943. On the back of the watch were the following inscriptions: "3-23-43, Y. K. Wu, from patients of Koch Hospital." (Reprinted from [11] with permission from Excerpta Medica Inc.)*

## 1943–1980: Unique Achievements in a Unique Time

Ying-Kai Wu left Philadelphia in August 1943. It took him 6 weeks to arrive India by a British ordnance ship, and another 2 weeks to catch a plane for China. Despite the poor working conditions during wartime, Wu struggled and made his contribution to thoracic surgery in his own country. In 1944, soon after he became the head of Department of Surgery at the Central Hospital in Chongqing (Fig. 10), Wu

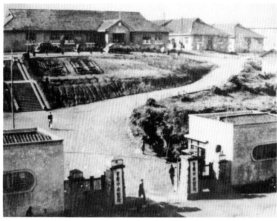

(A)

*Fig. 10. [A] The Central Hospital in Chongqing, China (1944); [B] Dr. Wu in Chongqing.*

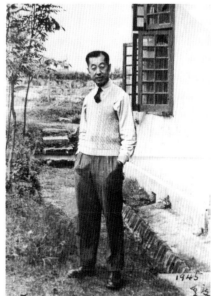

(B)

performed the first ligation of patent ductus arteriosus in (PDA) China [12] (Fig. 11). In 1947, Wu and his colleagues did the first successful pericardectomy in China for chronic constrictive pericarditis, after the hospital was re-located in Tianjin [13] (Fig. 12).

Dr. Wu returned to PUMC in May 1948 as an associate professor of surgery. Dr. Loucks left China two years later and Wu was soon appointed Chief of Surgery. Major political and economic changes took place after the founding of the People's Republic of China in 1949. This was followed by the Korean War and the so-called "Cultural Revolution." Communications between China and the USA essentially ceased during the next two decades.

In 1974, Dr. Lyman A. Brewer III, a former fellow under Graham and the fifty-fourth president of the American Association for Thoracic Surgery (AATS), invited Wu to join the Association's annual meeting. The trip was, unfortunately, not possible for Dr. Wu under the political circumstances then. Few who know the modern history of China would deny that the "Cultural Revolution" from 1966 through 1976 was a disaster to many in China. Dr. Wu was not an exception. His clinical practice was totally stopped during this period. He had even been forced to do some labor work unrelated to medicine for four years, despite being the founding president of the Military Thoracic Hospital and the Cardiovascular Institute of Chinese Academy of Medical Sciences. The latter institution is also known as Fuwai Hospital, the biggest cardiovascular medical center in China where Wu (Fig. 13) and his associates carried out some pioneering cardiac and thoracic projects some years earlier. Open heart surgery with the use of hypothermia and extracorporeal circulation started early in 1960 at this institution [14, 15], but was almost discontinued afterwards for ten years. Despite the setback, the work initiated by Dr. Wu on carcinoma of the esophagus has gained momentum.

Wu once said, "the only systematic scientific research I have done is the study on carcinoma of the esophagus." It indeed represents a long journey in his professional life, step by step since 1940. In fact, Wu and his colleagues had performed close to one thousand operations for patients with esophageal cancer through 1948 to 1958. Dr. Wu noticed that many patients came from the Taihang Mountain

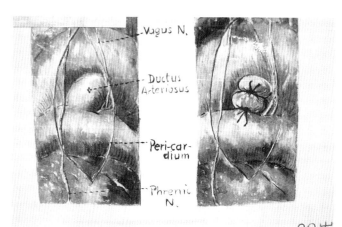

重庆中央医院住院号2715　　男　　20岁
手术日期: 1944.10.7.　手术者: 吴英恺

*Fig. 11. Wu performed the first PDA ligation in China for a 20-year-old male patient at the Central Hospital in Chongqing on October 7, 1944.*

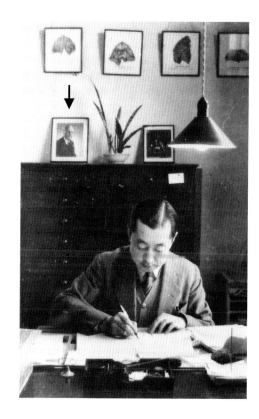

*Fig. 12. Wu at the Central Hospital in Tianjin in 1947. Note the picture of Dr. Graham (arrow).*

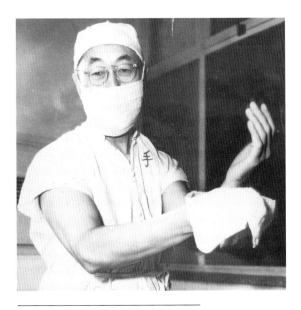

*Fig. 13. Dr. Wu at Fuwai Hospital in 1962.*

Range in North China. From April 1959 to August 1961, a survey of the prevalence and mortality of esophageal cancer was conducted in Beijing and four provinces of North China. Total populations of 17 million were studied. The incidence and mortality in some regions were found to be exceptionally high. For example, in Linxian of Henan Province, a county of half a million population, more than 500 cases of this malignant disease were diagnosed each year and four-fifths of those patients died. This represented that more than one patient died each day from esophageal cancer in that small county. Based on epidemiological, pathological, and clinical investigations, Wu and his colleagues, including Drs. Guo-Jun Huang, Ling-Fang Shao, Yu-De Zhang, proposed that the natural history of esophageal cancer consist of initial, developing, overt, and terminal phases. They concluded that emphasis should be directed to the first two phases: prevention in the initial phase and early detection/surgery in the developing phase. The first part includes avoiding carcinogenic substances such as nitrosamine, changing harmful habits such as eating too coarse, hard, and hot food and swallowing hastily [16].

The use of a cytologic screening technique, which was developed by the pathologist Dr. Qiong Shen, has been the most effective method for early detection of esophageal cancer in the high incidence region and contributed to the improved long-term survival of Stage I patients. In the hands of an experienced team in Linxian of Henan Province, headed by Dr. Shao, the five-year survival rate had reached 90% in more than 200 Stage I patients by 1977 [16, 17].

The political situation in China had improved by late 1970s. Dr. Wu had visited the USA in total 8 times since April 1979. In fact, he visited Dr. Loucks home near Philadelphia during his first trip (Fig 14). He became an honorary member of the American Surgical Association in 1979, an honorary Fellow of the American College of Surgeons in 1980 (Figs. 15A and 15B), and an honorary member of the Lyman A. Brewer III International Surgical Society in 1981. Wu was able to accept an invitation by another president of AATS, Dr. Thomas B. Ferguson, to deliver an honored lecture at the association's 62nd annual meeting in Phoenix, Arizona, on May 4, 1982. He was awarded an honorary member of the AATS after the address. The topic of his speech, naturally, was the 40-year Chinese experience on surgical treatment of esophageal cancer [16] (Fig. 16).

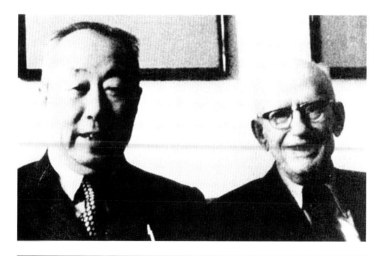

*Fig. 14. Wu visited Dr. Loucks home near Philadelphia in May 1979. (Reprinted from [11] with permission from Excerpta Medica Inc.)*

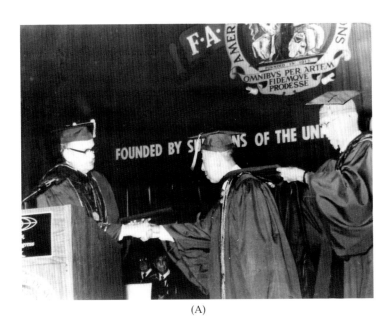

(A)

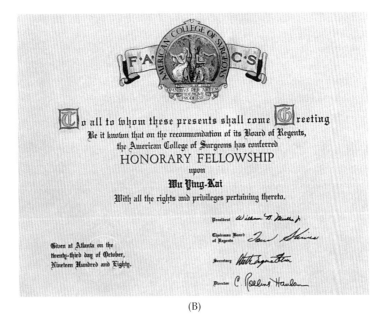

(B)

Fig. 15. *[A, B] Wu was conferred the Honorary Fellowship of American College of Surgeons in 1980.*

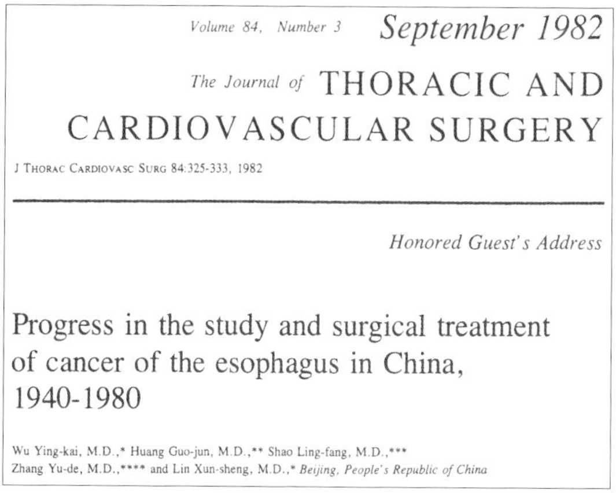

*Volume 84, Number 3* *September 1982*

*The Journal of* THORACIC AND
CARDIOVASCULAR SURGERY

J Thorac Cardiovasc Surg 84:325-333, 1982

*Honored Guest's Address*

Progress in the study and surgical treatment
of cancer of the esophagus in China,
1940-1980

Wu Ying-kai, M.D.,* Huang Guo-jun, M.D.,** Shao Ling-fang, M.D.,***
Zhang Yu-de, M.D.,**** and Lin Xun-sheng, M.D.,* *Beijing, People's Republic of China*

*Fig. 16. Wu delivered an
Honored Guest's Address
at the AATS in 1982.*

## 1980: The Second Decision

As the president of the Cardiovascular Institute of Chinese Academy
of Medical Sciences and Fuwai Hospital, Dr. Wu spared no effort to
promote open-heart surgical projects in the late 1970s, inasmuch as
the development of cardiac surgery was severely baffled during the
years of "Culture Revolution." However, he was forced to retire in
1980 when he approached his seventh decade. Many might have been
happy to do so having worked all their lives, but not for Dr. Wu.

"I was not prepared," Wu recalled, "I was still full of energy and,
most importantly, I wanted to make good for the loss of more
than 10 years" [8]. Despite being forced to retire at Fuwai Hospital,
he decided to start all over again and found a new center of
cardiovascular medicine which should provide not only clinical
services, teaching, scientific research, but also community health care,
prevention, as well as international exchange. The Beijing Heart Lung
Blood Vessel Medical Center was inaugurated in September 1981 at
Chaoyang Hospital. Two years later, the center moved to its current
location and became the Anzhen Hospital.

Aiming at high standards from the very beginning, Wu organized
an international symposium on cardiothoracic surgery in October
1981. Supported by Chinese Medical Association and the Lyman A.
Brewer III International Surgical Society, it was the first dedicated

meeting in China for exchanging knowledge on cardiothoracic surgery among more than one hundred experts from all over the world (Fig. 17). Moreover, the meeting became a foundation of continued collaboration. Four years later, the second international symposium on cardiothoracic surgery was held at Anzhen Hospital to celebrate the publication of a 111-chapter textbook entitled *International Practice on Cardiothoracic Surgery* [18]. Edited by Drs. Wu and Richard Peters (Fig. 18), with contributions from 157 distinguished authors in 12 countries, this book immediately became and has remained a classic reference for many Chinese cardiothoracic surgeons.

With the importance of teamwork in mind, Dr. Wu sent some of his assistants including cardiac surgeons, anesthesiologists, intensivists and perfusionists, for training abroad. The first open heart operation by this young team was done on December 27, 1982, and marked the launching of the cardiac program at Beijing Heart Lung Blood Vessel Medical Center. This program has grown rapidly thereafter at Anzhen Hospital: 528 open heart operations were performed in 1986, and the annual pump cases have exceeded a thousand since 1994.

Dr. Wu was also instrumental in developing a national cardiovascular community control program [19], which he called "my second specialty." A collaborating study, as part of the multinational monitoring of trends and determinants in cardiovascular disease — the MONICA project of the World Health Organization (WHO), has been carried out in 16 provinces in China since 1982, with a total population being monitored over 5.5 million. The data collected from this study are of particular importance since few other Asian countries were involved in this kind of epidemiological study. Although the trend in cardiovascular disease is increasing in this part of the world, the patterns of coronary heart disease and stroke in China are quite different from many western countries and these are probably related to the different ways of life [20]. Such a timely investigation also provided a reliable database for future internal evaluation as well as international comparison. The quality control of this project was ranked No. 1 by WHO in 1987, among 39 collaborative centers from

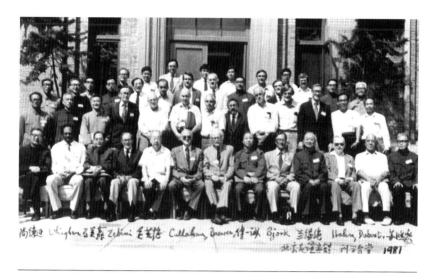

*Fig. 17. First International Symposium on Thoracic and Cardiovascular Surgery in 1981 at Beijing Friendship Hotel. Y. K. Wu (front row, 5th from left) and other distinguished speakers.*

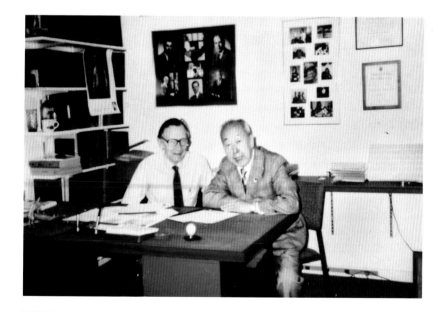

*Fig. 18. Drs. Wu and Richard M. Peters.*

27 countries. A comprehensive program in the prevention of hypertension, stroke, and coronary heart disease for a population of more than 50,000 in Beijing, was established in 1987. Wu and his associates have also vigorously fought for an anti-smoking campaign since 1984. "Where there is a will, there is a way" remarked the septuagenarian.

Dr. Wu enjoyed happy family life with his wife (Fig. 19). The Golden Anniversary of their marriage took place in 2000. They have 3 children and 6 grandchildren.

A one-week exhibition was held in the Chinese Revolution Museum in Beijing in June 1996, in honor of Ying-Kai Wu's seventy-year dedication to medicine. Dr. Wu was asked, regarding his two decisions in 1943 and 1980, whether he would do the same again if given the choice. The answer was a predictable yes (Fig. 20).

Irrespective of being 34 or 70, his prime concerns in life were for his patients, his country, and not himself.

## Acknowledgements

Part of this chapter is reproduced from: Wan S, Yim APC (1999) A Chinese thoracic surgeon and his two decisions. Ann Thorac Surg 67:1190–1193, with permission from the Society of Thoracic Surgeons and Elsevier Inc.

## References

1.  Wu YK, Miltner LJ (1936) The operative treatment of tuberculosis of the knee joint. Chin Med J 50:253–258.
2.  Wu YK, Miltner LJ (1937) A procedure for stimulation of longitudinal growth of bone: an experimental study. J Bone Joint Surg 19:909–921
3.  Wu YK, Loucks HH (1941) Surgical treatment of carcinoma of the esophagus. Chin Med J 60:1–33.
4.  Marshall SF (1938) Carcinoma of the esophagus. Successful resection of lower end of esophagus with reestablishment of esophageal gastric continuity. Surg Clin North Am 18:643–648.
5.  Adams WE, Phemister DB (1938) Carcinoma of the lower thoracic esophagus. Report of a successful resection and esophagogastrostomy. J Thorac Surg 7:621–632.

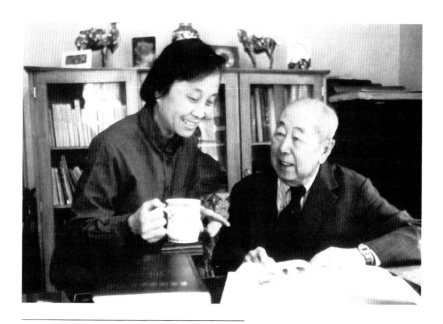

Fig. 19. *Wu and his wife, Shi-Yan Li, at home (1992).*

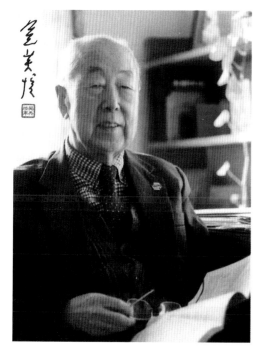

Fig. 20. *Y. K. Wu: a great surgeon, innovator, and investigator.*

6.    Ferguson TB (1984) Evarts A Graham—the man. J Thorac Cardiovasc Surg 88: 803–809.

7.    Lischer CE (1979) Discussion on: Wu YK, Huang KC. Chinese experience in the surgical treatment of carcinoma of the esophagus. Ann Surg 190:365.

8.    Wu YK (1997) Seventy years (1927–1997) of studying, practicing and teaching medicine. Beijing: China Science & Technology Press (in Chinese); 2006 (in English, O'Neal LW, Suen HC, Gao VH, editors)

9.    Wu YK, Loucks HH (1942) Resection of the esophagus for carcinoma. J Thorac Surg 11:516–528.

10.   Wu YK, Pianetto ME (1943) The problem of wound infection in thoracoplasty. J Thorac Surg 12:648–652.

11.   Wu YK (1980) Reminiscence of personal association with American thoracic and cardiovascular surgery. Am J Surg 139:765–770.

12.   Wu YK (1947) Ligation of patent ductus arteriosus. Chin Med J 65:71–76.

13.   Wu YK, Huang KC (1953) Surgical treatment of constrictive pericarditis. Chin Med J 71:247–286.

14.   Chang TH, Wang YC, Wu YK (1962) Open heart surgery under selective hypothermia and extracorporeal circulation. Chin Med J 81:207–211.

15.   Hou YL, Shang TY, Wu YK (1964) Surgical treatment of aneurysm of thoracic aorta. Chin Med J 83:740–749.

16.   Wu YK, Huang GJ, Shao LF, Zhang YD, Lin XS (1982) Progress in the study and surgical treatment of cancer of the esophagus in China, 1940–1980. J Thorac Cardiovasc Surg 84:325–333.

17.   Wu YK, Huang KC (1979) Chinese experience in the surgical treatment of carcinoma of the esophagus. Ann Surg 190:361–365.

18.   Wu YK, Peters RM (eds) (1985) International practice on cardiothoracic surgery. Beijing: Science Press.

19.   Wu YK (1979) Epidemiology and community control of hypertension, stroke and coronary heart disease in China. Chin Med J 92:665–670.

20.   Wu ZS, Hong ZG, Yao CH, et al. (1987) Sino-MONICA-Beijing study: report of the results between 1983–1985. Chin Med J 100:611–620.

# Dr. Norman Bethune in China: 1938–1939

*Larry Hannant*

**D**r. Norman Bethune, born in 1890 in Canada, may be better known in the country of his death, China, than in his birthplace. And while his political practice in China has helped to cement his fame (at least up to the dramatic reversal in political direction that arrived with the death of Ze-Dong Mao), his medical contributions in that country are also justly cited for renown. A considerable number of Westerners visited and lived in China in the 1930s, when Bethune was there, and more than a few of them were medical specialists. But few possessed Bethune's unique combination of political internationalism, zealous dedication to the Chinese people and medical expertise. In part for this reason, perhaps few of the Westerners who were Bethune's compatriots in China in the 1930s enjoy his prestige today.[1]

Medicine, then, is an important reason why Bethune has a high reputation in China. Moreover, assessing his medical contribution in China is also an effective way to address some important aspects of Chinese medical and general history in the first half of the 20th century. We can learn much about China in that unique and desperate historical moment by examining the medical challenges Bethune encountered in his time in China, from late January 1938 to his death on November 12, 1939 (Fig. 1). Through Bethune's eyes and his lengthy reports—from both urban and rural China, southern and

northern districts, Guomindang-controlled regions and those held
by the communists—we see China's actual situation in graphic detail.
It is a tale of backwardness caused by political stagnation and
corruption, an account of wretched poverty in which rudimentary
sanitation and health standards could not be met, a cry of desperation
borne out of foreign exploitation and, after 1931, Japanese invasion.
All these problems Bethune saw and described. All these problems
also manifested themselves in illness, trauma and death, which
Bethune worked medically to alleviate. Thus China's infirmity as a
country manifested itself in and mirrored the ailments of its 400
million people.

Bethune's initial survey of the medical situation in China, written
while he stopped over for three weeks in Guomindang-controlled
Hankou in February 1938, reveals the immense problems that China
faced. And this was in the relatively developed and central parts of
the country. He wrote that the Guomindang army's own medical

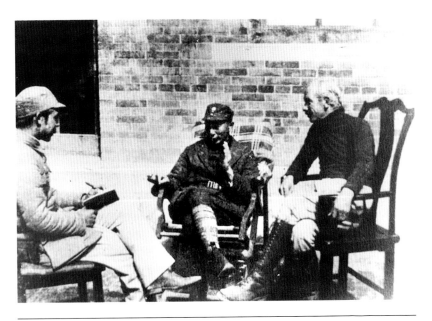

*Fig. 1. Bethune with General Rong-Zhen Nie (centre) and a Chinese journalist at Wutaishan in June 1938. (Source: Roderick Stewart)*

service at the time of the Japanese attack on Shanghai in 1937 was "very primitive, inadequately staffed and terribly under-supplied." The wounded "die because of a lack of proper surgeons" and the medical officers of what hospitals existed "are often inexperienced in surgical affairs. Many are incompetent through lack of training." In this situation of dire emergency, orderlies, nurses and medical students all were pressed into service and "are given the rank of medical officers and their partial training employed as best it may be."[2]

It should also be said that these problems did not originate only in the Japanese assault. In northeast China before Japan's all-out offensive on China proper, the Canadian nurse Jean Ewen (who, on her second trip to China, accompanied Bethune there in 1938) observed a similar inefficiency and lack of commitment to basic health care by the Guomindang government. Out of a spirit of adventurousness and international concern, Ewen had left Canada and signed up to work within the Franciscan mission system in Shandong Province and other parts of northeast China, where she remained from 1933 to early 1937. According to her, the Chinese government did next to nothing to address the great medical needs of the Chinese people. For example, "[t]here were no sanitation or public health programmes. The government simply wasn't responsible for anything."[3]

This inefficiency in the Guomindang medical and administrative system was not due solely to simple incompetence or, after 1937, the savagery of the Japanese assault on China. Some of it resulted from the fact that the Nationalist Party's patriotism took second place to its anti-communism. From the moment he became Guomindang leader in 1928, Jie-Shi Jiang's strategy was to hoard his resources for the real fight against communism in China. The Guomindang's dubious patriotic attachment, coupled with the influence of the communist Agnes Smedley, helped to confirm Bethune in his determination to travel beyond Hankou and reach the arena where he could directly assist the communists, who were actually battling the Japanese military forces occupying China.[4]

Even at the communist headquarters of Yan'an and on the frontlines of the military campaign against Japan north and east of Yan'an, Bethune saw plenty of confusion, inefficiency and suffering. In fact, his letters from the front to the Chinese Communist Party leaders at Yan'an did not fail to criticize what he saw as ineptitude and lackadaisical practice in health care. But he recognized one key difference between the problem in the communist-liberated areas and in the Guomindang regions—the activists in the liberated areas were marked by a genuine desire to serve the Chinese people and a willingness to improve. Again and again in his communications he noted the cohesiveness and spirit among the partisans. Describing Yan'an, for instance, he noted that "Everyone in the community is given equal treatment no matter what rank. There is an excellent spirit of diligence and friendliness."[5]

It does seem that when he first saw the medical conditions at Yan'an Bethune himself was appalled. Jean Ewen reported that when he was ushered to the operating rooms of the border-region hospital at Yan'an, which she, familiar with China from four years of experience in the mission system, considered "as well equipped as they could be," he "declared himself on strike" and "said he damned well wouldn't work in a place like that." But after that brief rebellion he performed his scheduled operations "like the soldier he was supposed to be."[6] This brief act of rebellion illustrates a common pattern with Bethune. His western medical chauvinism was shocked by methods and conditions that clearly threatened patients' very survival. But he did not remain dismayed for long, and he was soon elbows-deep in resolving the problem.

Mark Gayn, a journalist sent to China by the New York tabloid *PM Daily* and who visited what he described as "Bethune's hospital" in Yan'an in February 1947, eight years after Bethune died, gave a very graphic illustration of the rustic conditions: "There was a case with surgical instruments but very few of them were modeern [sic] steel scalpels, etc. Most seemed to be long nails, hammered flat and then sharpened to razor sharpness." Curiously, Gayn attributed this inadequacy to Bethune himself: "Why Bethune did not bring with him enough to this main base hospital that he himself had created is beyond me."[7]

What Gayn did not appreciate was the immense difficulty of obtaining supplies and equipment in the remote area of China that Bethune served. Medical missionaries knew what Gayn did not. Even before the Japanese invasion in 1937 and the catastrophic destruction and disruption of basic medical care it brought to China, rural mission clinics in northeast China had considerable difficulty obtaining vital supplies, Jean Ewen reported. Knowing this, she and Bethune spent more than a month at Hankou in early 1938 "frantically collecting surgical equipment and medical supplies to last at least three months" in northern China.[8] Bethune brought everything he could from North America to Yan'an, some of which was destroyed or pilfered en route. Unfortunately, what he brought was but a drop of blood, when the patient needed a transfusion.

The severe supply problem persisted long after Bethune died. In 1942 a Dutch engineer who escaped from the Japanese in Beijing was able to visit the Jin-Cha-Ji border region in northeastern China. This man, C. Brondgeest, reported that "Dr. Bethune's hospital" was scattered throughout homes in several hamlets in the district, each ready to shift its location on a moment's notice. And on one key issue nothing had changed from before Bethune's death. Brondgeest's assessment about the state of medical supplies was blunt: "They have nothing."[9]

The supply shortage was so critical that Bethune's letters from the front were filled with laments and tirades about and proposals to resolve it. In letter after letter to the China Aid Council in New York and other comrades in Canada and the United States of America, Bethune appealed for instruments and money to buy them. Most often the response was silence. By January 1939, so desperate was he that he devised a plan to go in disguise into Beijing to make purchases from stores there, a plan the Eighth Route Army command decisively rejected.[10]

Bethune was not alone in his urgent need for medical provisions. Acquiring supplies was one of the foremost problems of all medical personnel in the region in the 1930s. Kathleen Hall, a nurse from New Zealand who headed the Anglican medical mission at Songjiazhuang, in the Jin-Cha-Ji region, was well aware of the challenge. As a British subject in 1938–1939, she had a certain level of protection from Japanese harassment, she had an established network of suppliers in Beijing and elsewhere, and she could command far greater resources than the communists and Bethune. But like Bethune, she recognized how acutely dependent the very survival of her mission was upon obtaining medicine and equipment. For a short time she was able to overcome the problem by making the journey back and forth to Beijing, at considerable danger to herself. And beginning in 1939 she also began secretly to help replenish Bethune's pathetically-small stock of drugs and equipment, but this only caused the Japanese to burn her mission.[11]

Medical care in China at this time was indeed at a low level. But this low state of development was due to more than just lack of equipment. Training was also entirely rudimentary. As Bethune pointed out in July 1938, having reached the Jin-Cha-Ji border district, "[i]n this great area of 13,000,000 people and with 150,000 armed troops I am the only qualified doctor!" By his count "there are no more than 5 or 6 fully qualified doctors in the entire 8th [Route] Army."[12] With all his considerable energy he plunged into the effort to rectify this shortcoming, but he understood that surmounting it would take some time. Even his own exertions sometimes led to wrong turns. For example, his plan to construct a fixed model hospital at Sung-yen K'ou, whose purpose was to train new doctors and nurses, failed dramatically when the Japanese destroyed it in September 1938.[13]

Lack of formal medical education was compounded by another problem in China in the 1930s, continued reliance on unscientific folk cures. Jean Ewen reported that at the door of one sick room in the district north of Yan'an she was "transported back a few centuries in superstition" when she came upon a distressed family who had a desperately sick boy. At their wit's end, they summoned an exorcist, charm in hand, to attend to their son. When a fascinated and aghast Ewen asked what was in the charm, the medicine man cheerfully revealed its contents—feathers from a newly hatched chick, a couple of bones, teeth from a dog, a frog's leg, and shredded paper.[14]

Photos sent by Bethune to A. A. MacLeod, head of the Canadian

League for Peace and Democracy, in 1938–1939 reveal much about both poor medical conditions in the remote regions of China and the resources that Bethune envisioned as the means to overcome the primitiveness (Figs. 2–6). These previously-unpublished photos depict Bethune's International Peace Hospital at Wutaishan, which was established in October 1938. They may have been taken by Bethune himself, as the writing on the back of them is his. The extreme deprivation of the situation is very evident. On one photo of a hospital ward filled with wounded, Bethune wrote: "This is a typical hospital, rather better than most as [the patients] all have litters, in many [hospitals] they are lying on mats on the floor."[15] Shortages are also evident in the attached note that the International Peace Hospital in Wutaishan had 300 beds and served approximately 1,000 patients. Three patients to a bed! But if that seemed exceptionally inadequate, a report on medical conditions throughout China at the time offered a caveat: "2–3 patients per bed" was also the standard situation "found in the Chinese Hospitals of Hong Kong."[16]

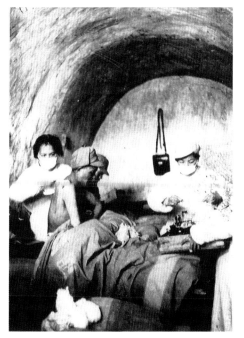

But while these photos clearly illustrate challenges, they also depict the new resources Bethune and the comrades were drawing upon to overcome their disadvantages. One new initiative was to advance the status of women, who feature prominently in several photos performing

*Fig. 2. Dressing heavily wounded cases in the ward of the International Peace Hospital, Wutaishan, 1938–1939. (Source: Archives of Ontario, F126-4-0-17)*

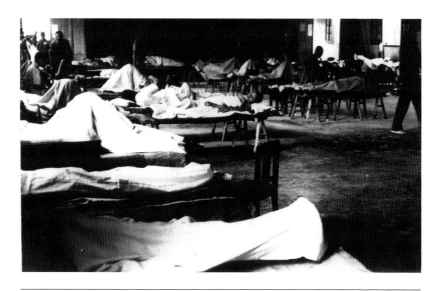

Fig. 3. *International Peace Hospital, Wutaishan, 1938–1939. The caption on the rear of this photo, which might have been taken by Bethune, reads: "This is a typical hospital, rather better than most as they all have litters, in many of them they are lying on mats on the floor." (Source: Archives of Ontario, F126-4-0-17)*

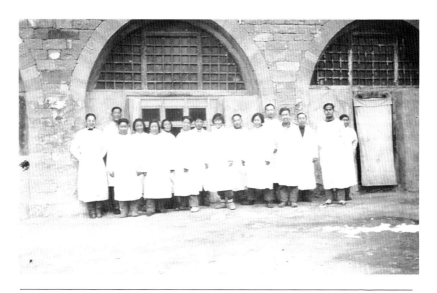

Fig. 4. *Staff of the International Peace Hospital, Wutiashan, 1938–1939. Note the high proportion of women, and the youthfulness of the staff. (Source: Archives of Ontario, F126-4-0-10)*

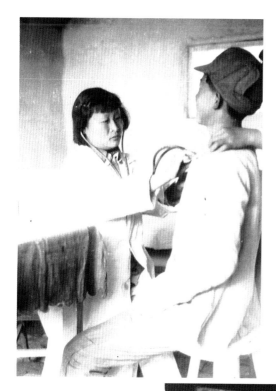

Fig. 5. *A female doctor examines a patient at the International Peace Hospital, Wutaishan. (Source: Archives of Ontario, F126-4-0-10)*

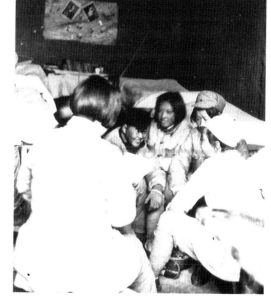

Fig. 6. *Dormitory discussion among young nurses at the International Peace Hospital, Wutaishan. These medical professionals appear to be very young, and their enthusiasm is evident. (Source: Archives of Ontario, F126-4-0-10)*

work of varied kinds. Some are nurses dressing wounded soldiers, but another photo shows a female doctor or nurse giving a wounded soldier a medical exam. This effort to draw women towards equality was a sign of change and hope. Throughout most of China at the time women had second-class status. In the liberated areas of China their talents were not ignored but instead were advanced and used to alleviate broader shortcomings. Now women could aspire to become nurses, even doctors. Thus, in a dialectical way, China's medical backwardness became an opportunity for a neglected element of China's population to leap forward and help overcome the country's backwardness. The same went for young people. The photos illustrated the youthfulness of Bethune's associates. One photo of nurses of the International Peace Hospital engaged in a dormitory political discussion shows young women and a man who are barely more than children. Bethune obviously viewed China's youth as a key strength in its fight against Western imperialism and Japanese militarism, a theme that also is seen in his writing from the time. A third theme evident in the photos is free treatment for combatants and civilians alike. One photo portrays two men receiving a free prescription at a pharmaceutical dispensary (Fig. 7).[17] This was in keeping with the communists' philosophy of ensuring fair treatment of civilians, which nurtured the critical relationship between the people and a people's army.

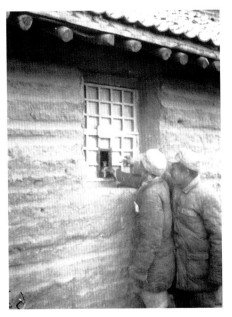

*Fig. 7. Two men obtain drugs at a dispensary at the International Peace Hospital, Wutaishan. (Source: Archives of Ontario, F126-4-0-10)*

One of the great medical innovations credited to Bethune in China was the mobile surgical unit that was the epitome of simplicity. Although he received accolades for this advance, front-line battle experience had previously acquainted the Eighth Route Army with the need for such units. Bethune himself took several months to see the folly of fixed medical facilities and the virtue of mobility. When Bethune and Jean Ewen first met Ze-Dong Mao at Yan'an, about midnight on March 31, 1938, Bethune presented the communist leader with his plan to improve the hospital at Yan'an. But Mao argued that the need for medical services was far greater at the front, in the Wutai Mountains on the border between Shansi and Hebei provinces. Bethune agreed to lead a team there. But even in this shifting military environment Bethune's first instinct was to build a permanent teaching hospital in the district, which was accomplished by September 1938 at Sung-yen K'ou. But it survived only weeks before being destroyed by the Japanese. Mobility was thus imposed, dramatically and immediately, on Bethune. For the month of October 1938 he reported: "This month we have been practically on the move for the entire month as a Mobile Unit." Out of this was born Bethune's mobile operating theaters. Guerrilla warfare against the Japanese thus created the objective conditions; Bethune's reception of the conditions helped produce the innovation.[18]

Once established, the mobile units proved themselves to be very effective. They consisted of two surgeons and three nurses; one of the three nurses was experienced in anaesthetics and one in drugs. The unit either carried with it a portable operating table or procured a local table. Surgical instruments, simple sterilizers, bandage cloth and dressings, anaesthetics and drugs were part of the unit's equipment. One unit was attached to each military brigade and was stationed 20 to 30 *li* (one *li* is half a kilometer) in the rear, so that wounded could be treated within 3 to 4 hours. After one engagement, Bethune reported that one third of the wounded he had treated (77 cases operated on over 40 hours) had no infection or fever, one third had slight infection and one third had the fever usually expected if the soldiers had waited to be treated until they reached the hospital.[19] This was a great improvement in treating the wounded, who frequently died of simple wounds because they did not receive medical care in time.

Although his renown might create an impression that Bethune was the only western doctor in China at the time, Bethune was in fact not alone. He had two types of colleagues, one politically inspired, the other religiously motivated. Among the former, the politically-committed medical personnel working among the communists in north China, were the Canadian nurse Jean Ewen and Dr. Hai-De Ma (George Hatem, a Lebanese American from Yonkers who went to China about 1935) and the five Indian doctors recruited by the Indian National Congress in 1938. All but one of the five Indians, the surgeon D. S. Kotnis, left China after two years. Dr. Kotnis remained and made his way north to work with the communists in the Jin-Cha-Ji border region, where he was still operating in 1942.[20] Another doctor who was politically motivated was Dr. Ianto Kaneti, a Bulgarian who served both the republicans in Spain and the Chinese anti-fascist cause. In fact, Kaneti was one of 17 doctors from the fascist-occupied countries who were selected to join a medical team to aid China after Franco's reactionary forces overwhelmed the republican government of Spain in 1939. [21]

The presence of these politically-motivated medical professionals helping China should not be overlooked. Thus my declaration in *The Politics of Passion* that, in going directly to the fighting front in north China, Bethune "became one of the very few people in the world who made their way to two centres of conflict between right-wing militarism and democracy in the 1930s," needs some modification. While Bethune certainly was one of a very few, the fact is that there were others who took up the cause of democracy in both Spain and China.

Yet two key aspects distinguished Bethune's contribution. One was that in going to both Spain and China to fight fascism and militarism, he acted individually. He pushed to go, he was not recruited by an existing organization. The second was that in his internationalist individualism he forcibly gave birth to internationalist collective organizations. In fact, in each case he was instrumental in helping to create organizations to sustain him and his work. For example, the Canadian Committee to Aid Spanish Democracy, which supported Bethune's blood transfusion work in Spain, was, in the words of its founder, Graham Spry, "a figment of my imagination" until Bethune seized it, gave it a specific goal and compelled it to begin the task of raising tens of thousands of dollars to initiate and sustain the blood transfusion unit. And nothing more than a scattered China-support effort existed in Canada in early August 1937 when Bethune set his sights on helping China fight the Japanese invasion.[22] The same may be true for the China Aid Council (CAC) based in New York, which became the foremost agent of pre-war American popular assistance to China. There is no printed history of the CAC (an historical oversight that needs to be corrected soon), but from what sketchy details are available, it could well be that Bethune's precipitous decision to go to China in the summer of 1937 kick-started its creation. Records show that by November 1937 Bethune was in New York raising funds, accumulating equipment and attempting to recruit other medical personnel to go with him to China. The next month, the China Aid Council was established in New York to collect money to provide medical aid to the victims of the war, including the wounded of the Chinese armies fighting Japanese in northern China. The first project of the CAC was to send out, in January 1938, the "American-Canadian Medical Unit"— comprised of Bethune, nurse Jean Ewen and the American doctor Charles Parsons. Of the three, we know that two, Ewen and Parsons, were dragooned into the project. And Parsons, a drunkard, jumped ship—or was pushed—from the unit at Hankou and returned in disgrace to the USA. Ewen, too, was separated from Bethune after the two reached Yan'an, so he alone proceeded to the front lines in 1938 while she served with the New Fourth Army in Anhui Province until 1939.[23] Thus the entire project to aid the Eighth Route Army seems to have been launched by Bethune and carried through to completion by him.

It could be that Bethune's example also stimulated Europeans to connect the struggles in Spain and China and, once the cause of Spain seemed lost by 1938, to devote themselves to giving medical assistance to the new front line in the anti-fascist struggle, in China. In February

1938, the month after Bethune landed in China with the "American-Canadian Medical Unit," an International Conference to Aid China held in London decided to establish an International Peace Hospital in China. After almost a year of work the hospital was established in Wutaishan under Bethune. Hilda Selwyn-Clarke, who headed the China Defence League in Hong Kong, advised the Canadian activist and friend of Norman Bethune A. A. MacLeod in April and July 1939 about various efforts in Europe to raise funds and doctors to provide medical assistance to Bethune's International Peace Hospital.[24] Was this burst of solidarity effort due to Bethune's path-breaking? Or did international events—especially the fascist toppling of the Spanish republican government on April 1, 1939—stimulate similar responses in like-minded people? It's hard to say authoritatively, and it's likely that a combination of factors gave birth to it. What we know for sure is that while other activists were planning actions and had made some preliminary steps towards accomplishing them, Bethune was already in the field and sending out a barrage of letters and cables demanding assistance from his western comrades.

A second group of medical professionals who offered medical service in China in the late 1930s were spiritually-motivated Christian missionaries. Bethune's personal background made him intensely suspicious of Christians. He was raised in a psychologically-troubled household where both his mother and father were zealous Christians; his mother did mission work in her youth. His view of his father was summed up with the contemptuous phrase "[w]hat hypocrites these professed religious are." And we know that when, at a tense moment under bombardment in China, Jean Ewen bluntly told him he was "nothing but a bloody missionary," he "blew his fuses."[25] Thus his dislike of Christians was deep and still strong in 1937.

In other circumstances than China, he might well have refused to work with missionaries. But in China this was simply not possible or sensible. Firstly, Western Christian mission clinics and hospitals existed in China long before he arrived. In the midst of appalling conditions, these missions were key elements of the medical system in China, rudimentary though it was. Western medical mission work had begun in China in 1861, and it was greatly advanced in 1906 when six British and American Protestant missions in China founded the Peking Union Medical College (PUMC). Its efforts to train Chinese medical personnel were significantly improved the next decade by assistance from the Rockefeller Foundation. In 1919 the PUMC Medical School was opened, including a new hospital, a pre-medical school and a school of nursing. Ironically, in a country marked by intense poverty, the PUMC in the 1920s and 1930s was one of the best and most modern medical centers in the world. Kathleen Hall, an Anglican missionary who trained as a nurse in New Zealand and arrived in China in 1922, described PUMC facilities as "at least twenty years ahead of anything in New Zealand."[26] But that was Beijing. In the provinces, the story was much different. Rural medical missions were far below the standard of the PUMC. Still they were significant additions to the inadequate medical system in China at the time. Ewen, who worked as a nurse in a Franciscan mission in Shandong Province and other parts of northeast China from 1933 to 1937, recalled that "we treated everything from ingrown toenails to leprosy."[27]

Seeing China under assault by Japanese militarism, Western political activists and Christians, who might normally have been at odds, had to throw themselves into a united front in medical work (Fig. 8). In this regard they were copying the united front that had been established among rival Chinese political parties following the Sian Incident of 1936. For Bethune, this medical united front specifically existed in his co-operation with the medical missionaries Kathleen Hall and Dr. Richard Brown (Fig. 9). In each case he saw dedicated professionals who used their medical know-how to benefit the Chinese people. As Ewen put it, "in these times no one was in a position to refuse help, especially in the medical field." In fact, the Christian missions indirectly performed a valuable role for the communists. As Ewen noted, "[a]n amazing number of people in the Eighth Route Army Medical Corps had at one time or another been connected with foreign missions"—in their schools, trained in mission hospitals or contacted in jails by missionaries.[28] In 1938, Bethune could not help celebrating the propaganda that could be made from Dr.

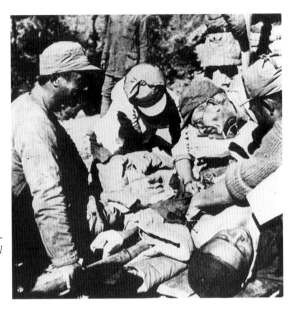

*Fig. 8. Bethune and medical workers examine a patient outdoors. (Source: Roderick Stewart)*

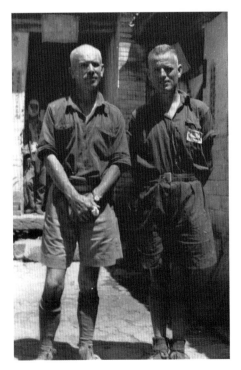

*Fig. 9. Bethune and Dr. Richard Brown, 1938. (Source: Library and Archives Canada, PA-161837)*

Brown joining him at Yan'an. In a communication to the China Aid Council on March 23, he crowed: "Think of the tremendous publicity value of having a medical missionary in charge of a combined Canadian and American Medical unit to the Communist Red Army. The terrible bandits! It's simply perfect."[29] By early 1939, however, desperation had taught him humility, and his genuine concern about the dangers of making such announcements to the world gave his thoughts on working with medical missionaries a new tone. After Kathleen Hall helped Bethune by purchasing essential supplies for him in Beijing, the Japanese retaliated by burning her mission clinic. Bethune's response was extreme solicitude:

> I have always felt and expressed some months ago that too much should not have been asked of these sympathetic missionaries.... Miss Hall can not be used again. Her life is already in danger owing to her help to the Region. The same applies to other missions such as the American Board Mission in Pao Ting.

Indeed, so much did he value Hall's dedication to China that Bethune asked her to join his unit.[30] Just as the Chinese Communist Party argued that joint work with the Guomindang depended only on the latter's strength of patriotic commitment to combating Japan's assault on China, so, too, did Bethune judge missionaries by the same standard—would they use their medical skills to aid the Chinese people?

Bethune's main frustration in China was not the rudimentary conditions, the lack of trained Chinese doctors and nurses or the shortage of supplies. These, he was convinced, could be overcome. However, doing so required assistance from North America. And that was where things broke down. By July 1938 he calculated that he had sent over a dozen letters and cables to the China Aid Council in New York, but had received just one response. By March 1939 he had received just three letters from the CAC. No less important, the money that he had left North America expecting to receive never did begin to flow, and he had to fall back on the Eighth Route Army itself to pay his personal expenses and those of his unit, which was a severe humiliation.[31]

At this remove, it's hard to assess the cause of the breakdown in the assistance that Bethune expected. But several factors stand out as contributing causes. One was that Bethune was simply too far from his supporting system. When it came to the anti-fascist struggle in Spain in 1936–1939, North American aid from the Canadian Committee to Aid Spanish Democracy, the North American Committee to Aid Spanish Democracy and the American Friends of Spanish Democracy did get through. But Spain and China were leagues apart, geographically, culturally and politically. Moreover, Japan's all-out invasion of China effectively cut off a great part of the latter country. In his enthusiasm Bethune was too optimistic about how well the mental and physical chasms between North America and Asia could be crossed. In *The Politics of Passion*, I have written that "negligence [at the China Aid Council] in New York is the primary reason for the failure to support Bethune. Once having sent the team to China, senior CAC members appear to have ignored it."[32] Until a detailed history of the CAC is written using its records, this must remain a preliminary assessment. But it does appear that the CAC in New York was not a pipeline but in fact the plug in the conduit pipe that was intended to direct cash from North America to Bethune. Yet at least some of his North American comrades did not abandon him. The Canadian support committees certainly remained active and sent significant sums intended for Bethune to both New York and to China. For example, A. A. MacLeod, who was head of the Canadian League for Peace and Democracy, wrote to Bethune on July 12, 1938 expressing great relief that "I have an address for you at last…. None of the letters [you] sent to the American League for Peace and Democracy have ever been forwarded to us." In his letter he detailed the monies that had been raised to aid the struggle in China. A support committee in the northern Ontario mining town of Timmins had raised enough money for an ambulance, and the money would be sent soon. A Vancouver support group had also raised $1,100 and had sent it to New York several weeks before. "I am, therefore, distressed to learn that you have not been receiving your regular allowance." In October 1938, MacLeod reported that the Canadian League for Peace and Democracy would "soon be sending 20,000 blankets and eight trucks to China." In February 1939 the CLPD sponsored a meeting featuring Colonel M. Thomas Tchou, former secretary to Jie-Shi Jiang, which generated $700 that was sent to Madame Jie-Shi Jiang. Then in March 1939 the CLPD raised a further $6,300 from the Canadian tour of Chinese student leader Loh Tsei's tour and forwarded this to the China Defence League to aid the International Peace Hospital. Other sums were sent by local committees in Ontario and British Columbia.[33] In short, the funds raised from Canada alone to aid Bethune's work in China were rather impressive. Yet Bethune never seems to have received any of it. Why? Leaving aside failings at the China Aid Council in New York, Tom Newnham has one explanation for the mystery. It is that the Guomindang systematically blocked and appropriated the shipments and money intended for the communists in north China. This was confirmed by Hilda Selwyn-Clarke, who, as head of the China Defence League, was on the scene in Hong Kong. She advised A. A. MacLeod not to send money to Madame Jie-Shi Jiang, the wife of the Guomindang leader. The problem, she wrote, was not Madame Jiang's patriotism or integrity but more the fact that the money might get diverted into Guomindang projects such as the New Life Movement, whose value Selwyn-Clarke doubted. "They have the best of intentions but they are not organized through a corps of qualified doctors such as you have in Dr. Bethune's Hospital ..."[34] Thus Bethune's irritated demand—"What in hell is that damned American Committee doing?"—was a legitimate expression of irritation with the CAC from his perspective in north China.[35] But "that damned American Committee" might not have been exclusively responsible for him being cut off from vital North American funds.

As much as Bethune influenced the delivery of medical care in China, practicing medicine in China also transformed him (Fig. 10). Bethune was clearly a disturbed and difficult man at the time he went to China. And the accounts of Westerners who knew him there suggest that he was also troubled during his first months in China.[36] But there is some evidence to suggest that the conditions of China changed Bethune. That the liberation war in China sometimes made this possible was illustrated by the life of De Zhu, one of the great

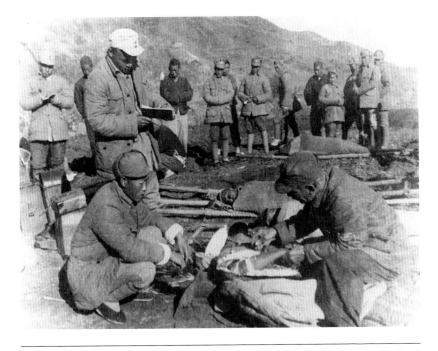

*Fig. 10. Bethune examines a patient outdoors, observed by staff and students. (Source: Roderick Stewart)*

military commanders produced by the Communist Party of China. Born in 1886, he came of age, took military training and rose as an officer in the years of China's democratic revolution in the first decade of the century. But his own despair at China's predicament led him, in the years from 1917 to 1922, down the path taken by too many of China's elite—into warlordism and opium addiction. Yet in 1922, answering the call to help transform and unite China, Zhu overcame his opium addiction and began to use his military skills to help China. Ultimately he would join the Communist Party and play a significant role in defeating the Japanese and the Guomindang.[37] Similarly, Bethune's personality appeared to change in the revolutionary conditions of China. Hai-De Ma has said that this occurred in part because Bethune witnessed, thousands of times, selflessness among the Eight Route Army fighters.

So of course he would want to get rid of every vestige of individual-ism.… He had always been highly individualistic [but in China] he knew that his job was to get rid of the accretions of the past. In normal circumstances, this takes a long time. In conditions of a people's war it doesn't take that long.[38]

Conditions in China also transformed Bethune's medical practice. It was not just a matter of him coming to see the necessity of mobile medical care that operated adjacent to the battle front or his inspired response to that, the mobile operating theaters. More than that, his entire orientation towards medicine was shattered and a new one was created. In China he became the people's doctor in a way that would previously have been unthinkable. Certainly throughout his early medical career he had been focused on people rather than, as for many other doctors, on profit or social status. In Detroit in the 1920s he had attended to working class clients for a minimal fee. In the 1930s in Montreal he had held a free open surgery every Saturday afternoon for the unemployed. In Spain, a considerable part of his waking hours was occupied in attending to anti-fascist fighters, although he also devoted special attending to children who had been made orphans or refugees because of the fascist onslaught on civilians. But in each case, he reserved part, or even much, of himself for the satisfaction of his considerable ego, his lust for fine art, fine food, fine women.[39] His patients were important but they remained secondary to his ego. In China, he became "the compleat people's doctor." He took no salary for his work. As he pointed out, why should he, when all his needs were met?[40] At times he gave his own blood to his patients. Medicine became intertwined with life so as to make the two inseparable. Bethune's medical practice had previously been altruistic, but altruism is an act of charity. His medical practice in China saw him, for the first time, literally embody the quote he had long before adopted from Walt Whitman—"I do not pity the wounded. I become the wounded."[41] This dialectical transformation meant the destruction of the Bethune of old and the construction of a new Bethune, the destruction of the old doctor and the creation of a new one.

It also meant the end of Bethune the man. In November 1939,

like millions of Chinese before and after him assailed by the blows of imperialism, Bethune was literally driven into the grave. Yet while they would die in their multitude, unremembered, Bethune, a western doctor, would be memorialized (Fig. 11). His dedicated approach towards medicine is a great part of why his fame has endured. When people today ask "What is the meaning of medicine?" Doctor Norman Bethune's name is sure to be invoked.

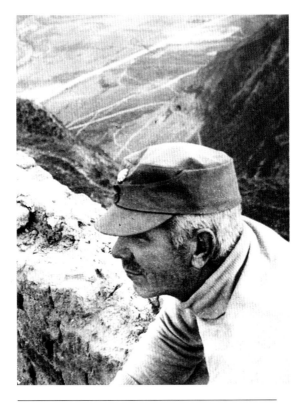

Fig. 11. *Bethune at the Great Wall, likely about 1939. (Source: Canadian Parks Service)*

## Notes

1   The reasons why Bethune attained such prominence in China are complex and perhaps reflect politics in China as much as they do Bethune's real contribution. If one is to believe journalist Mark Gayn, for instance, Bethune was virtually ignored in China at the time of Gayn's visit to Yan'an in 1947. (See Thomas Fisher Rare Book Library, University of Toronto, Mark Gayn Manuscript Collection, Fonds 215, Box 56, Folder 7 [Bethune, Chiang Ching], Bethune, Nov. 9, 1975.) Certainly Bethune does appear to have risen greatly in stature in China during and after the Great Proletarian Cultural Revolution, 1966–1976. But his martyrdom also accounts for some of this acclaim.

2   Larry Hannant (ed.), *The Politics of Passion: Norman Bethune's Writing and Art* (Toronto: University of Toronto Press, 1998), pp. 202, 204.

3   Jean Ewen, *China Nurse 1932–1939* (Toronto: McClelland and Stewart, 1981), p. 20.

4   Bethune's wife, Frances, was convinced that Agnes Smedley alone "was responsible for him [Bethune] going to Wutaishan." But this subjective factor, which certainly had some weight, does not take into account the broader objective factors, plus Bethune's own determination, that took Bethune to Yan'an. See Archives of Ontario, F126, MU7590 File 12 League for Peace and Democracy— Norman Bethune, Frances Coleman to MacLeod, September 29 [1940].

5   Hannant (ed.), *Politics of Passion*, p. 230.

6   Ewen, *China Nurse*, p. 90.

7   Thomas Fisher Rare Book Library, University of Toronto, Mark Gayn Manuscript Collection, Fonds 215, Box 56, Folder 7 (Bethune, Chiang Ching), Bethune, November 9, 1975. It is not clear that the hospital at Yan'an that Gayn saw was in fact "Bethune's hospital" or was at all influenced by Bethune during his 20 months in China. Although his goal in going to Yan'an was to reorganize the hospital there, Mao convinced him that working at the front, in the Jin-Cha-Ji liberated area, was more important. Consequently, Bethune quickly moved on to the battle front and left Yan'an. In the Jin-Cha-Ji liberated area there were eight "hospitals," seven of them smaller "base hospitals," all of them ill-equipped and poorly staffed, plus the International Peace Hospital at General Rong-Zhen Nie's headquarters at Wutaishan.

8   Ewen, *China Nurse*, pp. 34, 55.

9   T. A. Raman and Anup Singh, "China's International Peace Hospitals," *Far Eastern Survey*, Vol. 12, No. 8 (April 19, 1943), p. 79.

10   Hannant (ed.), *Politics of Passion*, p. 333.

11   Tom Newnham, *Dr. Bethune's Angel: The Life of Kathleen Hall* (Auckland, N.Z.: Graphic Publications, 2002), pp. 75–76.

12  Hannant (ed.), *Politics of Passion*, pp. 270, 279.

13  Ibid., p. 297.

14  Ewen, *China Nurse*, pp. 101–102. Not all folk medicine, of course, is quackery. Some elements of traditional medical care, developed over the course of centuries of practice, are practically sound and helpful.

15  Archives of Ontario, F126-4-0-17.

16  Archives of Ontario, F126, MU7590 File 13 League for Peace and Democracy— China, International Peace Hospital report n.d. [1939].

17  Archives of Ontario, F126-4-0-10, and F126-4-0-17.

18  Hannant (ed.), *Politics of Passion*, pp. 228, 297–298.

19  Archives of Ontario, F126, MU7590 File 18 League for Peace and Democracy— China, report by Dr. Robert Brown of July 1, 1939.

20  For a contrary view on Hai-De Ma, see Otto Braun, *A Comintern Agent in China 1932–1939*, trans. Jeanne Moore (London: C. Hurst and Company, 1982), p. 252. Concerning Kotnis, see Braun, p. 255, Agnes Smedley, *Battle Hymn of China* (New York: Alfred Knopf, 1943), pp. 229–230 and T. A. Raman and Anup Singh, "China's International Peace Hospitals," *Far Eastern Survey*, Vol. 12, No. 8 (April 19, 1943), p. 79.

21  Len Tsou, "Dr. Ianto Kaneti 1910–2004," *The Volunteer*, Vol. XXVI, No. 3 (September 2004), p. 19.

22  Hannant (ed.), *Politics of Passion*, pp. 197 and 119.

23  Ewen, *China Nurse*, pp. 44–46, 51–52 and 137–138; Smedley, *Battle Hymn of China*, p. 229; Hannant (ed.), *Politics of Passion*, pp. 192, 195–197. Tom Newnham declares it probable that once Bethune was joined by Dr. Richard Brown, a Methodist medical missionary who spoke Chinese, the former thought he did not need Ewen's services and asked that she be transferred to other duties. Newnham, *Dr. Bethune's Angel*, p. 101.

24  Archives of Ontario, F126, MU7590, File 13, International Peace Hospital report n.d. [1939] and File 24, Selwyn-Clarke to MacLeod, April 20, 1939 and July 2, 1939.

25  Hannant (ed.), *Politics of Passion*, p. 38; Ewen, *China Nurse*, p. 67.

26  Newnham, *Dr. Bethune's Angel*, pp. 25–26.

27  Ewen, *China Nurse*, p. 17.

28  Ibid., pp. 83, 110.

29  Hannant (ed.), *Politics of Passion*, p. 222.

30  Ibid., pp. 351–352.

31  Ibid., pp. 273, 355–356, 243.

32  Ibid., p. 273.

33  Archives of Ontario, F126, MU7590, File 12, A. A. MacLeod to Bethune July 12, 1938 and MU 7591, File 10, MacLeod to Phillip Noel-Baker, October 31, 1938;

MU7590, File 24, MacLeod to Selwyn-Clarke, March 7, 1939; MU7590 File 24, Virginia MacLeod to Selwyn-Clarke May 13, 1939 and Selwyn-Clarke reply May 18, 1939; A. A. MacLeod to Selwyn-Clarke, June 16, 1939.

34   Newnham, *Dr. Bethune's Angel*, 135; Archives of Ontario, F126, MU7590, File 24, Selwyn-Clarke to MacLeod, April 1, 1939.

35   Hannant (ed.), *Politics of Passion*, p. 294.

36   Ewen, *China Nurse*, pages 46 to 96 set out in vivid, engaging detail Ewen's five months of contact with Bethune, an experience that certainly did not endear him to her. And she claimed that Dr Richard Brown's "opinion of Dr. Bethune was not very high." (p. 119) Even Kathleen Hall's first impression was that he was "a most difficult man," although her assessment of him rose over time. (Newnham, *Dr. Bethune's Angel*, p. 110).

37   Agnes Smedley, *The Great Road: The Life and Times of Chu Teh* (New York: Monthly Review Press, 1956), pp. 128–144.

38   Ted Allan, "The Making of a Martyr: How Chairman Mao's China Transformed Norman Bethune," *Canadian Magazine*, July 12, 1975, p. 22

39   Roderick Stewart, *Bethune* (Toronto: New Press, 1973), pp. 17, 71, 105.

40   Hannant (ed.), *Politics of Passion*,

41   Allan, "The Making of a Martyr," p. 20.

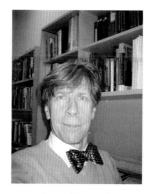

Larry Hannant

## *Editorial Comments*

Although Norman Bethune has been a truly legendary figure in China for almost 70 years, I was not fully aware of his multiple talents until reading an award-winning book entitled *The Politics of Passion: Norman Bethune's Writing and Art* by Larry Hannant (University of Toronto Press, 1998). Logically Mr. Hannant was invited to contribute to our book—with the only chapter in this volume written by a historian rather than a physician.

To help readers understand Bethune better, we also include below some additional background material, such as Bethune's art works (Figs. 1, 2, 3B, and 5 are selected from *The Politics of Passion* with permission), and several previous comments by people from different parts of the world on this Canadian thoracic surgeon.

The more I know about Dr. Bethune, the stronger I personally believe—a great surgeon is always a great person in the first place!

(S. W.)

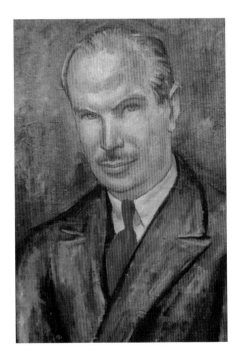

*Fig. 1. Self-portrait (this oil painting was completed in 1934, two years after Bethune was appointed chief of thoracic surgery at the Sacre Coeur Hospital in Quebec, Canada, and one year before he became the council member of the American Association for Thoracic Surgery).*

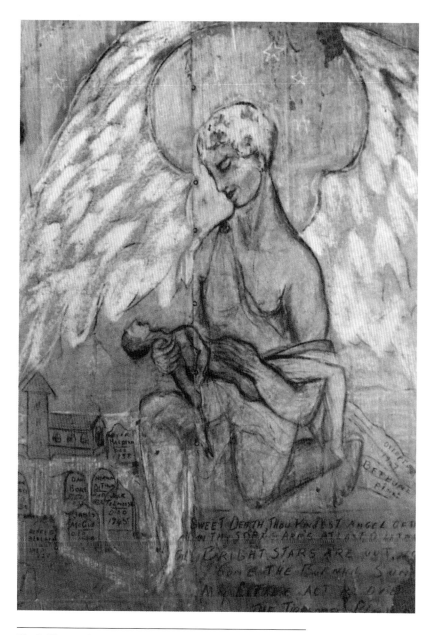

*Fig. 2. The T. B.'s progress—Scene IX (by Norman Bethune in 1921).*

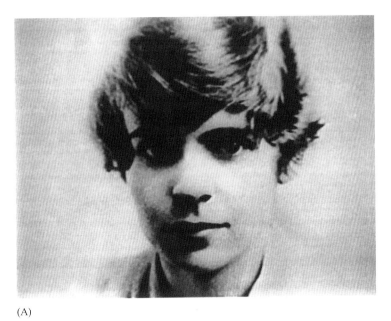

(A)

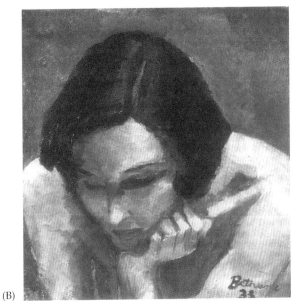

(B)

*Fig. 3.  The picture (A) and the portrait in oils (B, by Norman Bethune in 1933) of Frances Penney, Bethune's ex-wife, with whom he married twice.*

## *Appendix:*

### Alexander J. Walt, FACS, FRCS:

Henry Norman Bethune was born in Ontario in 1890 and was to become the best-known physician in the world. Bethune spent his professional life in Detroit and Montreal, with these periods separated by a year spent as a patient in a tuberculosis sanatorium. This was where his interest in pulmonary disease was stimulated. Pioneer thoracic surgeon, councilor to the American Association for Thoracic Surgery, artist, poet, polemist, conservative-turned-communist, iconoclast, and soldier, Bethune was a highly complex individual. Diverting his energies from surgery to social issues during the depression, Bethune participated in the Spanish Civil War, at which time he designed the world's first mobile blood transfusion unit. Eight months later, Bethune joined Mao Tse-tung [Ze-Dong Mao]'s Eight Route Army in China. In 1939 he died of septicemia acquired from a sliver of infected bone while he was operating on a wounded Chinese patient. Bethune's fame today derives principally from the popularization of his accomplishments by Mao, whom he met once and who subsequently decreed that all in China should learn about him. Bethune's posthumous influence played an important role in the reopening of relations between China and the West.

(Walt AJ. The world's best-known surgeon.
*Surgery* 1983;94:582–590)

### Iain Macintyre, FRCS, and Iain MacLaren, FRCS:

There are few famous surgeons even among those of the highest professional and scientific distinction whose achievements have won for them general, popular acclaim in their own countries, and fewer still have gained widespread international celebrity. Only one has ever become a posthumous national hero and nearly seven decades after his death he not only retains his herotic stature, but is held up as a role model to the schoolchildren of the most populous nation on earth.

*(Macintyre I, MacLaren I, eds.* Surgeons' lives. *pp 201–203,*
*Royal College of Surgeons of Edinburgh, UK, 2005)*

## Leo Eloesser, MD (President of the American Association for Thoracic Surgery in 1936–1937):

What better end could any man have than this fellow member of ours, who spent his life and met his death in the service of his ideals— Humanity and Freedom.

(Eloesser L. In memoriam: Norman Bethune 1890–1939.
*J Thorac Surg* 1940;9:460–461)

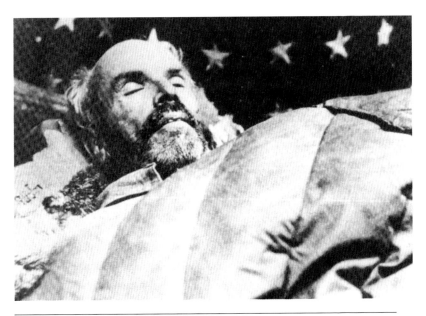

*Fig. 4. It was described that before his death on November 12, 1939, Bethune said, "My only regret is that I shall now be unable to do more."*

## Editor's Note (*J Thorac Surg* 1940;9:461–462):

In a letter to Dr. Louis Davidson, New York, which was reprinted in the *Baltimore Evening Sun,* January 13, 1940, Bethune, writing from China, said:

"The work I am trying to do is to take peasants (boys) and young workers and make doctors out of them. They can read and write and most have a knowledge of arithmetic. None of my doctors has ever been to college or universities, and none has ever been in a modern hospital (most of them have never been in any hospital), much less a medical school. With this material, I must make doctors and nurses out of them—six months for nurses and one year for doctors. We have 2,300 wounded in hospitals all the time. These hospitals are merely the dirty one-story mud-and-stone houses of out-of-the-way villages set in deep valleys, overhung by mountains, some of which are 10,000 feet high."

Bethune described himself as having traveled during the last year 3,165 miles, performing 762 operations, and examining 1,800 wounds. In addition, he reorganized the army's sanitary service, wrote three textbooks, and established a medical training school.

"It's a fast life," he wrote. "I miss tremendously a comrade to whom to talk. You know how fond I am of talking. I don't mind the conventional hardships—heat and bitter cold, dirt, lice, unvaried unfamiliar food, walking in the mountains, no stoves, beds, or baths. I find I can get along and operate as well in a dirty Buddhist temple with a twenty-foot high statue of the impassive-faced, gilded god staring over my shoulder, as in a modern operating room, with running water, nice green glazed walls, electric lamps, and a thousand other accessories.... They [the wounded] have no mattresses, no sheets. They lie in their old, stained uniforms with their knapsacks as pillows and one padded cotton blanket over them. They are grand. They certainly can take it."

Of his physical condition Bethune said: "My health is pretty fair—teeth need attention, one ear has been completely deaf for three months, glasses for eyes need correction, but apart from these minor things and being pretty thin, I'm OK." He added, "I dream

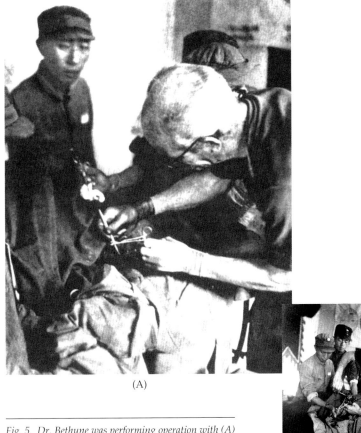

(A)

(B)

*Fig. 5. Dr. Bethune was performing operation with (A) or without (B) surgical gloves (due to lack of supply).*

of coffee, of rare roast beef, of apple pie, and ice cream. Books—are books still written? Is music still being played? Do you dance, drink beer, look at pictures? What do clean sheets in a soft bed feel like? Do women still love to be loved?"

## Ze-Dong Mao:

What kind of spirit is this that makes a foreigner selflessly adopt the cause of the Chinese people's liberation as his own? ... No one who returned from the front failed to express admiration for Bethune whenever his name was mentioned, and none remained unmoved by his spirit.... Now we are all commemorating him, which shows how profoundly his spirit inspires everyone. We must all learn the spirit of absolute selflessness from him. A man's ability may be great or small, but if he has this spirit, he is already noble-minded and pure, a man of moral integrity and above vulgar interests, a man who is of value to the people.

(Mao ZD. In memory of Norman Bethune.
This speech was delivered on December 21, 1939)

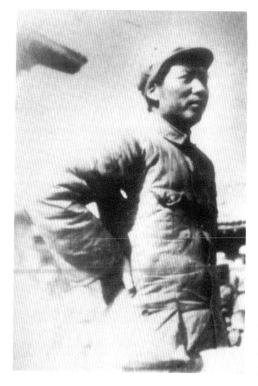

*Fig. 6. Ze-Dong Mao in 1938 (this picture was taken by Bethune after his only meeting with Mao. It was eventually sent back to Canada and published in a local newspaper).*

# The Evolution of Cardiovascular Surgery in China

*Song Wan, Anthony P. C. Yim*

> *"Things present are judged by things past."*
> — *A Chinese idiom*

The history of the development of cardiovascular surgery in China was little known to the West not only because the majority of the earlier reports were published almost exclusively in the Chinese language, but also because China was essentially closed to the West before the 1980s. We present here a brief account on how some Chinese surgeons struggled to establish a new specialty in their homeland.

## [1945, Chongqing]

Although the Chinese were the first to discover the concept of blood circulation some two thousand years before William Harvey [1], cardiovascular surgery did not exist in China until the time of World War II. The first successful cardiac operation ever recorded in China—a direct repair of a right ventricular stab wound—was carried out in October 1940 by Dr. Chao-Mei Zhang [2]. As happened similarly in the United States and Europe, subsequent developments in cardiovascular surgery in this country started with extracardiac anomalies. A leading Chinese thoracic surgeon, Dr. Ying-Kai Wu [3], performed the first ligation of patent ductus arteriosus at the Central Hospital of Chongqing in October 1944 (six years after the groundbreaking operation by Robert Gross) [4] and the first successful pericardectomy for constrictive pericarditis in 1947 [5] after the hospital was relocated to Tianjin.

In the early 1940s, the city of Chongqing (previously known as Chungking) was the wartime capital of China. Several famous Chinese universities were forced to move from the other major cities just before their occupation by Japanese troops to Chongqing and Chengdu, two large cities in Sichuan Province, China. Many Chinese physicians and surgeons who were to become leaders in their fields received their medical or surgical training there during this time of turmoil. Among them was Dr. Mei-Hsin Shih (Fig. 1), one of the foremost pioneers in cardiac surgery in China.

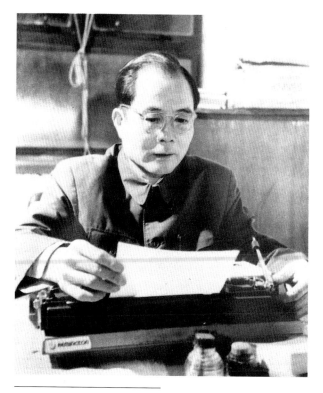

*Fig. 1. Dr. Mei-Hsin Shih in 1978.*

Shih's pursuit of cardiac surgery was stimulated by a talk in 1945 in Chongqing. As a second-year surgical resident at the Teaching Hospital of National Shanghai Medical College (which was later moved back to Shanghai in 1946), Shih was among the audience one day for a special lecture by Professor Leo Eloesser from Stanford University who visited China under the United Nations' Relief and Rehabilitation Administration [6]. With great enthusiasm Eloesser introduced to the Chinese surgeons the Blalock-Taussig operation, which has been first performed only months previously at the Johns Hopkins Hospital on November 29, 1944. The combination of a brilliant concept and its technical success brought hopes to those "blue babies" who were formerly considered incurable. "If anyone of you can perform such an operation," Eloesser teased the audience at the end of his talk, "I will cut my head off." Probably trying to enliven the atmosphere, he even made a gesture to imitate cutting off his head. Without his realizing it, this condescending remark became a powerful stimulus to the budding surgeons in the audience. Decades later Shih could still recall the exact words.

## *Rising to the Challenge*
## *[1953 to 1958, Shanghai]*

Mei-Hsin Shih performed the first Blalock-Taussig shunt in China at Zhongshan Hospital of the Shanghai First Medical College on March 2, 1953. Few of us today can even come close to imagine the hardship facing Shih at that time. He returned to Shanghai shortly after the Korean War and under the political and socioeconomic circumstances at the time it was impossible to acquire any Western-made surgical materials or instruments. This however did not deter Shih from pursuing his goal. He spent all his spare time in the week before surgery converting some ordinary sewing needles (the smallest he could find) into improvised curved surgical needles. These "homemade" needles turned out to be quite satisfactory during the operation on a 13-year-old boy with tetralogy of Fallot (Fig. 2; the picture was taken 38 years after the operation when the grateful patient returned to visit the surgeon who saved his life).

Over the next few years, Shanghai as the biggest city in China witnessed many breakthroughs in cardiovascular surgery (Table 1). Xi-Chun Lan (previously spelled as Hsi-Ch'un Lan, Fig. 3) and his team at the Shanghai Second Medical College performed the first closed mitral commissurotomy (using the index finger through the left atrial appendage) in February 1954, which marked the beginning of intracardiac surgery in China. Within a year they were able to report their experience with 32 patients and only one death (secondary to cerebral embolism) [7].

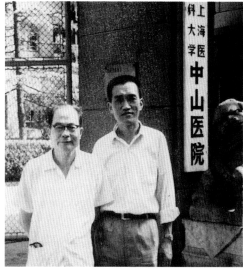

*Fig. 2. The patient who underwent the first Blalock-Taussig procedure in China visited Dr. Shih at Zhongshan Hospital in Shanghai 38 years later.*

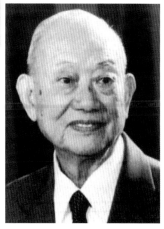

*Fig. 3. Dr. Xi-Chun Lan*

## Table 1   Reported First Cardiovascular Procedures in China

| Year | Surgeon | Procedure |
|------|---------|-----------|
| 1940 | Chao-Mei Zhang | Direct repair of a right ventricular stab wound |
| 1944 | Ying-Kai Wu | Ligation of patent ductus arteriosus |
| 1948 | Ying-Kai Wu | Pericardectomy for constrictive pericarditis |
| 1953 | Mei-Hsin Shih | Blalock-Taussig shunt |
| 1954 | Xi-Chun Lan | Closed mitral commissurotomy |
| 1955 | Pei-Bin Fu | Homograft replacement of huge innominate artery aneurysm |
| 1956 | Tao-Ying Xie | Resection of thoracic aortic aneurysm under hypothermia |
| 1957 | Qi-Chen Liang | Direct-vision pulmonary valvotomy under hypothermia |
| 1957 | Kai-Shi Gu | Aortic aneurysm repair using vascular prosthesis |
| 1958 (Apr) | Mei-Hsin Shih | Atrial septal defect repair under hypothermia |
| 1958 (Jun) | Hong-Xi Su | First CPB procedure (ventricular septal defect repair) |
| 1958 (Jul) | Kai-Shi Gu | Correction of RVOTO using Chinese made heart-lung machine |
| 1958 (Sep) | You-Lin Hou | Mitral valve repair for regurgitation under hypothermia without CPB |
| 1959 | Mei-Hsin Shih | Homograft replacement of aortic arch aneurysm |
| 1960 | Mei-Hsin Shih | Direct repair of ruptured sinus of Valsalva under CPB |
| 1962 | Zhuo-Rong Feng | Excision of left atrial myxoma |
| 1965 | Yong-Zhi Cai | Valve replacement with Chinese made mechanical prosthesis |
| 1972 | Jia-Qiang Guo | Resection of post-infarction ventricular aneurysm |
| 1974 | Jia-Qiang Guo | Coronary artery bypass grafting using saphenous vein |
| 1974 | Wen-Xiang Ding | Pediatric (< 2-year-old) open-heart surgery |
| 1976 | Xiao-Dong Zhu | Valve replacement with Chinese made bovine pericardial prosthesis |
| 1977 | Zheng-Xiang Luo | Valve replacement with Chinese made porcine prosthesis |
| 1978 | Shi-Ze Zhang | Orthotopic heart transplantation |
| 1979 | Zeng-Wei Wang | Complex congenital cardiac operations |
| 1985 | Yan-Qing Sun | Bentall operation |
| 1986 | Wen-Xiang Ding | Senning operation and arterial switch operation in infants |
| 1988 | Shu-Hsun Chu | Heterotopic heart transplantation |
| 1992 | Xiao-Cheng Liu | Heart-lung transplantation |

CPB: cardiopulmonary bypass; RVOTO: right ventricular outflow tract obstruction.

In the meantime, Pei-Bin Fu and associates at Guangci Hospital of the Shanghai Second Medical College excised a huge syphilitic aneurysm of the innominate artery (with a diameter of 15 cm) on October 13, 1955 [8]. To connect the right internal carotid artery to the left subclavian artery, they had to implant 2 pieces of arterial homografts as no single available graft was adequate enough in length. The operation lasted more than 13 hours. The 49-year-old patient was able to sit up and talk comfortably within a day after surgery. However, the patient died suddenly on postoperative day 15 while he was having dinner. The autopsy showed rupture at the anastomosis of the homograft to the left subclavian artery [8]. Seven months later, this group of surgeons performed another operation on a 38-year-old man with a similar pathology. They waited more than a month for suitable arterial homografts, which had been stored in the modified "Tyrode" solution for 3 days prior to the operation. The surgeons certainly had learned from their experience as this operation went uneventfully and was 4 hours shorter than the previous one. The patient was successfully discharged home weeks later after having finished a full course of anti-syphilitic therapy [8].

In January 1957, Qi-Chen Liang and Yi-Shan Wang at Renji Hospital of the Shanghai Second Medical College performed the first two cases in China of pulmonary valvotomy for stenosis under direct vision using hypothermia (28 to 30°C) without extracorporeal circulation [9]. One of the patients had undergone a closed pulmonary valve dilatation (through the right ventricle using the Brock valve knife) two and a half years earlier by the same group of surgeons. However, her pulmonary valve became stenotic again within months. The patient demonstrated sustained relief of symptoms after the second operation [9].

On April 10, 1958, Shih and colleagues closed an atrial septal defect (ASD) under moderate hypothermia at 30°C on a 21-year-old student. This first direct repair of ASD in China lasted 7 minutes and 15 seconds, without the use of cardiopulmonary bypass (CPB). By the end of 1959, Shih's group had collected a series of 20 patients who underwent this operation. All patients except one survived the operation and remained in excellent condition on follow-up [10].

Although one of the ASD repairs in Shih's series [10] was eventually done with the use of a heart-lung machine, the first successful open-heart operation under CPB in China was performed a few months earlier by another group of surgeons in Xi'an.

## First Cardiopulmonary Bypass Procedure in China [1958, Xi'an]

Dr. Hong-Xi Su (Fig. 4) was born in 1915. He graduated from the Medical College of National Nanjing Central University in 1943 (the same year as Mei-Hsin Shih) in Chengdu, the neighbor city of Chongqing. He served more than a year in the war before returning to his university to complete his surgical training. After his chief residency year, Su was sent to the United States in 1949 for further training in thoracic and cardiovascular surgery. He spent the next seven years in Chicago at Northwestern University and the University of Illinois. During this period, Su not only personally experienced the rapid development of cardiac surgery, he also met Jane H. McDonald, who was to become his wife.

During his visit to the University of Illinois, Su had a chance to participate in the experimental studies on extracorporeal circulation. This experience had a tremendous impact on his future career and life. He used up his own savings to buy the expensive Dewall-Lillehei heart-lung machine and shipped it back to China in January 1957 for his use upon returning home [11]. Under the political circumstances at the time the return journey to China for the young couple was not straightforward. Pretending to be a tourist, Jane flew through Canada to England. Meanwhile Su spent a week on a British ship crossing the Atlantic Ocean. The couple met again in Liverpool and finally arrived together in Beijing five weeks later at the end of February 1957. Mrs. Jane Su (known to many Chinese friends as "Su Jane") spent the next few decades in China with her husband and played a strong supporting role in his career (Fig. 5).

Su became the chief of cardiovascular surgery at the Fourth Military Medical University (former Medical College of National Nanjing Central University) in Xi'an, where the animal research

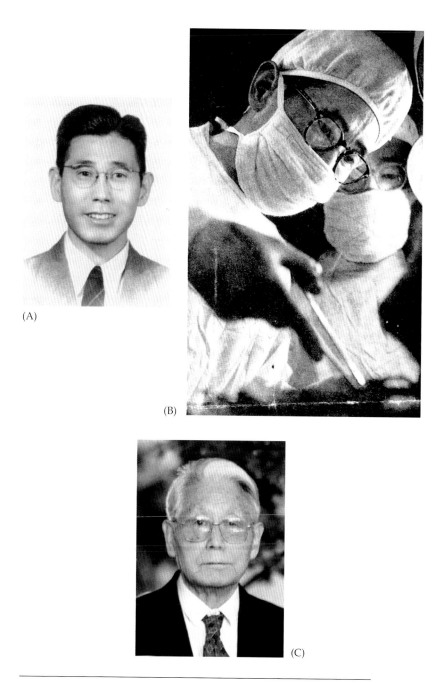

*Fig. 4. Dr. Hong-Xi Su in the late 1940s [A], in 1958 [B] and in the early 2000s [C].*

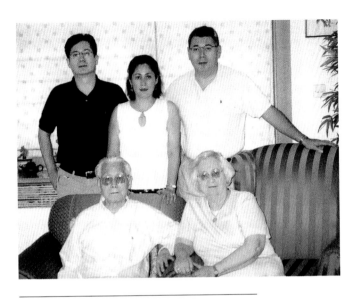

Fig. 5. Dr. Hong-Xi Su, his wife Jane, and their children.

project on extracorporeal circulation began in July 1957. In total, Su and his colleagues performed various procedures under CPB in 168 dogs with an overall survival rate of 76%. This preceded the clinical application of a newly learnt technique.

On June 26, 1958, five years after John Gibbon's landmark operation, Su and his team set out to close a ventricular septal defect (VSD) on a 6-year-old boy (Fig. 6A) under CPB [12]. However, an unexpected event happened. Convulsion suddenly developed in the patient just when the cannulas were inserted into his right atrium. As such an unforeseen convulsion was considered due to fever resulting from the high room temperature and heavy surgical drapes (air-conditioning did not exist then), the decision was made not to abandon the procedure. The convulsion subsided as soon as the patient went on CPB. Naturally, the success of this operation (Figs. 6B, 6C) hit the headlines in over 40 newspapers across China.

Within a month, Kai-Shi Gu (Fig. 7) and his associates at the Shanghai Chest Hospital had also performed a surgical correction of congenital right ventricular outflow tract obstruction under CPB [13].

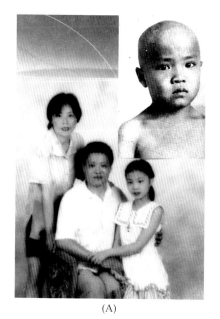
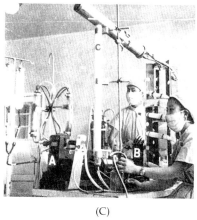

(C)

(A)

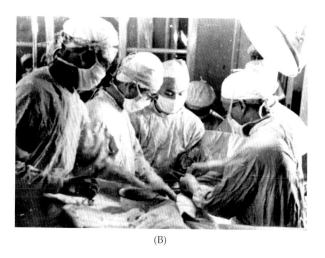

(B)

Fig. 6. [A] The patient who underwent the first cardiopulmonary bypass procedure in China in 1958 (inset) and in 1998 (with his wife and daughter); [B] Dr. Su (second from left) and colleagues at the operation. Courtesy of Dr. Wei-Yong Liu (third from left); [C] The heart-lung machine used in Xi'an in 1958.

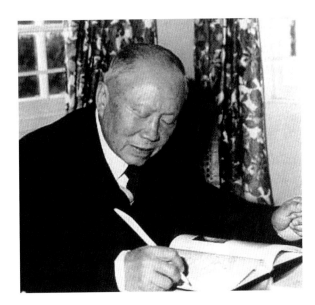

*Fig. 7. Dr. Kai-Shi Gu*

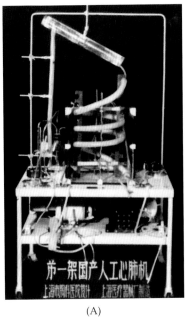

第一架国产人工心肺机
上海市胸科医院设计　上海医疗器械厂制造

(A)

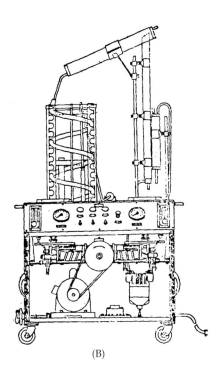

(B)

*Fig. 8. [A, B] The first Chinese-made heart-lung machine used at the Shanghai Chest Hospital in July 1958.*

This operation marked the first clinical use of an entirely Chinese-made heart-lung machine. The extracorporeal circuit consisted of a roller pump and a bubble oxygenator (Fig. 8), which was designed by the surgeons at the Shanghai Chest Hospital and produced by the Shanghai Medical Equipment Factory [13]. The continued collaboration between these two teams soon led to another important accomplishment—a Chinese-made mitral valve dilator. This device was first used clinically in December 1960 by Kai-Shi Gu and colleagues to perform the closed mitral commissurotomy through the left ventricle for the first time. This novel approach rapidly gained wide popularity in China [14].

## In the Ascendant
### [1959 to 1966, Shanghai and Beijing]

By the end of 1959, hundreds of direct vision intracardiac operations under hypothermia without the use of CPB had been performed at 30 hospitals in 13 provinces across China, although the majority of such cases (with a small number of CPB procedures) were carried out in Shanghai and Beijing [15].

Several milestones in the history of cardiovascular surgery in China were linked with Shanghai over this period (Table 1). From August 1957 through February 1960, Kai-Shi Gu and his team [16] performed different types of aortic aneurysm repair in 17 patients (ascending 4, arch 7, descending 5, and abdominal 1), remarkably with 14 survivors (Fig. 9). Using temporary left heart bypass followed by a temporary shunt of synthetic vascular prosthesis between the ascending and descending aorta (Fig. 10), Mei-Hsin Shih and colleagues [17] performed two cases of complete resection of the syphilitic aortic arch aneurysm with homograft replacement in July and September of 1959. Both aortic arch homografts were stored in liquid nitrogen and supplied by the surgical colleagues at Guangci Hospital in Shanghai. Unfortunately, the first patient died 3 days later owing to respiratory failure (ventilators were not widely available then) [17].

Meanwhile another locally made heart-lung machine was applied

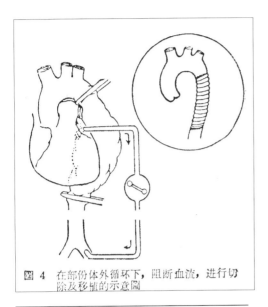

图 4　在部份体外循环下，阻断血流，进行切
　　　除及移植的示意圖

Fig. 9. *Repair of descending aortic aneurysm by Gu and colleagues with the use of partial left atrial-femoral bypass (Reprinted from [16] with permission).*

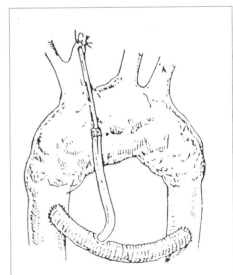

Fig. 10. *A temporary shunt of vascular prosthesis between the ascending and descending aorta for resection of an aortic arch aneurysm with homograft replacement in 1959 (Reprinted from [17] with permission).*

Fig. 3. Case 1. Temporary shunt established before occlusion and resection of aortic arch.

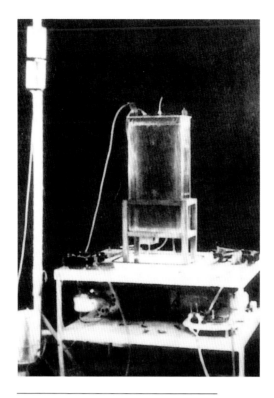

Fig. 11. The heart-lung machine used in 1959 at
Zhongshan Hospital in Shanghai.

clinically in 1959, once again the result of the collaboration by six
hospitals and six factories in Shanghai. A vertical screen oxygenator
was developed (Fig. 11), in combination with the use of a roller pump.
After more than a year and a total of 191 animal experiments, the
first case was carried out at Zhongshan Hospital in Shanghai on
September 21, 1959. In the next 10 weeks, 9 out of 11 patients with
congenital cardiac defects survived direct intracardiac repairs under
CPB [18]. Using this device, Shih and associates performed complete
correction of tetralogy of Fallot in December 1959 and repair of
ruptured sinus of Valsalva in January 1960 [19].

Two years later Zhuo-Rong Feng and colleagues at the Shanghai
Chest Hospital excised a left atrial myxoma from a patient under

CPB [20], about seven years after a similar operation was first described by Crafoord and others. This 48-year-old male patient was initially diagnosed to have mitral stenosis and underwent a closed mitral commissurotomy through a left thoracotomy on November 27, 1961. However, a mobile soft tissue mass was felt as soon as the surgeon's index finger entered the left atrium, while the patient's mitral valve appeared normal on palpation. Realizing it was a left atrial myxoma, the operation was then abandoned as no CPB device was prepared. A rescheduled operation was later performed on January 24, 1962. A 5x4x3 cm myxoma was successfully excised under

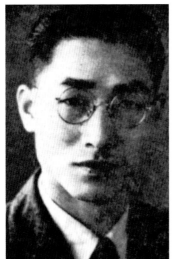

CPB via a right hemiclam shell incision (the left pleural cavity was not entered this time) [20].

Another important breakthrough occurred on June 12, 1965, when Yong-Zhi Cai (1917–1989, Fig. 12) and associates at Changhai Hospital of the Second Military Medical University in Shanghai performed the first successful mitral valve replacement

Fig. 12. [A, B] Dr. Yong-Zhi Cai.

(A)

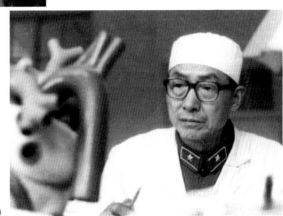

(B)

with a locally made ball and cage mechanical prosthesis (Fig. 13A) [21], five years after the world's first artificial mitral prosthesis implantation. Over the 2-year period prior to this operation, Cai and his team had conducted more than 100 valve implantations in dogs and cows. This event (Fig. 13B) marked the beginning of the era of valvular replacement in China (Fig. 13C). At Changhai Hospital alone, more than 6,500 valvular operations performed during the next four decades.

At the same time, a relatively new hospital in Beijing started to attract attention. Founded in 1956, Fuwai Hospital grew to become the biggest cardiovascular center in China. Intracardiac operations under hypothermia without CPB (Fig. 14), such as repairs for atrial and ventricular septal defects and pulmonary commissurotomy, had been conducted since early 1958 at Fuwai [22]. Using this hypothermic approach, You-Lin Hou (1917–1971, Fig. 15) and colleagues performed the first direct mitral valve repair for regurgitation in China in September 1958, aortic valve commissurotomy in March 1959, and total arch replacement in December 1961 [22, 23]. They also successfully repaired a ruptured sinus of Valsalva under hypothermia before their "homemade" CPB device became available [22, 23]. The CPB pump initially used in Fuwai Hospital (Fig. 16) was designed by a group of investigators at the Chinese Academy of Medical Sciences, with a modified Dewall-Lillehei bubble oxygenator made in the same hospital by the anesthetists and the technicians. After experimentation on more than 100 animals, the device was first utilized clinically in late 1959. However they soon switched in the 1960s using the Shanghai heart-lung machine. A total of 3,021 CPB cases were performed at Fuwai Hospital using only this type of device (which was later modified) up till 1980, when more sophisticated CPB equipment from the United States or Europe became available [24].

## Striving Against the Stream [1967 to 1980]

During the first few years of the "Cultural Revolution" period (1967 to 1976), cardiovascular surgery in China came to a complete halt. However by the early 1970s, cardiac surgery reemerged in a few major

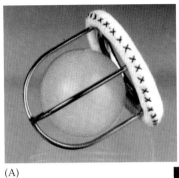

(A)

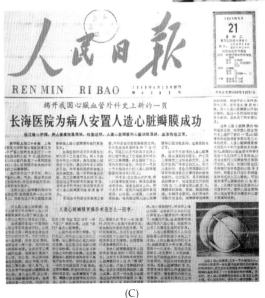

(B)

(C)

*Fig. 13. [A] The first Chinese made mechanical valve prosthesis; [B] The patient (left) with Drs. Bao-Ren Zhang (2nd from left) and Yong-Zhi Cai (3rd from left) after the first mitral valve replacement at Changhai Hospital; [C] The operation hit the headline in national newspaper in 1965.*

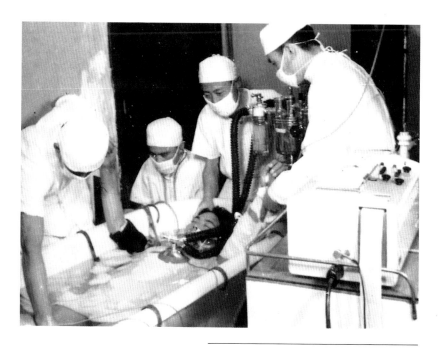

Fig. 14. *Whole-body cooling during a hypothermic open-heart operation at Fuwai Hospital in 1958.*

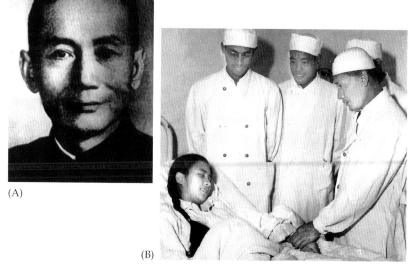

(A)

(B)

Fig. 15. *[A] Dr. You-Lin Hou, the founding Chairman of Department of Cardiac Surgery, Fuwai Hospital, Beijing; [B] Dr. Hou (first from right) in ward round.*

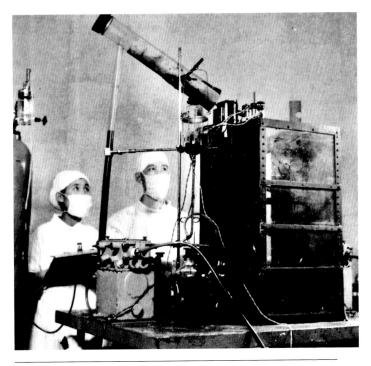

Fig. 16. *The heart-lung machine used in late 1959 at Fuwai Hospital, Beijing.*

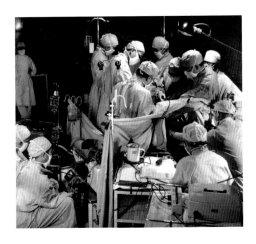

Fig. 17. *The first-in-China CABG operation by Dr. Jia-Qiang Guo on November 18, 1974 at Fuwai Hospital, Beijing.*

centers in Beijing, Shanghai, Xi'an, Guangzhou and Shenyang [25].

At Fuwai Hospital in Beijing, Jia-Qiang Guo and colleagues performed the first resection of post-infarction ventricular aneurysm in 1972 and the first coronary artery bypass operation (Fig. 17) using saphenous vein as graft conduits on November 18, 1974 [22]. After more than four years of experimental study, Xiao-Dong Zhu and Jia-Qiang Guo performed the first aortic valve replacement with a bovine pericardial prosthesis made in Fuwai in May 1976 (Fig. 18), which marked the first use of tissue valve in China [23]. Over the following year, Zheng-Xiang Luo (Fig. 19) and his team from Guangzhou also reported their clinical experience of porcine valve implantations [25]. Soon after, Yong-Zhi Cai and coworkers from Shanghai and Lanzhou successfully developed the first entirely Chinese-made single-leaflet disk prosthesis (the "C-L valve", Fig. 20) in 1978 [14]. For the first time, this type of mechanical prosthesis became commercially available in the national market. As valvular replacement operations gained momentum, there were 2,051 documented prostheses implantation (439 mechanical and 1,612 biological) between 1978 and 1982 in China [25].

For complex congenital heart surgery like the surgical correction of tetralogy of Fallot, however, the learning curve was steep. Between 1959 and 1979 the mortality rate at Fuwai Hospital was prohibitively high by today's standard at 32%. This later dropped to 11% between 1980–88, 5% in 1989–90, and less than 3% in 1991–95, in a total of 2,896 cases [23]. The best published result of this procedure before 1979 in China came from Zeng-Wei Wang (Fig. 21) and his colleagues at the Army General Hospital in Shenyang. They reported 150 cases with a mortality rate of 6% in 1979 (for the 82 patients who underwent surgery in 1978, the mortality rate was only 2.4%) [25].

## The Dawn of a New Era
## [1981 Onward]

A total of 6,444 open-heart operations were recorded in China for the year 1982. The number increased to about 15,000 cases a year by 1990 [26]. In 1999 cardiac surgical programs were available in over 600

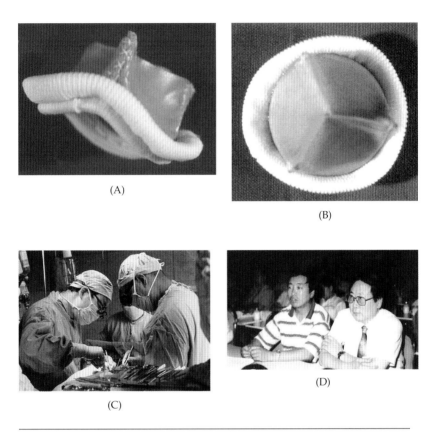

*Fig. 18. [A, B] The first Fuwai-made tissue valve prosthesis; [C] Drs. Xiao-Dong Zhu and Jia-Qiang Guo performing tissue valve implantation in 1976 at Fuwai Hospital; [D] The patient who received the first Fuwai-made tissue valve 19 years after operation with Dr. Zhu (right).*

centers in China. Among them, more than 50 centers have a workload of over 250 cases a year. The number of annual open-heart operations is over 500 in some 20 centers in China and the highest workload remains at the Fuwai Hospital in Beijing. For example, there were 3,856 cardiac operations performed at this institution in 1997, and the number has approached nearly 7,000 in 2005.

Although by now, valvular replacement is theoretically available at every hospital with a cardiac surgical program in China, this

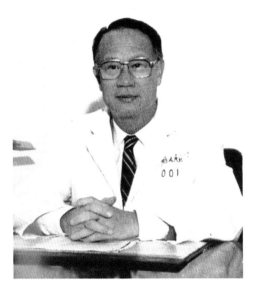

Fig. 19. Dr. Zheng-Xiang Luo

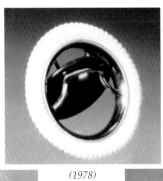

(1978)

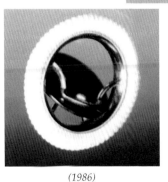

(1986)

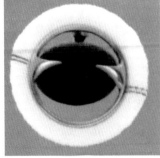

(1989)

Fig. 20. The Changhai-made mechanical prostheses: the C-L valves.

procedure is concentrated in centers in the major cities. For instance, large series of valvular replacements for rheumatic heart disease were reported in 1997 in 3,656 patients by Bao-Ren Zhang (Fig. 22) and colleagues at Changhai Hospital in Shanghai, and in 4,960 patients at Fuwai Hospital in Beijing (the overall mortality rate was less than 6% in both series) [14]. Owing to the high incidence of chronic rheumatic heart disease in China, about 30% of the patients received multiple valvular replacements [14]. In May 1985 another mechanical prosthesis (the "G-K valve") also became available in China, which was developed by the investigators at Fuwai Hospital led by Xiao-Dong Zhu. However, more complex operations such as the Ross procedure or homograft implantations are only available in a few centers. In July 1987, Ming-Di Xiao and the Fuwai team reported the clinical use of homografts in repairing complex congenital valvular diseases or in reconstruction of the left ventricular outflow tract. New types of tissue valves or mechanical prostheses are currently under development in Beijing, Xi'an, Shanghai (Fig. 23), Guangzhou, and Chengdu.

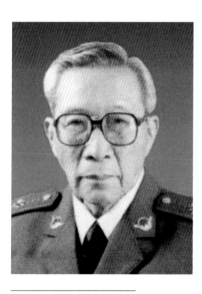

*Fig. 21.  Dr. Zeng-Wei Wang.*

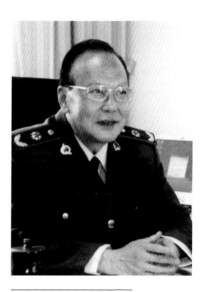

*Fig. 22.  Dr. Bao-Ren Zhang.*

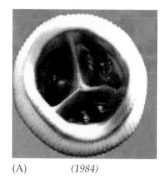

(A)          *(1984)*

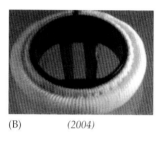

(B)          *(2004)*

*Fig. 23. The recent Shanghai-made [A] tissue and [B] bileaflet mechanical prostheses.*

The development of coronary surgery in China was somewhat slow until recent years. Between 1974 and 1990, 238 CABG operations had been performed at Fuwai Hospital and the mortality rate was 6.5% in 1990 [14]. In the 10 year period of the 1980s, Zhi Pan (Fig. 24A) and associates at the Shanghai Chest Hospital performed 98 CABG operations with an overall mortality rate of 8.2% [14]. According to a survey conducted by the Chinese Society for Thoracic and Cardiovascular Surgery, only five centers in 1998 performed more than 50 CABG operations annually while there were about 1,000 CABG cases performed that year [26]. From 1996 through 2000, Qing-Yu Wu and Sheng-Shou Hu and their colleagues at Fuwai Hospital performed the largest series of CABG operations in China (n = 2,315) with an early success rate of 98.7% [27, 28]. In 2002 this team performed 1,034 CABG operations with an overall mortality rate of 0.97% [29]. With the maturation of the younger generation of Chinese cardiac surgeons, complete arterial grafting and off-pump beating heart CABG have also rapidly gained popularity in China. It was estimated that at least 10,000 CABG cases were carried out across the country in 2005 (Professor Qiang Zhao, Zhongshan Hospital, Shanghai, personal communication).

Open-heart surgery for children younger than 2 years of age was first conducted by Wen-Xiang Ding (Fig. 24B) and colleagues at Xinhua Hospital of the Shanghai Second Medical College in May 1974 [25, 26]. In the early 1990s they summarized their experiences in surgical correction of transposition of great arteries using either Senning operation [30] or arterial switch operation [31]. From 1973 through 1988, Zeng-Wei Wang and his associates at Army General

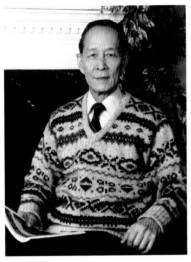

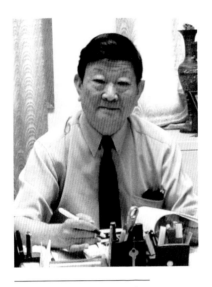

*Fig. 24A. Dr. Zhi Pan.*

*Fig. 24B. Dr. Wen-Xiang Ding.*

Hospital in Shenyang performed 1,895 complex congenital cardiac operations in 1,880 patients with tetralogy of Fallot, Ebstein malformation, double-outlet right ventricle, univentricle and tricuspid atresia, transposition of great arteries, and so forth [32]. The overall surgical mortality rate in this group of patients was 4.0% [32]. They also reported the first series (n = 14) in China of total cavopulmonary connection for complex Fontan operations [33]. In 1977 Wei-Yong Liu (Fig. 25) and colleagues at Xijing Hospital of the Fourth Military Medical University in Xi'an (the previous unit of Hong-Xi Su) developed a prosthetic conduit containing a locally made porcine valve. They first used this conduit in the surgical correction of double-outlet right ventricle and transposition of great arteries in early 1979 [34]. This group of surgeons also successfully operated on two patients with left ventricular outflow tract obstruction in March 1983 using a similar apicoaortic valved composite conduit [35].

In October 1977, long before Cyclosporin A was widely available, Shi-Ze Zhang (Fig. 26) and associates at Ruijin Hospital of the Shanghai Second Medical College were preparing to begin a new adventure. A total of 30 orthotopic and six heterotopic heart

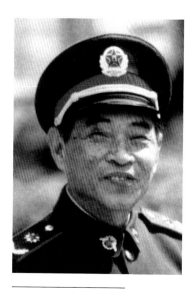

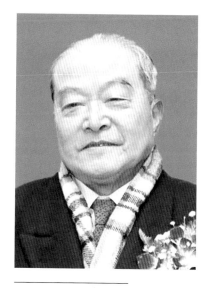

*Fig. 25. Dr. Wei-Yong Liu.*

*Fig. 26. Dr. Shi-Ze Zhang.*

transplantations were done in animals by this group of surgeons over a 6-month period. Subsequently they performed the first clinical orthotopic heart transplantation in China on April 21, 1978 [36]. The donor was a 23-year-old victim of a road traffic accident, who arrived in the same hospital with irreversible brain injury. The 38-year-old recipient who had end-stage heart failure due to chronic rheumatic valvular disease survived 109 days. In the following decade at least five additional cardiac transplant procedures were carried out in China and none of these recipients had a longer survival. Despite this setback, others were not deterred. In 1992 Bao-Tian Chen and colleagues at Anzhen Hospital in Beijing, Qiu-Ming Xia and associates at the Harbin University Hospital, and Xiao-Cheng Liu's team at Mudanjiang Cardiovascular Institute independently restarted their heart transplantation program with much improved results [37, 38]. In December 1992 Xiao-Cheng Liu and colleagues also performed the first heart-lung transplantation in China [39]. By the end of 1999, approximately 130 heart and nine heart-lung transplantations had been accomplished in more than 35 centers in China [37]. Among the heart transplantation recipients, the longest survivor has remained well for 14 years. On a separate note, the first clinical implantation of a heterotopic heart with long-term survival in China, as well as in Asia, was carried out in Taiwan by Shu-Hsun Chu and co-workers in 1988 [40].

The beginning of 1980s also witnessed the "door-opening" era in China. In particular, the progress of cardiovascular surgery in China over the next two decades was taken forward by the remarkable increase in scientific exchanges with colleagues worldwide as exemplified by the following photographs (Figs. 27A–27F).

The founding of the Chinese Society for Thoracic and Cardiovascular Surgery (CSTCS) in 1985 was another cornerstone in the development of this specialty in China. As a branch of the Chinese Medical Association, the CSTCS played an important leadership role in education and professional training through organizing national and international symposiums or workshops, as well as producing scientific publications in its official journal (Fig. 28). Past presidents of this society include Professors Hong-Xi Su (1985 through 1992), Yan-Qing Sun (1992 through 1996), and Xiao-Dong Zhu (1996 through 2006) (Fig. 29).

## Concluding Remarks

> *"The trend of time makes one a hero."*
> —*A Chinese idiom*

The great difficulty of establishing a new surgical subspecialty has been universally recognized and cardiovascular surgery is no exception. On top of various technical obstacles, socioeconomic factors can also significantly influence the whole process. The development of cardiovascular surgery in Europe was slowed down by the tragedy of World War II [41]. Compared with the United States and Europe, the growth of cardiovascular surgery was even more difficult in China over the first few decades after World War II under the ever-changing political and harsh socioeconomic conditions. This chapter presents only a few interesting frames from a movie of the

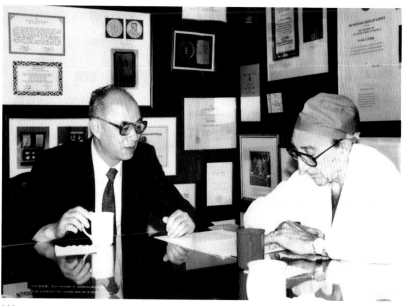

(A)

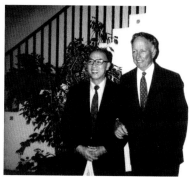

(B)

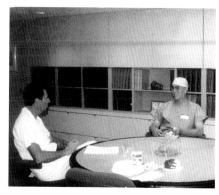

(C)

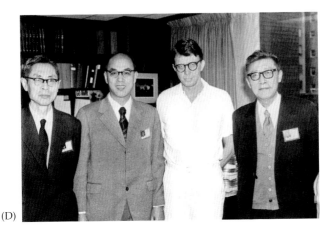

(D)

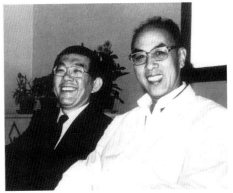

(E)

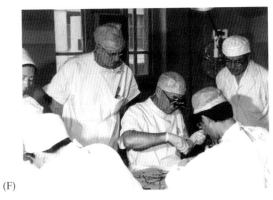

(F)

Fig. 27. [A] Dr. Jia-Qiang Guo with Michael E. DeBakey, MD; [B] Denton A. Cooley, MD; [C] Delos M. Cosgrove, MD; [D] Floyd D. Loop, MD; [E] Victor Y. H. Chang, MD; [F] Mark O'Brien, MD. (Courtesy of Professor Jia-Qiang Guo)

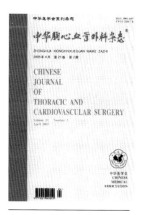

Fig. 28. *The Chinese JTCVS.*

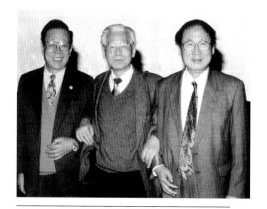

Fig. 29. *Three past presidents of CSTCS: Drs. Yan-Qing Sun (left), Hong-Xi Su (middle), and Xiao-Dong Zhu (right).*

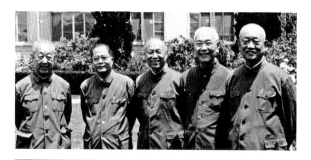

Fig. 30. *Some pioneering Chinese cardiothoracic surgeons in Shanghai in May 1981 (from left to right): Ying-Kai Wu, Mei-Hsin Shih, Kai-Shi Gu, Jia-Si Huang, and Xi-Chun Lan.*

unique history of cardiovascular surgery in China. In view of the rising incidence of cardiovascular diseases worldwide, the struggle to establish our specialty in a country with more than one-fifth of the world population is certainly one of the most important challenges in the last century. Through the continued perseverance, dedication, and hard work of many individuals working together, the evolution of cardiovascular surgery is still ongoing in China, with the expectation that this progress will accelerate with improvement in the country's economy. However, we should never forget it was the bold ventures of those pioneers (Fig. 30) that brought us to where we are today.

## *Acknowledgements*

A major part of this chapter is reproduced from: Wan S, Yim APC (2003). The evolution of cardiovascular surgery in China. Ann Thorac Surg 76:2147–2155, with permission from the Society of Thoracic Surgeons and Elsevier Inc.

## *References*

1.  Temple R (1986) The genius of China: 3000 years of science, discovery and invention. London: Prion Books.
2.  Lan XC (1984) The development of cardiac surgery in China. In: Lan XC (ed) Cardiovascular surgery (Vol. I). Beijing: People's Health Press, 1–12 (in Chinese).
3.  Wan S, Yim APC (1999) A Chinese thoracic surgeon and his two decisions. Ann Thorac Surg 67:1190–1193.
4.  Wu YK (1947) Ligation of patent ductus arteriosus. Chin Med J 65:71–76.
5.  Wu YK, Huang KC (1953) Surgical treatment of constrictive pericarditis. Chin Med J 71:274–286.
6.  Wang YS, Cheng TO (2001) Leo Eloesser: an American cardiothoracic surgeon in China. Ann Thorac Surg 71:1387–1388.
7.  Lan HC, Feng CJ, Huang MH, Yu KJ (1955) Surgical treatment of mitral stenosis. Chin Med J 73:278–292.
8.  Fu PB, Shen YK, Lin YJ, Zhang TX (1957) Surgical treatment of innominate aneurysm: excision and replacement with homograft. Chin J Surg 5:265–273 (in Chinese).
9.  Liang QC, Wang YS, Song XM, Ye CX (1958) Transpulmonary direct vision valvulotomy for pulmonary stenosis. Chin J Surg 6:974–978 (in Chinese).
10. Shih MH, Wan TH, Ling HS, Jen CY (1960) Surgical treatment of congenital atrial septal defect. Chin J Surg 8:234–238 (in Chinese).
11. Liu WY (1995) Professor Su Hong-Xi and his achievements at the Fourth Military Medical University. Proceedings of a scientific symposium in honor of Professor Su Hong-Xi's 80th birthday. Fourth Military Medical University, Xi'an, 1–5 (in Chinese).
12. Su HX, Liu WY, Lin CJ, et al. (1959) Direct repair of ventricular septal defect with the use of cardiopulmonary bypass: a case report. Chin J Surg 7:557–565 (in Chinese).
13. Su HX (1985) Cardiopulmonary bypass. In: Gu KS (ed) Cardiothoracic surgery [1st edition]. Beijing: People's Health Press, pp 201–212 (in Chinese).
14. Zhang BR (2003) The brief history of the development of cardiac surgery in China. In: Wang ZW, Liu WY, Zhang BR (eds) Cardiac surgery. Beijing: People's Military Medical Publisher, pp 3–8 (in Chinese).

15. Wu YK (1960) Cardiac surgery in China: current status and future directions. Chin J Surg 8:209–211 (in Chinese).

16. Gu KS, Wu SF, Wu SC, et al. (1961) Surgical treatment of aortic aneurysm. Chin J Surg 9:353–357 (in Chinese).

17. Shih MH, Wan TH, Ling HS, et al. (1960) Total resection and homograft replacement of the aortic arch. Chin Med J 80:505–513.

18. Shih MH, Wan TH, Ling HS, et al. (1960) Study on extracorporeal circulation: the clinical use of vertical screen oxygenator. Chin J Surg 8:211–213 (in Chinese).

19. Shih MH, Wan TH, Ling HS, et al. (1962) Surgical treatment of ruptured sinus of Valsalva. Chin J Surg 10:15–17 (in Chinese).

20. Feng ZR, Zheng DS, Lan XC (1963) Excision of left atrial myxoma under extracorporeal circulation. Chin J Surg 11:305–307 (in Chinese).

21. Cai YZ, Wei T, Geng ZJ, et al. (1965) Mitral valve replacement with a ball and cage mechanical prosthesis. PLA Med J 2:530–538 (in Chinese).

22. Zhu XD (1991) The evolution of cardiovascular surgical techniques at Fu-Wai Hospital. In: Xue GX (ed.) Proceedings of the 35th anniversary scientific symposium on cardiovascular surgery. Beijing: Cardiovascular Institute of Chinese Academy of Medical Sciences, pp 1–7 (in Chinese).

23. Xiao MD (1996) 40-year history of cardiac surgery at Fu-Wai Hospital. Proceedings of the 40th anniversary scientific symposium on cardiovascular surgery. Beijing: Cardiovascular Institute of Chinese Academy of Medical Sciences, pp. 1–9 (in Chinese).

24. Hu XQ (1996) The development of cardiovascular anesthesia and extracorporeal circulation at Fu-Wai Hospital. Proceedings of the 40th anniversary scientific symposium on cardiovascular surgery. Beijing: Cardiovascular Institute of Chinese Academy of Medical Sciences, pp 56–59 (in Chinese).

25. Lan XC, Gu KS, Wu YK (1985) History and present status of thoracic and cardiovascular surgery in China. In Wu YK, Peters RM (eds) International practice in cardiothoracic surgery. Beijing: Science Press, pp 23–27.

26. Yu YF (1999) A 50-year appraisal of cardiovascular surgery in China. Chin J Surg 37:554–557 (in Chinese).

27. Wu QY (2001) Current status of coronary artery surgery in China. In: Hu DY, Ma CS (eds) Practice in cardiology—2001. Beijing: People's Health Press, pp 445–448 (in Chinese).

28. Wu QY, Huang ZX, Hu SS, et al. (1999) Clinical analysis of 1539 cases undergoing coronary artery bypass grafting. Chin Med J 112:978–981.

29. Wu QY (2001) Cardiovascular Institute and Fu-Wai Hospital, Beijing. Presented at the 11th annual meeting of the Asian Society for cardiovascular surgery, Kuala Lumpur, Malaysia, 13 February.

30. Ding WX, Su ZK, Xu ZW. (1991) Senning operation for correction of transposition

of great arteries with intact ventricular septum. Chin J Thorac Cardiovasc Surg 7:1–3 (in Chinese).

31.  Ding WX, Su ZK, Xu ZW, et al. (1992) Arterial switch operation for transposition of great arteries in infants. Chin J Thorac Cardiovasc Surg 8:78–80 (in Chinese).

32.  Wang ZW, Fei CJ, Sun LZ, et al. (1989) Surgical treatment of complex congenital heart disease. Chin J Thorac Cardiovasc Surg 5:206–209 (in Chinese).

33.  Wang ZW, Fei CJ, Zhu HY, et al. (1992) Total cavopulmonary connection. Chin J Thorac Cardiovasc Surg 8:142–147 (in Chinese).

34.  Liu WY, Zhang WL, Shi WR, et al. (1981) Valve-containing prosthetic conduit for surgical correction of complex congenital heart disease. Chin J Cardiol 9:172–175 (in Chinese).

35.  Liu WY, Ju MD, Yang JX, et al. (1985) Surgical treatment of left ventricular outflow tract obstruction using apicoaortic valved conduit. Chin J Thorac Cardiovasc Surg 1:34–37 (in Chinese).

36.  Zhang SZ, Zhou SB, Fang LD, et al. (1980) Orthotopic heart transplantation: a case report. Chin J Surg 18:204–207 (in Chinese).

37.  Xia QM, Zang WF (2001) Heart transplantation. In: Hu DY, Ma CS (eds) Practice in cardiology–2001. Beijing: People's Health Press, pp 771–779 (in Chinese).

38.  Zhang ZG, Han L (2000) Heart and Lung transplantation: past, present and future. In: Sun YQ (ed) Modern cardiothoracic surgery. Beijing: People's Army Medical Press, pp 1571–1578 (in Chinese).

39.  Liu XC (2000) Heart-lung transplantation. In: Sun YQ (ed) Modern cardiothoracic surgery. Beijing: People's Army Medical Press, pp 1615–1635 (in Chinese).

40.  Chu SH, Tsai CH, Wang SS, et al. (1991) Heterotopic heart transplantation: a life-saving procedure with a size-mismatched donor. Jpn Circ J 55:1–4.

41.  Turina MI (2002) European Association for Cardio-Thoracic Surgery: carrying the torch. Eur J Cardiothorac Surg 22:857–863.

# The Historical Perspective of Surgery for Congenital Heart Disease

*Wen-Xiang Ding*

C hina is the most populous country in the world, with a population of 1,300,000,000, which accounts for one-fifth of the world's population. There are 25,000,000 live births per year. According to a survey involving 20,000 newborns, reported by Shanghai Children's Medical Institute, the incidence of congenital heart disease (CHD) is 6.7 per 1,000 live births. Thus there are 150,000 neonates born with CHD per year in mainland China. The majority of minor forms of CHD do not need specialized cardiologic care, and indeed many of these, such as the tiny ventricular septal defect (VSD) or atrial septal defect (ASD) and the small PDA, may either close spontaneously or never cause medical problems. Meanwhile, some severe cardiac anomalies cannot currently be repaired. Apart from these two categories, at least 100,000 neonates are born every year with CHD which needs surgical or interventional therapy.

To date, cardiac surgical programs for CHD are available in approximately 400 hospitals in mainland China. The total number of open-heart surgical operations performed is around 50,000 annually, including adults and children. Today, the number of operations has increased by 30% compared to 10 years ago. In most hospitals the surgical patients' age is over 5 years old. There are approximately 100 modern cardiac centers in the metropolises and most patients of less than 3 years old underwent open-heart surgery at these cardiac centers. Four hospitals perform more than 1,000 open-heart operations annually, 10 hospitals more than 500, 20 hospitals more than 250, 40 hospitals more than 100, and other hospitals less than 100.

Currently diagnostic equipment has been upgraded in many hospitals due to the improved socioeconomic conditions in our country. For example, two-dimensional Doppler echocardiography is more popular. Special instruments such as three-dimensional echocardiography, transesophageal echocardiography (TEE), angiographic equipment for cardiac catheterization, computed tomography (CT), and magnetic resonance imaging (MRI) are available in several cardiac centers. The set-up and devices in the operating room and intensive care unit are similar to those in sophisticated cardiac centers worldwide. The diagnostic accuracy rate of CHD is above 95%. Diagnostic cardiac catheterization can be performed for newborn patients.

In the surgical therapy field overall surgical mortality varies from 2% to 5%, according to previously published reports based on the major cardiovascular journals. The mortality of young patients and complex cases is relatively high. The mortality of CHD also differs greatly from study to study. Overall, the surgical survival rate ranged from 95% to 98% in patients older than 4 years old, 90% to 95% in patients younger than 2 years old, 85% to 90% in patients younger than 1 year old, and 80% to 90% in neonates. In fact the younger the patient, the more complex and critical the case. Therefore the mortality rate is high in these patients. Seven stages can reflect the level of surgery for CHD in mainland China: 1) the beginning era, 2) the developing era, 3) the stagnation era, 4) the second developing era, 5) the beginning and development of surgery for CHD in infants and young children, 6) research work, 7) specialized education.

## The Beginning Era (1944–1950)

It was not until the 1930s that cardiac surgery, as it practiced today, became a reality. At that time cardiac surgery was a minor specialty, perhaps even slightly esoteric, but that has all changed and it is now an important branch of major surgery in its own right. In China,

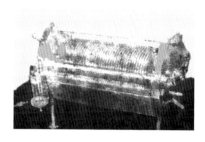

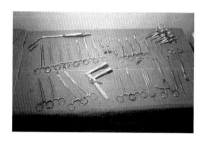

*Fig. 1. In 1974, the Disc oxygenator for children made in Shanghai.*

*Fig. 2. In 1976, the cardiac surgical equipment for children was made in Shanghai.*

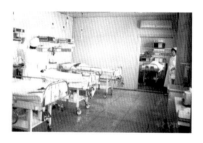

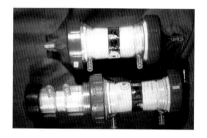

*Fig. 3. In 1985, CICU for pediatric cardiovascular surgery in Shanghai Xinhua Hospital.*

*Fig. 4. In 1981, the Hollo fiber oxygenator for children made in Shanghai.*

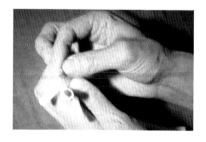

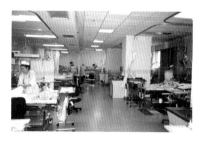

*Fig. 5. In 1980, the expanded Teflon artificial graft made in Shanghai.*

*Fig. 6. Now CICU for pediatric cardiovascular surgery in Shanghai Children's Medical Center.*

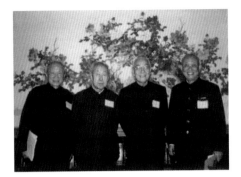

Fig. 7. *The pioneers and founders of cardiovascular surgery in China. (from left to right) Drs. Gui-Shi Gu, Ying-Kai Wu, Jia-Si Huang, Xi-Chun Lan.*

Fig. 8. *In 1974, the first VSD repair for a child using the artificial lung heart machine made by same group. In Shanghai Xin-hua Hospital.*

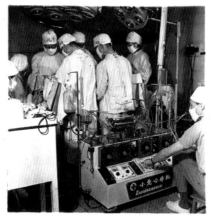

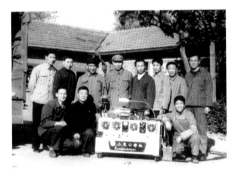

Fig. 9. *In 1974, the children artificial lung heart machine made in Shanghai, China by Dr. WX Ding and Dr. ZK Su and factory group.*

cardiac surgery was established at the early 1940s. Dr. Chao-Mei Zhang successfully sutured a stab wound to the right ventricular wall in 1940, which was first successful cardiac surgery in China. Dr. Ying-Kai Wu performed the first ligation. the patent ductus arteriosus (PDA) in 1944, which marked the beginniï. ᶜvascular surgery in China.

In 1947 Dr. Ying-Kai Wu performed the first successful pericardectomy for constrictive pericarditis. These were the pioneers of cardiovascular surgery, and this marked the beginning of cardiovascular surgery.

## The First Developing Era (1950–1965)

Since the People's Republic of China was established in 1949, the health care industry had been increasingly emphasized by the government because of basic changes in social policy. As a consequence, cardiovascular surgery also won great support. Despite a shortage of manpower, techniques, equipment and materials, the cardiovascular surgeons contributed much to the development of this fascinating and rapidly advancing field. Furthermore, their achievements were excellent. Centered on the training of specialists, a cardiac surgery specialty diagnosis and treatment system was established throughout the country. Departments of cardiac surgery were also established in many provinces and cities, except in Xinjiang and Tibet. Meanwhile the surgical treatment of CHD developed rapidly, based on what little experience there was in the 1940s.

In 1953 Dr. Mei-Xin Shi successfully performed the first Blalock-Taussig shunt for a patient with tetralogy of Fallot (TOF) at Zhong-shan Hospital in Shanghai. In 1954, closed pulmonary valvular dilation through the right ventricle performed by Dr. Qi-Shen Liang on a pulmonary stenosis case marked the beginning of ventricular operations.

In 1955 Dr. Mei-Xin Shi successfully dissected and sutured PDA using Potts clamp.

In 1956 Dr. Zhong Zhang and coworkers successfully performed Potts procedure for TOF case at Tongren Hospital in Shanghai.

In 1957, a closed pulmonary valve dilation (through the right ventricle using the Broke valve knife) was performed for a TOF case at Fuwai Hospital in Beijing. The closed banding procedure to repair ASD was also performed successfully.

In 1957 Dr. Xi-Chun Lan excised wedge the stenostic segment of coarctation. Dr. Yong-Zhi Cai performed end-to-end anastomosis between the left subclavian artery and descending aorta in which the stenostic segment was excised for coarctation repair.

In 1957 Dr. Qi-Shen Liang cut the stenostic pulmonary valve via pulmonary artery incision under hypothermia, which opened the door to open heart surgery.

In 1957 the closed operation to enlarge the pulmonary valve and right ventricular outlet via the right ventricle was successfully introduced by Dr. You-Lin Hou.

In 1957 Dr. Qi-Shen Liang cut the stenostic pulmonary valve via pulmonary artery incision (Swan procedure) using the transient arrest returned blood flow technique under hypothermia.

In 1958 Dr. Kai-Shi Gu performed anastomosis between the right pulmonary artery and superior vena cava for a TOF case at the Shanghai Chest Hospital.

In 1958 ASD was sutured primarily via open-heart field using arrest returned blood flow technique under hypothermia by Dr. Mei-Xin Shi at Zhongshan Hospital and by Dr. Xi-Chun Lan at Renji Hospital in Shanghai.

June 1958 was an extremely important month for the history of treatment for CHD in China, a milestone of open-heart surgery under cardiopulmonary bypass (CPB). Dr. Hong-Xi Su closed a VSD for a 6-year-old child under CPB at the Fourth Military Medical University in Xi'an, using an artificial heart-lung machine imported from the US. One month later the first artificial heart-lung machine was made in China. Meanwhile, Dr. Kai-Shi Gu cut the stenostic pulmonary valvular commissure under CPB for a 12-year-old child using this machine in Shanghai, which demonstrated the opening of a new era of open-heart surgery using CPB in China. New types of artificial heart-lung machines, which were utilized clinically, were made at Zhongshan Hospital, Renji Hospital in Shanghai, and Fuwai Hospital in Beijing.

In 1960 Dr. Xi-Chun Lan operated to correct a trilogy of Fallot case using arrest returned blood flow twice under hypothermia. Dr. Mei-Xin Shi performed a repair operation directly on a ruptured sinus of Valsalva.

In 1961 Dr. Kai-Shi Gu closed PDA using the patent ductus clamps made in Shanghai. During the 1960s a total of 1,065 cases were operated on. Only 11 cases were re-admitted, and 3 patients died (report published in 1977).

In 1963 Dr. Jia-Qiang Guo sutured or ligated PDA via extra-pleura.

The development of the first era marked the fact that treatment of CHD had become the common practice in China. It also built a solid foundation for the further development of congenital heart surgery.

## Stagnation Era (1965–1975)

Cardiac surgery in China came to a complete halt from the mid 1960s to the early 1970s, while the development of cardiac surgery flourished rapidly in developed countries. Therefore the gap in this speciality widened between China and other countries. It was not until the mid 1970s that China's professional status recovered.

## The Second Developing Era (1975 Onward )

During this stage cardiac surgery further flourished in China, especially the development of congenital heart surgery. In the early 1970s surgical treatment for simple CHD and TOF became popular. Some clinical reports involved more than 1,000 cases with common CHD, such as ASD, VSD and PDA, and TOF, in the late 1970s and the early 1980s. The outcome was similar to that in previous overseas reports. The study of the morphology of the pulmonary vasculture of VSD with severe pulmonary hypertension demonstrated the optimal operative indications and the features of perioperative management. The mortality rate was lowered below 5% at General Hospital of Shenyang Military Region and Fuwai Hospital in Beijing.

In the early 1980s, the mortality rate for corrective operations for TOF cases averaged about 15.5%. In 1979 Dr. Zeng-Wei Wang reported that the mortality rate for corrective operations for 150 patients with TOF was 6% (1964–1974). In 1983 the mortality rate was lowered to 3.6% among 555 cases.

In 1977 Dr. Jia-Qiang Guo reported 1,755 corrective operations on TOF cases, with a mortality rate of 3.4%.

In 1983 122 children with TOF underwent corrective operations at Shanghai Second Medical University, which was affiliated to Xinhua Hospital, and the mortality rate was 5.9%. In 1995 the mortality rate was lowered to 3.6% in 721 cases (1986–1995).

In 1988 Dr. Zhi-Liang Zhang reported a mortality rate for corrective operations for adult patients with TOF of 2%.

Surgical treatment for complex CHD was initiated at 1973. The study of the pathoanatomy and pathophysilogy of complex CHD was first introduced by Dr. Zeng-Wei Wang and coworkers at General Hospital of Shenyang Military Region. Based on these studies, they developed surgical strategies for various types of complex CHD. By the late 1980s approximately 2,000 operations for complex CHD cases had been performed in this cardiac center, including TOF, Ebstein anomaly, double-outlet right ventricle (DORV), single ventricle (SV), tricuspid atresia (TA), corrected transposition of the great artery associated with intracardiac anomaly, total anomalies of the pulmonary veins connection (TAPVC), aortic stenosis (AS), transposition of the great artery (TGA) with VSD and pulmonary stenosis (PS), and pulmonary atresia (PA) with intact ventricular septum. The total hospital mortality rate was 4%, which facilitated the implementation of complex CHD surgery countrywide.

In 1960s surgical treatment of complex CHD was initially introduced at Fuwai Hospital in Beijing, which contributed to the improvement of therapy for complex CHD. For instance, in 1962 Dr. Gan-Xing Xue repaired a partial endocardial cushion defect for five patients under CPB. Among them, two patients had mitral valve cleft. In 1978 Dr. Jia-Qiang Guo and his colleagues successfully operated on TGA cases using homografts.

In 1980 Zhi Pan and coworkers reported 53 cases with endocardial cushion defect between 1972 and 1980, of which 50 cases were partial type and three cases were complete type. The patients underwent corrective operations under CPB. Four patients died during hospitalization.

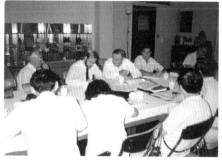

*Fig. 10. In 1989, the chairman of Project HOPE in US Dr. William Walsh endorsed the treaty of establishment of Shanghai Children's Medical Center at Shanghai Second Medical University.*

SHANGHAI DAILY

Little Lu Ziyi looks healthy yesterday after heart surgery in July at the Shanghai Children's Medical Center.

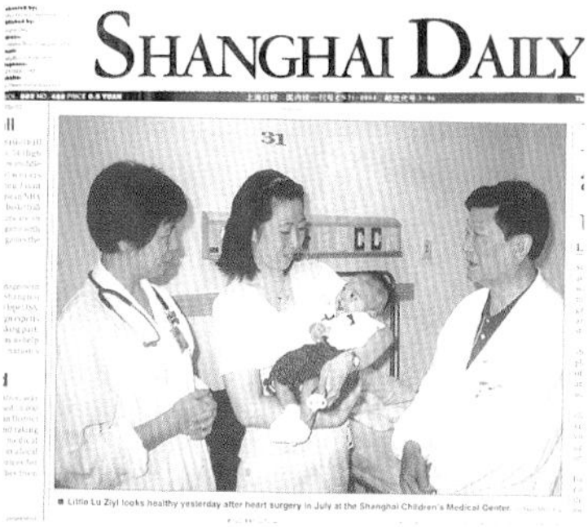

*Fig. 11. The infant who underwent mitral valve replacement visited Dr. Wei-xiang Ding one month later.*

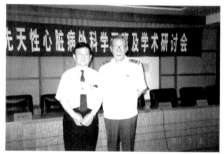

*Fig. 12. The pioneers of congenital heart surgery in China. Dr. Wen-Xiang Ding (left), Dr. Zeng-Wei Wang.*

This valuable experience laid a solid foundation for the implementation of complex CHD surgery in large hospitals in different cities in China after 1990.

The surgical skills required for complex CHD are now widespread throughout the country and so various kinds of common forms of complex CHD can be treated in cardiac centers.

## The Beginning and Development of Surgery for CHD in Infants and Young Children

Surgical treatment of CHD for adults and children had gradually

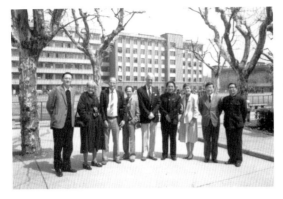

Fig. 13. In 1983, Dr. Tusler (Chief of cardiac surgery, the Hospital for Sick Children, Toronto, Canada) and his group visited Xinhua Hospital in Shanghai.

Fig. 14. In 1999, the first Sino-American symposium on new developments in the care of children with congenital heart disease was held in Shanghai Children's Medical Center.

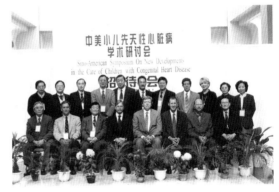

matured since the 1970s. Meanwhile, Dr. Baratt Boyes in New Zealand contributed a new philosophy to the development of surgical treatment for infant CHD, which advocated open-heart surgery for neonates, infants, and young children. No toddlers, infants and neonates were operated on China, which lagged behind the developed countries, until the mid 1970s.

In May 1974 Dr. Wen-Xiang Ding and his colleagues closed VSD for a 4-year-old child under CPB using an artificial heart-lung machine made by themselves in Shanghai Second Medical University, affiliated to Xinhua Hospital, which opened the door for surgical treatment of infant CHD in China. In the early 1980s the same group introduced the deep hypothermia cardiac arrest (DHCA) and deep hypothermia low flow (DHLF) for infants with complex CHD.

This group developed polypropylene hollow fiber membrane oxygenators in collaboration with the surgeons at the First Pulmonary Hospital and engineers at Shanghai Fudan University, which provided important equipment for infancy open-heart surgery. Thereafter they continued to evolve the Mustard, Senning, and Jatene procedures to treat the infants with TGA. They also carried out the Fontan procedure for young patients with TA, SV, and PA, with excellent results.

The number of congenital heart surgery operations on infants and neonates has increased rapidly over the last 10 years and the patients have tended to be younger and of lower weight. However surgical operations for young infants still lag behind those of advanced developed countries in terms of both quantity and quality. Great progress has been made within the last five years. For example, in Shanghai Second Medical University, affiliated to Shanghai Second Medical Center (SCMC), the number of operations on infants under 2 years old increased from 20% to 50% within two years, during which time the total number of operative cases increased from 1,500 to 1,700. Similar ratios have been reported by Fuwai Hospital in Beijing, Anzhen Hospital in Beijing, General Hospital of Shenyang Military Region, Guangdong Cardiovascular Disease Institute, Nanjing Children's Hospital, Zhejiang University affiliated Children's Hospital, and Beijing Children's Hospital. The total surgical mortality rate was lowered from 5%–17% to 2%–5%. The operative mortality rate for CHD is less than 3% at Fuwai Hospital in Beijing and SCMC. However the mortality rate for low-weight neonates with complex and critical CHD remains high. In SCMC, 115 patients weighing between 2.3 kg and 4.5 kg underwent open-heart surgery. Among them 4 cases were neonates, and 71 cases had complex CHD. The mortality rate was 16.5%.

It has been reported that corrective operations have been conducted for patients of TOF associated with pulmonary atresia, aortic coarctation, absence of left pulmonary artery, and atrioventrivencular valve defect at Fuwai Hospital in Beijing, SCMC, and General Hospital of Shenyang Military Region. Emergency operations for patients with severe TOF can be performed at those cardiac centers. During this period departments of pediatric cardiac surgery have been established at more than 20 children's hospitals in China.

## Research Work

There has recently been a lot of research focusing on the mechanisms, surgical techniques, pathophysiology and materials related to congenital heart surgery. The papers related to congenital cardiac surgery published in the *Journal of Chinese Cardiovascular Surgery* in the 15 years are listed in the following (Table 1).

A total of 259 papers related to congenital heart surgery were published in the *Journal of Chinese Cardiovascular Surgery* from 1989 to 2003. 149 papers were published in the first 10 years and 110 papers in the latter five years. The number of published papers in the latter five years was almost equal to those published in the earlier 10 years. Among those papers, 203 were related to surgery, 8 were related to postoperative intensive care, and 24 were related to basic and clinical research.

## Specialized Education

Specialized education involves both undergraduate and postgraduate teaching. Many pediatric cardiac surgeons, cardiologists, intensivists, perfusionists, and nurses have received specialized training in th last 30 years. About 15 medical universities have been approved by the government as teaching hospitals for master of medical science students and PhD students. Currently in China, about 30% of cardiac surgical staff hold PhD degrees and 50% of staff hold MD degrees.

Continuing medical education includes specialized teaching courses twice per year, teaching courses for MD and PhD students, specialized training programs, overseas training projects, and international specialized mentors' teaching programs. Many excellent cardiac centers around the world have provided valuable training opportunities and enlightened mentorship for our young cardiac surgeons and physicians in order to further narrow down the gap between China and overseas in this specialty. For example, Project

Table 1    Papers Related to Congenital Cardiac Surgery
Published on *Journal of Chinese Cardiovascular Surgery*
within the 15 Years

| Diagnosis/Procedure | No. | Date | Hospital no. | Total cases |
|---|---|---|---|---|
| TOF | 24 | 1989–2003 | 14 | 664 |
| PTA | 5 | 1991–2003 | 4 | 28 |
| Homograft | 8 | 1991–2003 | 5 | 823 |
| Fontan Procedure | 12 | 1992–2003 | 5 | 486 |
| TGA | 12 | 1989–2003 | 6 | 115 |
| Glenn Procedure | 3 | 2000–2003 | 3 | 141 |
| Minimal Incision | 7 | 1999–2003 | 6 | 242 |
| DORV | 10 | 1989–2003 | 7 | 161 |
| Ebstein's Anomaly | 9 | 1990–2003 | 9 | 300 |
| CAVC | 6 | 1989–2002 | 4 | 159 |
| PAVC | 4 | 1991–2002 | 4 | 59 |
| VSD | 28 | 1992–2002 | 22 | 1614 |
| Others | 32 | 1989–2002 | 22 | |
| CHD with PH | 4 | 1989–2002 | 4 | 578 |
| DCRV | 4 | 1989–2002 | 4 | 99 |
| CoA | 7 | 1993–2001 | 6 | 125 |
| TAPVC | 3 | 1998–2001 | 3 | 33 |
| APW | 4 | 1991–2001 | 4 | 37 |
| IAA | 2 | 1990–2000 | 2 | |

TOF, Tetralogy of Fallot; PTA, Persistent Truncus Arteriosus; Homograft, application of Homograft as extracardiac conduit; TGA, Transposition of Great Artery; DORV, Double-Outlet Right Ventricle; CAVC, Complete Atrioventricular Canal; PAVC, Partial Atrioventricular Canal; VSD, Ventricular Septal Defect; CHD, Congenital Heart Disease; PH, Pulmonary Hypertension; DCRV, Double Chamber of Right Ventricle; CoA, Coarctation; TAPVC, Total Anomalies of the Pulmonary Veins Connection; APW, Aortopulmonary Window; IAA, Interrupted Aortic Arch.

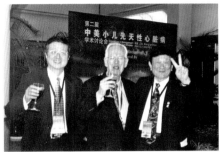

*Fig. 15. In 2004, the famous cardiac pathologist Dr. Van Praaph visited Shanghai Children's Medical Center.*

*Fig. 16. The patients who underwent the first arterial switch operation in China visited Dr. Wen-Xiang Ding and his coworkers 12 years later.*

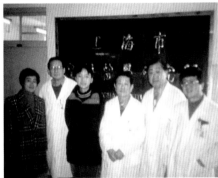

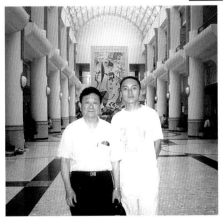

*Fig. 17. The patients who underwent the first arterial switch operation in China visited Dr. Wen-Xiang Ding 17 years later.*

HOPE and Shanghai Second Medical University collaboratively set up the Pediatric Cardiovascular Program in 1984, which was subsequently established in SCMC in 1998. Dr. Richard Jonas has assisted us for the last 20 years, not only in technology but also in program and evolution direction. The teams that traveled to Shanghai each year were sent to target subspecialty areas within the children's hospitals where particular instruction was required. The American teams educated their Chinese peers, and these individuals subsequently become the instructors for the local staff at Xinhua Hospital in Shanghai, SCMC, Fuwai Hospital in Beijing, Anzhen Hospital in Beijing, and Shanghai Children's Hospital. Meanwhile, exchange fellowship programs have enabled numerous physicians and nurses to spend time at cardiac centers in the advanced developed countries.

The cardiac center in SCMC is a training center for pediatric cardiac surgeons, cardiologists, intensivists and perfusionists from all over China. About 200 cardiac surgeons and cardiologists have received training from our cardiac center, and continuing medical education for surgeons, physicians and nurses who will specialize in pediatric cardiac surgery and cardiology has been scheduled regularly each year. Due co-operation with sophisticated cardiac centers worldwide, remarkable improvements have been achieved in comparison to the last 20 years in the fields of clinical diagnosis and treatment, scientific research, and specialized education.

## References

1. Cai DP, Shi YM, Zhang CT (1989) Stress response of adrenal cortex after congenital heart surgery in children. Chin J Thorac Cardiovasc Surg 5:11–13.
2. Su ZK, Ding WX, Xu ZW (1989) The primary report of surgical treatment of D-transposition of the great arteries. Chin J Thorac Cardiovasc Surg 5:150–152.
3. Wang ZW, Fei CJ, Sun LZ, et al. (1989) Surgical treatment of complex congenital heart disease. Chin J Thorac Cardiovasc Surg 5:206–209.
4. Lin XS, Tian YX, Song RQ, et al. (1989) Postoperative management of left to right shunt congenital heart disease with pulmonary hypertension. Chin J Thorac Cardiovasc Surg 5:202–205.
5. Zhong FT, Sun PW, Zhang X, et al. (1990) Surgical treatment of Ebstein's anomaly. Chin J Thorac Cardiovasc Surg 6:14–15.
6. Zhang ZL, Zhu HS, Feng ZR, et al. (1989) Early results and risk factors of low cardiac output syndrome after repair of tetralogy of Fallot (Report of 100 consecutive cases). Chin J Thorac Cardiovasc Surg 5:195–198.
7. Chen XF, Zhu XD (1990) Statistical analysis for surgical treatment of 1267 adult congenital heart diseases. Chin J Thorac Cardiovasc Surg 6:209–211.

8.  Ding WX, Su ZK, Xu ZW (1991) Senning procedure for D-transposition of the great arteries with intact ventricular septum. Chin J Thorac Cardiovasc Surg 7: 1–3.

9.  Zhu YL, Liu YT, Shi JY, et al. (1991) Surgical treatment of atrioventricular septal defect (Report of 30 cases). Chin J Thorac Cardiovasc Surg 7: 69–70.

10.  Wang JQ, Zhang ZS, Ma HL, et al. (1991) Congenital vent dysfunction of left atrium: supra valvular stenosis of mitral valve and cor triatriatum. Chin J Thorac Cardiovasc Surg 7:142–144 .

11.  Ding WX, Su ZK, Shi ZY (1991) Surgical treatment for congenital heart defect in children: a report of 2392 cases. Chin J Pediatr Surg 12:5.

12.  Wang ZW, Fei CJ, Zhu HY, et al. (1992) Clinical application of modified Fontan procedure (Report of 63 cases). Chin J Thorac Cardiovasc Surg 8:11–13.

13.  Sun DH, Zhang BR, Chen RK, et al. (1992) Repair of ventricular septal defects (Report of 319 consecutive cases without death). Chin J Thorac Cardiovasc Surg 8:8–10.

14.  Zhang RF, Wang ZW, Fei CJ, et al. (1992) Surgical treatment of tetralogy of Fallot with complete atrioventrical septal defect. Chin J Thorac Cardiovasc Surg 8:80–82.

15.  Ding WX, Su ZK, Xu ZW, et al. (1992) Arterial switch procedure for D-transposition of the great arteries in infants. Chin J Thorac Cardiovasc Surg 8: 78–79.

16.  Wu DM, Chen Q (1992) Clinical analysis of congenital subpulmonary ventricular septal defect (Report of 249 cases). Chin J Thorac Cardiovasc Surg 8:281–282.

17.  Luo Y, Yang NS, Liu CS (1992) Deep hypothermic cardiac arrest for congenital heart disease in young children. Chin J Thorac Cardiovasc Surg 8:240–241.

18.  Guo B, Guo Q, Shi L, et al. (1993) Surgical treatment of ventricular septal defect with pulmonary hypertension. Chin J Thorac Cardiovasc Surg 9:15–17.

19.  Chen Q, Wang ZH, Pan Z, et al. (1993) Clinical analysis of congenital heart surgery less than 5 years old (Report of 606 cases). Chin J Thorac Cardiovasc Surg 9:75–77.

20.  Chen G, Chen WQ, Xu KJ (1993) Clinical values of hemodynamic parameters for young children undergoing open heart surgery. Chin J Thorac Cardiovasc Surg 9:23–25.

21.  Zhao XW, Yang GC, Zhang XQ, et al. (1993) Surgical treatment of Ebstein's anomaly (Report of 20 cases). Chin J Thorac Cardiovasc Surg 9:157.

22.  Liu JF, Su ZK, Zhu DM, et al. (1993) Surgical treatment of aortic coarctation in children (Report of 21 cases). Chin J Thorac Cardiovasc Surg 9:142–144.

23.  Ding WX, Su ZK (1993) Retrospection and prospection of pediatric thoracic cardiac surgery. Chin J Pediatr Surg 14(2).

24.  Cao DF, Su ZK, Zhu DM, et al. (1993) Cardiac surgery undergoing deep hypothermia cardiac arrest in young children (Report of 200 cases). Chin J Thorac Cardiovasc Surg 9:207–209.

25. Xu ZW, Su ZK, Ding WX (1993) Surgical treatment of heterotaxy syndrome. Chin J Thorac Cardiovasc Surg 9:289–291.

26. Cao DF, Su ZK, Ding WX, et al. (1994) Surgical treatment of complete atrioventricular septal defect in children. Chin J Thorac Cardiovasc Surg 10:20–22.

27. Zhang RF, Wang ZW, Fei CJ, et al. (1994) Surgical treatment of hypoplastic right ventricle. Chin J Thorac Cardiovasc Surg 10:100–102.

28. Cao DF, Ding WX, Su ZK (1994) Application of modified Fontan procedure for complex congenital heart disease in children. Chin J Thorac Cardiovasc Surg 10:103–105.

29. Chen L, Su ZK, Ding WX (1994) Long-term outcome of corrective operation for tetralogy of Fallot in children (Report of 47 cases). Chin J Thorac Cardiovasc Surg 10:109–111.

30. Jiang ZB, Ren CY, Wang MS, et al. (1994) Surgical treatment of aortic coarctation (Report of 35 cases). Chin J Thorac Cardiovasc Surg 10:145.

31. Gao XM, Jiao J, Shen K, et al. (1994) Surgical treatment of ventricular septal defect with aortic valvular prolapse and insufficiency. Chin J Thorac Cardiovasc Surg 10:202–204.

32. Huang HM, Ding WX, Su ZK, et al. (1994) Use of Aprotinin during cardiopulmonary bypass in pediatric heart surgery. Chin J Thorac Cardiovasc Surg 10:205–207.

33. Mao ZF, Gao SZ, Lin DM, et al. (1994) Surgical treatment of tricuspid valvular disease (Report of 37 cases). Chin J Thorac Cardiovasc Surg 10: 217–219.

34. Ding WX, Su ZK, Xu ZW (1994) Anatomic corrective operation for D-transposition of the great arteries. Chin J Thorac Cardiovasc Surg 10:293–295.

35. Ding WX, Su ZK, Xu ZW (1995) Experimental observation and clinical application of expanded polytetrafluoroethylene (Gore-Tex) made in China. Chin J Thorac Cardiovasc Surg 11:30–31.

36. Zhang RF, Wang ZW, Sun LZ, et al. (1995) Surgical treatment of congenitally corrected transposition of the great arteries with cardiac anomaly. Chin J Thorac Cardiovasc Surg 11:196–197.

37. Li XH, Guo B, Shi J, et al. (1996) Video-assisted thoracoscopic closure of patent ductus arteriosus (Report of 12 cases). Chin J Thorac Cardiovasc Surg 12:5–6.

38. Fu WD, Cao DF, Su ZK, et al. (1996) Surgical treatment of persistent truncus arteriosus. Chin J Thorac Cardiovasc Surg 12:68–70.

39. Chen Q, Wang ZH (1996) Surgical treatment of double outlet of right ventricle with atrioventricular discordance. Chin J Thorac Cardiovasc Surg 12:160.

40. Yu YF, Li GS, Zhu LB, et al. (1996) The diagnosis and surgical repair of aortic coarctation. Chin J Thorac Cardiovasc Surg 12:129–131.

41. Xu ZW, Su ZK, Sun AM (1996) Surgical repair in congenital ventricular septum defect in children: a clinical analysis of 2085 cases. Chin J Pediatr Surg 3:143.

42. Gu XL, Dai Y, Quan LB, et al. (1996) Prevention and outcome of residual ventricular septal defect. Chin J Thorac Cardiovasc Surg 1996;12:282–283.

43. Gong HD, Wang ZW, Zhang RF (1997) The diagnosis and surgical repair of common atrium with associated anomalies. Chin J Thorac Cardiovasc Surg 13:5–7.

44. Li XB, Yang GT, Sun XG, et al. (1997) Surgical treatment of Ebstein's anomaly. Chin J Thorac Cardiovasc Surg 13:176–177.

45. Zhuang J, Zhang JF, Chen wd, et al. (1997) One-staged surgical repair of aortic coarctation with intra-cardiac anomalies. Chin J Thorac Cardiovasc Surg 13:146–147.

46. Zheng JH, Xu ZW, Su ZK, et al. (1997) Surgical treatment of ventricular septal defect with pulmonary hypertension in infants less than 8 kg. Chin J Thorac Cardiovasc Surg 13:260–261.

47. Zhu XK, Hu SL, Xue PY, et al. (1998) Surgical repair of ventricular septal defect in infancy. Chin J Thorac Cardiovasc Surg 14:1–3.

48. Yang CH, Lan HJ, Zhang KL, et al. (1997) Modified Senning procedure for d-transposition of the great arteries. Chin J Thorac Cardiovasc Surg 14:103.

49. Xing QS, Zhang ST, Chen ZG, et al. (1998) Surgical outcome of ventricular septal defect with aortic insufficiency in children. Chin J Thorac Cardiovasc Surg 14: 71–73.

50. Ding WX, Su ZK, Xu ZW (1998) Surgical treatment of atrioventricular canal (Report of 130 cases). Chin J Thorac Cardiovasc Surg 14:68–70.

51. Zhu XD, Sun HS, Wu QY, et al. (1998) The pathologic anatomy and surgical repair of abnormally atrioventricular connection. Chin J Thorac Cardiovasc Surg 14(4).

52. Zhang SY, Liang FY, Qin TC, et al. (1998) Surgical repair and results of total anomalous pulmonary veins connection. Chin J Thorac Cardiovasc Surg 14:152–154.

53. Zhang RF, Wang ZW, Sun LZ, et al. (1998) Surgical treatment of d-transposition of the great arteries. Chin J Thorac Cardiovasc Surg 14:136–138.

54. Wang JQ, Rong YB, Cui XD, et al. (1998) Reconstruction of right ventricular outlet tract with aortic homograft for tetralogy of Fallot. Chin J Thorac Cardiovasc Surg 14:334–336.

55. Zhang RF, Wang ZW, Sun LZ, et al. (1999) Surgical treatment of single ventricle (Report of 56 cases). Chin J Thorac Cardiovasc Surg 15:87–89.

56. Liu KY, Chen YC, You B, et al. (1999) Surgical repair of Ebstein's anomaly (Report of 44 cases). Chin J Thorac Cardiovasc Surg 15:144–146.

57. Chen CC, Shen ZL (1999) Surgical treatment of ventricular septal defect in children less than 10 kg. Chin J Thorac Cardiovasc Surg 15:141–143.

58. Liu YL, Su JW, Yu CT, et al. (1999) Corrective repair of tetralogy of Fallot via small right thoracotomy in children. Chin J Thorac Cardiovasc Surg 15:200–202.

59. Wu QY, Chu JM, Yan J (1999) Modified Senning procedure for d-transposition of the great arteries. Chin J Thorac Cardiovasc Surg 15:287.

60. Liu JF, Zhu HB, Zhu DM, et al. (1999) Surgical repair of tetralogy of Fallot (Report of 115 consecutive cases without death). Chin J Thorac Cardiovasc Surg 15:263–265.

61. Xu ZW, Su ZK, Ding WX (1999) Surgical treatment of double outlet of right ventricle. Chin J Thorac Cardiovasc Surg 15:327–329.

62. Li XM, Zhang RF, Wang ZW, et al. (2000) Surgical repair of interrupted aortic arch with intra-cardiac anomaly. Chin J Thorac Cardiovasc Surg 16:46.

63. Sun K, Chen SB, Zhang YQ, et al. (2000) Application of transesophageal echocardiography during pediatric open heart surgery. Chin J Thorac Cardiovasc Surg 16:43.

64. Yu YF, Zhu LB, Li GS (2000) Surgical correction of Ebstein's malformation in 39 cases. Chin J Thorac Cardiovasc Surg 16:275–276.

65. Chen CC, Shen ZL, Ji SY (2000) Surgical repair of congenital heart disease in young infants: a report of 160 cases. Chin J Thorac Cardiovasc Surg 16:327–329.

66. Wang MH, Cao SW, Xu ZH (2001) Surgical repair of congenital heart disease in children via right small thoracotomy: a report of 90 cases. Chin J Thorac Cardiovasc Surg 17:53–54.

67. Liu YL, Zhang J, Xie N, et al. (2001) The application of cryopreserved homografts for complex congenital heart disease. Chin J Thorac Cardiovasc Surg 17:9–10.

68. Wang SY, Hu SS, Wu QY, et al. (2001) Surgical treatment of aortopulmonary septal defect in 21 cases. Chin J Thorac Cardiovasc Surg 17:71–73.

69. Zhang J, Liu YL, Xie N, et al. (2001) Long-term result of right ventricular outflow tract reconstruction with an allograft conduit. Chin J Thorac Cardiovasc Surg 17:68–70.

70. Xu ZW, Su ZK, Wang SM, et al. (2001) Repair of double-outlet right ventricle with Taussig-Bing by arteries Switch operation. Chin J Thorac Cardiovasc Surg 17:132–134.

71. Zheng QJ, Cai ZJ, Wang G (2001) Results of the modified Fontan operation. Chin J Thorac Cardiovasc Surg 17:332–334.

72. Liu F, Luo HZ, Yin BL, et al. (2002) Surgical treatment of congenital heart disease in infant less than 7 kilogram. Chin J Thorac Cardiovasc Surg 18:51–52.

73. Chen HS, Zhong HQ, Chen JW, et al. (2002) Corrective repair of Tetralogy of Fallot in 102 cases. Chin J Thorac Cardiovasc Surg 18:37–38.

74. Liu YL, Zhu XD, Wu QY, et al. (2002) Surgical and transcatheter coil embolization treatment of 94 cases of congenital coronary artery fistula. Chin J Thorac Cardiovasc Surg 18:153–154.

75. Xu ZW, Ding WX, Su ZK (2002) Arterial Switch operation for complete transposition of great arteries in neonates. Chin J Thorac Cardiovasc Surg 18: 147–149.

76. Xu ZM, Chen L, Shi ZY, et al. (2002) Postoperative management of congenital heart defects in young infants. Chin J Thorac Cardiovasc Surg 18:208–210.

77. Yang SC, Zhou QW, Chen YC, et al. (2002) A long-term follow-up investigation for the repaired congenital heart defects with severe pulmonary hypertension. Chin J Thorac Cardiovasc Surg 18:199–201.

78. Fang MH, Wang ZW, Zhang RF, et al. (2002) The analysis of risk factors for the modified Fontan operation (159 cases). Chin J Thorac Cardiovasc Sur 18:193–195.

79. Su ZK, Zhu ZQ, Xu ZW, et al. (2002) Two staged operation for transposition of the great artery. Chin J Thorac Cardiovasc Surg 18:278–280.

80. Weng GX, Xie Q, Wang H, et al. (2002) Video-assisted thoracoscopic surgical closure of patent ductus arteriosus in 86 cases. Chin J Thorac Cardiovasc Surg 2002;18:374.

81. Wang Z, Gu JR, Wang JM, et al. (2002) Corrective repair of Tetralogy of Fallot in 100 infants. Chin J Thorac Cardiovasc Surg 18:347.

82. Cao DF, Su ZK, Ding WX (2002) Surgical repair of complete artioventricular cancal defect in children: a report of 50 cases. Chin J Thorac Cardiovasc Surg 18: 340–341.

83. Liu YL, Zhu XD, Yu CT, et al. (2002) Update on surgical treatment for congenital heart disease in children in the past 10 years. Chin J Thorac Cardiovasc Surg (2002) 18:321–324.

84. Liu YL, Zhu XD, Yu CT, et al. (2002) Update on surgical treatment for congenital heart disease in children in the past 10 years. Thorac Cardiovasc Surg 18:321–324.

85. Zhang HJ, Liu YL, Feng JP et al. (2003) Change of plasma level cardiac troponin I in myocardiol ischemia reperfusion injury during the operation for congenital heart disease. Chin J Thorac Cardiovasc Surg 19:21–24.

86. Zhang RF, Wang ZW, Zhu HY, et al. (2003) Surgical corrective of Ebstein's malformation in 139 cases. Chin J Thorac Cardiovasc Surg 19:10–12.

87. Yang JF, Hu DX, Hu JG, et al. (2003) Surgical treatment of double outlet of right ventricle: a clinical analysis of 72 cases. Chin J Thorac Cardiovasc Surg 19:7–9.

88. Liu YL, Yu CT, Wei B, et al. (2003) Bi-directional cavopulmonary anastomosis without cardiopulmonary bypass: a report of 68 cases. Chin J Thorac Cardiovasc Surg 19:4–6.

89. Chen HW, Su ZK, Xu ZM, et al. (2003) Age influences the early effect of bidrectinal cavopulmonary anastomosis on cyanosis. Chin J Thorac Cardiovasc Surg 19: 69–71.

90. Mo XM, Gu XL, Qian LB, et al. (2003) Surgical correction for transposition of great arteries in 24 cases. Chin J Thorac Cardiovasc Surg 19:181–182.

91. Xu ZM, Chen L, Su ZK, et al. (2003) Inhaled nitric oxide in patients critical pulmonary perfusion after bi-directional cavopulmonary shunt. Chin J Thorac Cardiovasc Surg 19:142–144.

92. Xu ZW, Su ZK, Ding WX, et al. (2003) The double-switch operation used in cardiac anomalies with atrioventricular and atrioventricular discordance. Chin J Thorac Cardiovasc Surg 19:134–135.

93. Cao DF, Qiu LS, Su ZK, et al. (2003) Surgical correction of 19 children with persistent truncus arteriosus. Chin J Thorac Cardiovasc Surg 19:131–133.

94. Wei B, Liu YL, Yu CT, et al. (2003) Effects of pulmonary artery perfusion with hypothermic protective solution on pulmonary vascular endothelial cell injury during cardiopulmonary bypass. Chin J Thorac Cardiovasc Surg 19:220–222.

95. Chen L, Xu ZM, Shi ZY (2003) Postoperative management of congenital heart defects in neonates: a report of 50 cases. Chin J Thorac Cardiovasc Surg 19:212–214.

96. Wang X, Chen X, Yang JX et al. (2004) Using inhaled nitric oxide after surgical treatment of congenital heart disease. Chin J Thorac Cardiovasc Surg 20:173–174.

97. Lan XC, Feng ZR (eds) (2002) Cardiovascular surgery. 2nd edn. People's Health Press.

98. Wang ZW, Liu WY, Zhang BR (eds) (2003) Cardiac surgery. People's Military Surgeon Press.

99. Gu KS (ed) (2003) Cardiothoracic surgery. Shanghai Science and Technology Press.

100. Wang ZW (ed) (1996) Surgery: cardiovascular surgery. People's Military Surgeon Press.

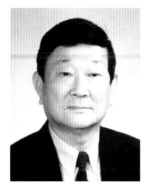

Wen-Xiang Ding

# The History, Current Status, and Future of Coronary Heart Disease

*Qing-Yu Wu, Ming-Kui Zhang*

**C**oronary heart disease has become a very serious health problem in the world. It has become the principal cause of death following the aging of the population in advanced countries. In China, the morbidity and mortality are increasing year after year. More work has been done on myocardial revascularization. The advent of the coronary artery bypass graft (CABG) was a landmark in treating coronary heart disease, and this has become the most common and effective method.

## History

In China, Jia-Qiang Guo (Fig. 1), a famous surgeon at Beijing Fuwai Hospital, performed the first coronary artery bypass grafting operation in 1974. Thereafter Guo and his colleagues [1] reported 24 cases of coronary artery bypass grafting. From 1980 to 1984, Zhi Pan of Shanghai Chest Hospital performed 21 cases of coronary artery bypass grafts [2]. The operation was then performed at

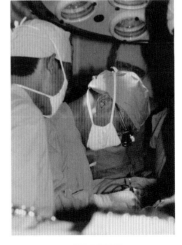

Fig. 1. Dr. Jia-Qiang Guo

Shanghai Renji Hospital, Shandong Provincial Hospital, and Xi'an Xijing Hospital [4–5]. In 1995 Qing-Heng Huang of Xi'an Medical University reported the first case of coronary artery bypass grafting without pump [6]. But the initial development of coronary artery surgery was very slow in China. Only a total of 60 operations were performed up until 1984. In 1992 the total rose to 500. To 1996 Dr. Jia-Qiang Guo and his colleagues performed 700 operations of CABG in Fuwai Hospital. But over the last 10 years Qing-Yu Wu, as the President of Fuwai Hospital, has trained a large group of youthful cardiac surgeons in his hospital. From 1993–1996 he performed 110 operations of CABG, using the left internal mammary artery in 60 cases. The success rate approached 99%. He was among the first to emphasize that full revascularization and perioperative treatment were very important [7]. The number of cases of CABG at Fuwai Hospital increased greatly from 84 cases in 1992 to 1,288 cases in 2003, and the mortality rate decreased from 7.1% in 1992 to 0.84% in 2003 [8] (Fig. 2). Simultaneously, he did his best to popularize the coronary artery surgical technique in China. He assisted surgeons in more than thirty provincial hospitals and affiliated hospitals of

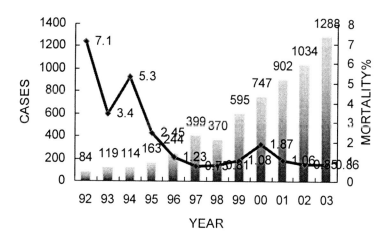

Fig. 2. The cases and mortality for CABG in Fuwai Hospital from 1992 to 2003.

medical colleges to perform the procedure, and held congresses of coronary artery surgery technique. For his contribution to coronary artery surgery, he was awarded the National Science Advancing Prize in 2002.

## *Current Status*

### The Effect of Coronary Artery Bypass Grafting

Today, coronary artery bypass grafting has become an effective method in treating coronary heart disease. In China there were approximately 2,000 cases of CABG in 1999, and 6,000 cases in 2004. Looked from the point of view of population statistics we have an apparent gap compared with advanced countries. But the effectiveness of our operations approaches that in advanced countries [9]. The results of the national key project for standardization and generalization of CABG technique, organized by Qing-Yu Wu, showed that the total mortality rate of CABG was 2.33% in 10,100 cases in 18 heart centers from 2000 to 2003. The mortality rates for elective operations and emergency operations were 1.88% and 4.77% respectively. The mortality rate for on-pump was 2.72%, but for off-pump was 1.08% [7] (Fig. 3). Wu reported [10] that of 1,100 CABG cases from 1996 to 1999, 1,048 procedures were performed on hypothermia cardiopulmonary bypass and 60 on beating hearts. The

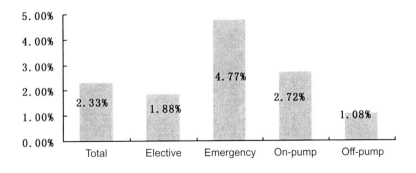

Fig. 3. Mortality of CABG in multi-center from 2000 to 2003 (10,100 cases).

hospital death rate was 0.81%. Wan reported [11] the multi-center early outcomes and clinical experience for 1,507 patients who had undergone coronary artery bypass grafting. Of these patients 1,198 were off-pump and 309 were on-pump. The total hospital mortality rate was 2.1%.

## Total Arterial Myocardial Revascularization

Coronary artery bypass grafting has been utilized as a beneficial treatment for myocardial ischemic disease for over three decades. Failure of coronary artery venous grafts occurs at a substantial rate and has a large impact on two main endpoints, survival and quality of life. The internal thoracic artery (ITA) graft has the best long-term patency rate of all the conduits currently used for myocardial revascularization. The ten-year patency rate for pedicled ITA grafts was 95%, but it was 50% for venous grafts. Today, the left internal thoracic artery is widely used as grafting material [3, 4, 10, 12–14] (Table 1). Use of the radical artery (RA) and right gastro-epiploon artery (RGEA) as the grafting material has been reported [10, 15–17] (Table 2).

## Off-pump Coronary Artery Bypass Grafting and Mini-Invasive Coronary Artery Bypass Grafting

In 1995 Huang [6] reported the first performance of the off-pump coronary artery bypass grafting procedure in China. In 1999 Wu reported [10] 60 cases of off-pump CABG with satisfactory clinical results. Off-pump CABG is widely used because it entails less blood transfusion, shortened ventilation time, shortened hospital time, and less expenditure. The percentage use of off-pump CABG has increased from 3.8% in 1996 to 46.04% in Fuwai Hospital in 2003 [8] (Fig. 4).

Off-pump CABG through limited lower sternotomy technique was reported in Fuwai Hospital in 2001 [18]. Video-assisted minimally invasive coronary artery bypass (VACAB) operations were performed in Nanjing Gulou Hospital, including preoperative PTCA (Hybrid technique) for RCA diseases in some patients with double vessel diseases [19].

## Table 1   ITA as the Grafting Material

| Author | Time | Case | Grafting Material | Target Vessel | Percent |
|--------|------|------|-------------------|---------------|---------|
| YH Su | 1982 | 1 | ITA | LAD | |
| HS Zhu | 1988 | 1 | ITA | LAD | |
| TY Wang | 1994 | 2 | ITA | LAD | |
| F Xiao | 1998 | 61 | ITA | LAD, LCX | |
| QY Wu | 1999 | 751 | ITA | LAD | 66.7% |
| CQ Gao | 1999 | 112 | ITA | LAD | 92.0% |

## Table 2   RA, RGEA as the Grafting Material

| Author | Time | Case | Grafting Material | Target Vessel |
|--------|------|------|-------------------|---------------|
| QY Wu | 1999 | 101 | RA | LAD,Diag,RCA |
| WJ Zhen | 2001 | 54 | RA | ? |
| QM Wang | 2004 | 93 | RGEA | OM,RCA,PDA |
| FJ Huang | 2005 | 32 | RGEA | PDA |

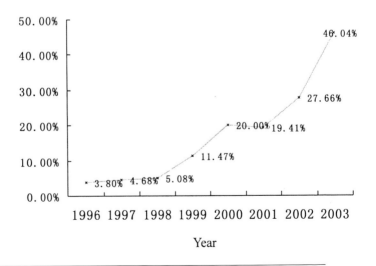

*Fig. 4. The percentage of off-pump CABG in Fuwai Hospital from 1996 to 2003.*

## Surgical Treatment in Complication of Myocardial Infarction

Left ventricular aneurysm and ventricular septal rupture are severe complications of myocardial infarction. From 1973 to 1980, Dr. Jia-Qiang Guo of Fuwai Hospital performed 19 cases of left ventricular aneurysmectomy (LVA), including 6 cases of CABG plus aneurysmectomy [1]. The technique was then perfomed in several hospitals [2, 7, 20, 21] (Table 3). Surgical treatment of ventricular septal rupture has been performed in Fuwai Hospital and Xijing Hospital [10, 22, 23].

The morbidity rate for ischemic mitral regurgitation (IMR) in coronary heart disease is 20%. Mammilla muscle rupture is the main cause of ischemic mitral regurgitation in acute postinfarction. In 1999 Wu (1999) performed [10] 24 cases of CABG plus mitral operations, including 8 cases of mitral valvuloplasty and 16 of mitral valve replacement, without in-hospital death. In 2005, Meng reported [24] 53 cases of IMR, 33 cases with CABG combined with mitral valvuloplasty, and 22 with mitral valve replacement. The total operative mortality rate was 15.09% (8/53)

## Transmyocardial Laser Revascularization (TMLR)

The development of the use of transmyocardial laser revascularization (TMLR) in treating ischemic heart disease in China

Table 3   The Surgical Treatment of Ventricular Aneurysm

| Author | Time | Case | Method | Result |
|--------|------|------|--------|--------|
| JQ Guo | 1984 | 19 | LVA or LVA + CABG | 3 cases death |
| Z Pan | 1984 | 5 | LVA + CABG | ? |
| MD Xiao | 1994 | 125 | LVA or LVA + CABG | 12 cases death |
| QY Wu | 1996 | 10 | LVA + CABG | 0 cases death |
| CQ Gao | 2003 | 42 | LVA + CABG | 0 cases deathleft |

ventricular aneurysmectomy = LVA

was in synchronization with developed countries. The technique was performed in Xijing Hospital, the Third Hospital of Beijing Medical University, Anzhen Hospital, and other hospitals [5, 25, 26]. There remains some disagreement about TMLR. In 1999 Qu reported [26] on the clinical experience of sole transmyocardial laser revascularization (TMLR) in treatment of coronary heart disease (CHD) in 50 cases. It showed that a sole TMLR is a safe and effective procedure for treatment of end stage CHD, especially for those not amenable to PTCA or CABG. The best result is achieved with full preoperative preparation, correct evaluation of myocardial ischemia, better anaesthesia, and successful perioperative management.

## Re-operation after Coronary Artery Bypass Grafting

As more CABG operations are performed and the time-lapse increases, the number of repeat-CABG cases will increase greatly. From 1996 to 2000 Wu performed [27] 5 cases repeat-CABG. There were no preoperative deaths or complications except for one case of re-thoracotomy for hemorrhage. This showed that repeated coronary artery bypass grafting can be achieved successfully if proper operative indications are chosen and reasonable management implemented.

## *Future*

First, as the population ages, the morbidity of coronary artery disease (CAD) is increasing year after year and there are more patients with severe diabetes, cerebrovascular disease, renal failure, and left ventricular dysfunction. Some reports show that CABG is helpful for these patients, even for some ischemic heart disease patients with EF<30%, but all of us know that it is still a problem. Secondly, because of CAD characteristics and venous graft occlusion, repeat-CABG is another clinical problem we have to face today.

Minimally invasive surgery was the greatest step made in the 1990s. The minimally invasive coronary artery bypass is less invasive and involves a shorter hospital stay and a quicker recovery time. Currently, minimally invasive coronary surgery includes minimally invasive direct coronary artery bypass surgery (MIDCAB), port-access bypass surgery, and robotically assisted coronary surgery. Robotic microsurgical systems have been developed to assist the surgeon in endoscopic coronary surgery and to enhance the surgeon's ability, dexterity and precision. The long-term effects remain unclear, but robot-assisted CABG with dexterity, precision and tele-manipulation is a new minimally invasive method.

## References

1.  Le XH, Guo JQ, Zhu XD, et al. (1984) Combined coronary artery bypass grafting with ventricular aneurysmectomy. Chin J Cardiol 12:165–168.
2.  Pan Z, Zhou YQ, Chen Q, et al. (1984) Experience of coronary artery bypass grafting. Chin J Cardiol 12:162–164.
3.  Su YH, Yang AM, Zhou YZ, et al. (1984) Application of left internal mammary artery for coronary artery bypass grafting. Chin J Cardiol 12:169–170.
4.  Zhu HS, Wang YS, Feng ZR, et al. (1984) The use of internal thoracic artery and saphenous veins for coronary artery bypass grafting. Chin J Cardiol 12:134–136.
5.  Liu WY, Cai ZJ, Yang JX, et al. (1994) Coronary artery bypass grafting and ventricular aneurysmectomy. Chin J Clin Thorac Cardiovasc Surg 1:2–4.
6.  Huang QH, Sun L, Li Zhao Z (1995) Coronary artery bypass grafting. Chin J Thorac Cardiovasc Surg 11:208.
7.  Wu QY, Song YH, Lu F, et al. (1996) Early results of CABG operation in 110 patients. Chin J Surg 34:670–672.
8.  Wu QY. The tenth 5-year national key technology R&D program: standardization and promotion of coronary artery bypass grafting. (2001BA703D12)
9.  Wu QY (2000) Current status and prospects of coronary artery bypass grafting in China. Chin J Clin Thorac Cardiovasc Surg 7:217–218.
10. Wu QY, Hu SS, Xu JP, et al. (1999) Early results of 1,110 cases of coronary artery bypass. Chin J Surg 37:666–668.
11. Wan F, Chen Y, Jiang L, et al. (2003) Clinical analysis of 1,507 cases after coronary artery bypass grafting. Beijing Med 25:34–41.
12. Wang TY, Sun YQ, Li WS, et al. (1994) Coronary artery bypass grafting. Chin Circulation J 9:532–534.
13. Xiao F, Zhang XT, Liu Y, et al. (1998) Use of the internal mammary artery for coronary artery bypass. Chin J Cardiovasc Med 3:395–397.
14. Gao CQ, Zhu LB, Li BJ, et al. (1999) Internal mammary artery for coronary artery bypass grafting in 112 elderly patients. Chin J Geriatric Cardiovasc Cerebrovasc Dis 1:15–17.

15. Zhen WJ, Tong HF, Wang YZ, et al. (2002) Coronary revascularization with radial artery and internal mammary artery grafts. Chin Med J 115: 55–57.

16. Wang QM (2004) Application of right gastroepiploic artery for coronary artery bypass grafting. Chin J Thorac Cardiovasc Surg 20:309.

17. Huang FJ, Yang JF, Lai YQ, et al. (2005) Use of right gastroepiploic artery for coronary artery bypass grafting in 32 cases. Chin J Surg 43:98–99.

18. Sun HS, Shao MP, Wu QY, et al. (2001) Off-pump coronary artery bypass grafting through limited lower sternotomy. Chin Circulation J 16:296–299.

19. Wang DJ, Cao B, Chen JB, et al. (2004) Video-assisted minimally invasive coronary artery bypass in 12 cases. Biomed Engin Clin Med 8:20–22.

20. Xiao MD, Shen XD, Zhu XD, et al. (1994) Surgical treatment of left ventricular aneurysm. Chin J Surg 32:732–734.

21. Gao CQ, Zhu LB, Xiao CS, et al. (2003) Left ventricular aneurysmectomy with geometric reconstruction. Chin J Surg 41:917–919.

22. Shen XD, Zhu XD,Xiao MD, et al. (1995) Surgical treatment of post-infarction ventricular septal defect. Chin Circulation J 10:60–61.

23. Xu JP, Wang LQ, Chen L, et al. (2002) Surgical Repair of Postinfarction interventricular septal defect. Chin Circulation J 17:138–140.

24. Zheng SH, Meng X, Zhang JQ, et al. (2005) Surgical management of ischemic mitral regurgitation. Nat Med J China 85:1473–1475.

25. Zhang MJ, Guo JX, Liu DD, et al. (1997) Successful laser myocardial revascularization with coronary bypass surgery grafting: a case report. J Beijing Med Univ 29:277–278.

26. Qu Z, Zhang ZG, Sun YQ, et al. (1999) Clinical experience of transmyocardial laser revascularization. Chin J Thorac Cardiovasc Surg 15:266–268.

27. Wu QY, Meng Q, Hu SS, et al. (2002) Redo coronary artery bypass grafting. Nat Med J China 82:927–928.

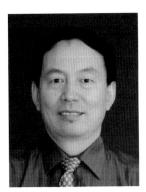

Qing-Yu Wu

# The Made-in-China Mechanical Valve Prostheses

*Bao-Ren Zhang, Zhi-Yun Xu, Jian-Zhou Xing*

I n early 1963, Professor Yong-Zhi Cai started his research on designing and making a mechanical heart valve prosthesis. After a series of experiments the first "home made" ball and cage prosthesis was successfully implanted in a patient with mitral valve disease by Cai at Shanghai Changhai Hospital in 1965 (Fig. 1). This was the first case in China. Subsequently many novel mechanical valve prostheses were produced in China, such as the Beijing GK valve, C-L standard tilting-disc valve, C-L short pole tilting-disc valve, CL-V valve etc. Up to date over 100,000 Chinese-made mechanical valve prostheses have been implanted inside and outside China, with excellent performances.

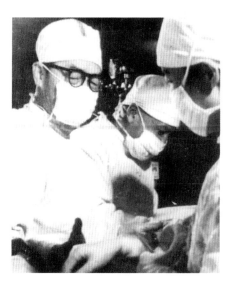

Fig. 1. Dr. Yong-Zhi Cai (left).

# Shanghai Ball and Cage Valve Prosthesis

The Shanghai ball and cage valve was designed and manufactured by the Shanghai Institute of Medical Instruments, Shanghai Changhai Hospital, and Shanghai Institute of Rubber Products. This type of prosthesis was used in the clinical setting in China from June 1965 until 1978. It is principally composed of a cage and a poppet (Fig. 2). The cage is made of a casting of OCr18Ni9Ti or OOcr17Ni14Mo$_2$ without weld. The ring of the cage prevents the ball from escaping and locking. The inner diameter of the ring (RID) is shorter than the ball diameter (BD), while RID/BD varies from 0.85 to 0.88. The proportions of the ring and the ball can keep the lowest pressure gradients. The four struts connected with the symmetry sites of the ring are joined at the apex to form the cage. The length of the struts greatly affects the function of the valve. If too long, the volume of regurgitating blood may increase. If too short, the pressure gradient would increase. Running distance of the ball is 1/2 of the ball diameter. When the ball opens by moving towards the roof of cage, it creates a circular primary orifice (CPO) and a ring shaped secondary orifice (RSSO) between the ball and the housing. RSSO/CPO ratio is between 1.2 and 1.4, which keeps the lowest pressure gradient and regurgitation volume. The sewing ring is made from knitted Dacron enwrapping silicon rubber sponge. The ball, of specific gravity 1.12 to 1.16, is a silicone rubber polymer impregnated with barium sulfate for radiopacity. The Shanghai ball and cage prosthesis had two models with five different inner ring diameters: 18 mm, 20.5 mm, 22 mm, 23 mm, and 23.5 mm.

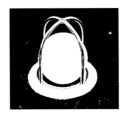

*Fig. 2. Shanghai ball and cage valve prosthesis.*

# The First Case

The first recipient of the Shanghai ball and cage valve was a 34-year-old woman (Fig. 3), who suffered from severe progressive rheumatic mitral valvular disease and was in New York Heart Association (NYHA) functional class IV. After the mitral valve replacement procedure she recovered fully and enjoyed a normal life in NYHA class I. She died of brain metastasis from colon cancer 28 years later without any complications related to the prosthesis. She was the longest survivor after valve replacement with this particular prosthesis.

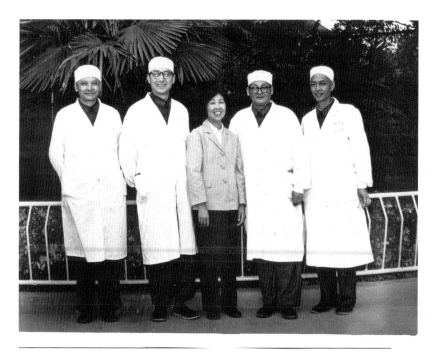

*Fig. 3. The patient (middle) who underwent the first valve replacement in China visits her surgeons 5 years after the operation (from left: Drs. Bao-Ren Zhang, Yong-Zhi Cai, Zhen-Jiang Geng, and Guo-Cui Long).*

# The First Fourteen Patients

From July 1965 to July 1970, 14 patients with severe rheumatic mitral valve disease received Shanghai ball and cage valve prostheses at Changhai Hospital (Fig. 4). All of them were in NYHA class IV and had low cardiac output and pulmonary hypertension before the operation. Most of the patients also had severe cachexia and weight loss. During that period this procedure was indicated only in those high-risk patients with severely diseased native valve not amenable to any repair, and in those were the operation could reasonably be postponed. Therefore the surgical mortality (within 30 days) was very high (6/14). The causes of death were heart failure, renal failure, and arrhythmia. There were 2 late deaths in this group of patients. One died of prosthetic valve endocarditis and the other from carcinomatous metastasis. The remaining six patients survived for more than 24 years in NYHA class I or II. One of them underwent redo MVR in 1997 because of repeating embolism.

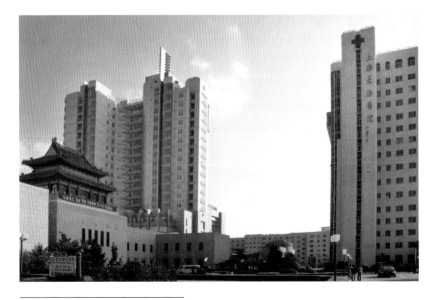

*Fig. 4. Changhai Hospital in Shanghai.*

# Shanghai Tilting-disc Valve

The Shanghai tilting-disc valve prosthesis was designed by the Shanghai Institute of Medical Instruments, Shanghai Changhai Hospital, and Lanzhou Carbon Factory. It has been applied clinically since 1978. The structure of the Shanghai tilting-disc valve basically resembles the Bjork-Shiley prosthesis. The disc holding was initially made of OOcr17Ni14Mo2 without welding, and later made of titanic alloy. The tilting-disc prosthesis had a carbon disc held in place by two "π"-shaped struts, one lying on the inlet of the valve and the other on the outlet. The disc floats between the two struts in such a way that it closes when the blood begins to flow backward and opens when blood begins to flow forward. The tilting-disc valve is vastly superior to the ball and cage design. It opens at an angle of 60° and closes at 2°. This tilting pattern provides improved central flow while still preventing backflow. The tilting-disc valve can reduce mechanical damage to the blood cells. Its improved flow pattern can also limit clot formation. However the problem with such a design was the tendency of the outlet struts to fracture due to fatigue resulting from repeated ramming of the struts by the disc. The sewing ring was made of knitted Dacron. The tilting-disc prostheses had aortic and mitral models. The total number of implantations of this prosthesis had reached over 10,000 in China by 1998.

The authors retrospectively analyzed the results of 1,360 patients undergoing MVR using the Shanghai tilting-disc valve. Follow-up period lasted over 10 years. The 30-day mortality was 6.6% (reduced to 2.0% after 1980). The actuarial 5-year survival was 89.8%, and 10-year survival was 81.7%. Late mortality was 1.7% patient/year. Thromboembolism rate was 0.4% patient/year. Bleeding events related to anticoagulation was 0.8% patient/year. Structural failure rate was 0.1% patient/year. Prosthetic endocarditis was 0.1% patient/year. Leakage rate was 0.1% patient/year. Five- and ten-year freedoms from valve-related complications were 89.9% and 78.5% respectively. The last follow-up showed that heart function of the survivors was NYHA class I in 64.4%, NYHA class II in 25.6%, and NYHA class III in 8.9%. Risk factors for postoperative cardiac dysfunction included tricuspid regurgitation and aortic regurgitation.

# C-L Standard Tilting-disc Valve

The C-L standard tilting-disc valve prosthesis was designed by Lanzhou Carbon Factory, Shanghai Changhai Hospital, and Lanzhou Instrument Factory. This prosthesis originated from the Shanghai tilting-disc valve (in which some strut fractures found since its use in 1986). The C-L standard tilting-disc valve greatly improved the structure design by increasing the diameter of the strut, thus decreasing stress on the strut. The integration of strut and ring was right-angled. Moreover contact area between disc and bearing was increased from 50% to 90% in order to make the disc move smoothly, which also had the merit of low regurgitation (Fig. 5). A novel polishing technique made strut, ring, and disc smoother. Titanic alloy was used for the strut and the ring. Graphite (Poco Co., USA) served as the main material of the disc. A novel coating technique was applied to coat carbon on the surface of the valve. It opens at an angle of 60° and closes at 2°. The sewing ring was made of knitted Dacron.

Over 15,000 C-L standard tilting-disc prostheses have been used in China. The results showed that this valve has good performance with low prosthesis-related complications. However fracture of a small strut was reported in a patient 6 years after aortic valve replacement.

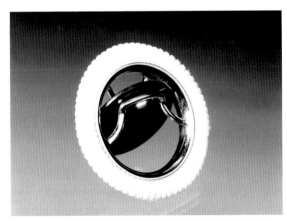

*Fig. 5. C-L standard tilting-disc valve prosthesis.*

# C-L Short Strut Tilting-disc Valve

The C-L short strut tilting-disc valve prosthesis was designed by Xinlan Instrument Factory, Shanghai Changhai Hospital, and Lanzhou Carbon Factory. This prosthesis has been widely used in China since 1991 and the number of implantations is well over 50,000. There is no report of structural failure. Its small "π"-shaped strut was substituted by a single pole whose transverse section was increased by 2.5 times, while design of streamline prism in the struts increases the strength of the struts which have an intensity 37.5 times that of the C-L standard tilting-disc valve. The big "π"-shaped strut of this prosthesis was substituted by two short struts like streamlined crab pincers. Compared with the C-L standard tilting-disc valve, the length of the struts in the C-L short strut tilting-disc prosthesis is significantly shorter, the ratio being 4:1. The joined area of strut and ring was 4 times greater than that of the C-L standard tilting-disc valve (Fig. 6). Thus potential for fracture of struts in the C-L short strut tilting-disc valve was reduced further. The stress point of the disc in the C-L short strut tilting-disc valve lies in the border of disc, while in the C-L standard tilting-disc valve it lies in the center, so a vaulted disc may now be used. Moreover pyrolytic carbon coating was greatly enhanced over the stress area of the disc. Join points of the three struts and the ring form a right-angled triangle. Such improvements not only increase intensity and smooth movement of the disc, they also produce better dynamics of the blood stream. Ring and struts are made from alloy of chromium and nickel cast without welding. It opens at an angle of 70° and close at 2°. Turbulence and vortex of blood have been greatly reduced. The ratio of big orifice to

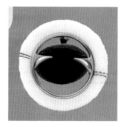

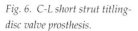

*Fig. 6. C-L short strut titling-disc valve prosthesis.*

small orifice in the C-L standard tilting-disc valve is 5:1 (3:1 in the C-L short strut titling-disc prosthesis), which makes blood flow easily through the valve with lower pressure gradient. The sewing cuff is made of knitted terylene fiber which allows endothelial ingrowth over it. The mechanical heart valve prosthesis can be rotated within its sewing cuff. Mitral and aortic configurations are the same in the C-L short strut tilting-disc valve as in the standard tilting-disc valve except for the sewing cuff.

The author studied 135 patients who underwent implantation of this valve from 1991 to 1995. In total 196 valves were implanted, including 128 mitral and 68 aortic. Indications for valve replacement included rheumatic valve disease in 119 patients, congenital valve disease in 5 patients, native endocarditis in 5 patients, and mitral prolapse in 2 patients. Most of the patients had poor heart function before operation—NYHA class III in 67% and class IV in 33%. The early mortality was 6.8% but there were no valve-related deaths. Mean follow-up time was 2.04 years. There were 2 late deaths due to heart failure and severe lung infection. There were no complications such as thromboembolism, bleeding, peravalvular leak, thrombosis, and hemolysis. Echocardiogram sixth months after operation confirmed excellent performances.

## GK-2 Valve

The GK-2 prosthesis was designed and manufactured by the Beijing Material and Technology Institute of the Aeronautics and Astronautics Ministry of China and the Fuwai Hospital. It is a tilting-disc valve. GK is the abbreviation for "gou kong" in Chinese. The disc has a small hole, allowing a J-shape strut to go through it. Three struts control the movement of the disc (Fig. 7). There are some important merits in the configuration of the GK-2 valve, which are aimed at decreasing potential for thromboembolism, thrombosis, turbulence of blood, and to limit pressure gradient. The special configurations of the valve are as follows:

1. Three struts lie in the inlet of the valve.
2. A main J-shape strut extends to the center of the valve.

3. There is a hole in the center of the disc.
4. Small orifice of the valve has no remora.
5. There is no blind spot and the simple configuration is easy to manufacture.
6. Disk opens at an angle of 70° in the mitral configuration and 75° in the aortic configuration.

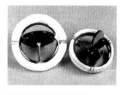

*Fig 7. GK-2 valve prosthesis.*

7. The prosthesis can be rotated within its sewing cuff.
8. The sewing cuff is supra-annular in the mitral configuration.
9. The sewing cuff is vertical collar in the aortic configuration.

More than 20,000 of these valve prostheses have been used and no structural failure has been reported. It is still widely used nowadays in China.

## CL-V Valve

The CL-V prosthesis is a bileaflet valve. Research on it can be traced back to 1995. It became available in early 2004, after thousands of experiments with hundreds of changes in design. The CL-V prosthesis passed national authentication and was put into clinical use in 2004. The scrutiny phase lasted over 6 months. The data suggests excellent performances and no structural failure.

The valve opens at 82° and closes at 25°, with a travel arc of 57°. The sewing cuff is made of knitted Dacron fiber allowing endothelial ingrowth. The prosthesis is rotatable. Compared with other tilting-disc prostheses, the CL-V valve possesses the following merits.

1. Larger orifice area and lower pressure gradient in this series of valve.
2. Blood may flow through the orifice more smoothly.
3. Weight of the valve is 1/3 that of tilting-disc valve prostheses.
4. Lower noise and almost no disc obstacle.
5. The special design distributes stress evenly between struts and disc.

6. Lower profile.
7. Lower regurgitation volume.
8. Better blood stream dynamics.
9. Improved biocompatibility with better polished surface which may minimize thromboembolism and thrombosis.

The CL-V prosthesis has 5 sizes available (19, 21, 23, 25, and 29 mm) for aortic position and 8 sizes (19, 21, 23, 25, 27, 29, 31, and 33 mm) for mitral.

## *References*

1. Zhang JH, Wang GM, Xue DS (2003) Development of the C-L Pugestrut heart valve prosthesis. Chin J Biomed Engin 22:527–532.

2. He ZM, Xi BS, Zhu KQ, et al. (2002) Visualization of cavitation on mechanical heart valve. Chin J Biomed Engin 21: 298–303.

3. http://www.cdnnews.com.tw/20050613/med/yybj/400000002005061223011 629.htm. Over 100,000 valve replacements in China. China Daily. June 12, 2005.

4. Shen YZ (1993) Thirteen years follow-up of China-made cage-ball valve substituting for mitral valve replacement in a patient. Acta Univ Med Tongji 22: 74.

5. Wu LJ (1988) Chinese-made tilting-disc valves in 14 patients. Acad J Sun Yat-Sen Univ Med Sci 2:61–63.

6. Zhu R (1984) Chinese-made tilting-disc valves substitute for six patients. Qian Wei Med J 4:31–32.

7. Cai YZ, Wei T, Geng ZJ, et al. (1975) Development of cage-ball valve and successfully mitral valve replacement. Med J Chin PLA 2 (6):530–534.

8. Cai YZ, Zhang BR, Long GC, et al. (1981) Experiment study and clinical application of Chinese-made isotropic pyrolytic carbon tilting-disc mitral valve. Shanghai Med J 13:211–214.

9. Zhu JL, Cai YZ, Zhang BR (1981) In vitro experiment of C-L tilting-disc valve and clinical applications. Med J Chin PLA 19:111–114.

10. Cai YZ, Zhang BR, Chen RK, et al. (1980) Experimental study and clinical application of Chinese-made tilting-disc valve with isotropic pyrolytic carbon. Shanghai Med J 7:1–4.

11. Cai YZ, Zhang BR, Chen RK, et al. (1985) The experience of no operative dearth in 124 consecutive mitral valve replacements. Clin J Thorac Cardiovasc Surg 2: 3–7.

12. Cai YZ, Zhang BR, Chen RK, et al. (1985) Chinese-made tilting-disc valves

substitute for 222 patients with mitral valve disease. Chin J Thorac Cardiovasc Surg 6:42–44.

13. Cai YZ, Geng ZJ, Zhang BR, et al. (1985) Long-term follow-up of the Chinese-made cage-ball valve used in the mitral position. Clin J Thorac Cardiovasc Surg 2:8–10.

14. Zhang BR, Cai YZ, Zhu JL, et al. (1987) Chinese-made tilting-disc valves substitute for native aortic valves. Clin J Thorac Cardiovasc Surg 4:5–9.

15. Zhu JL, Zhang BR, Cai YZ, et al. (1992) The experience of Chines-made tilting-disc valves used in 1,013 patients with valve diseases. Chin J Cardiol 20: 16–18.

16. Xu ZY, Zhang BR, Zhu JL, et al. (1995) Over 10-year follow-up of home-made tilting-disc valve used in mitral position. Chin J Thorac Cardiovasc Surg 11: 135–137.

17. Cai YZ (1986) Over 20-year follow-up of home-made cage-ball valve used in mitral position. Clin J Thorac Cardiovasc Surg 4: 193–195.

18. Cai YZ (1985) Chinese-made tilting-disc valves substitute in 22 patients. Chin J Cardiol 2: 81–83.

19. Zhang BR, Xu ZY, Zou LJ, et al. (2003) Long-term results of prosthetic mitral valve replacement with home-made tilting disc valve: a report of 125 cases. Chin J Surg 41:253–256.

20. Cai YZ, Zhang BR, Chen RK, et al. (1985) Experience with 124 consecutive elective mitral valve replacement with Shanghai-made tilting-disk prosthesis. Chin Med J 98:299–304.

21. Zhang BR (2001) Heart valve surgery in China: past and present. Chin J Surg 39: 21–24.

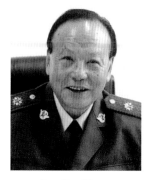

Bao-Ren Zhang

# The History of Cardiothoracic Surgery at the Shanghai Chest Hospital

*Ying-Ze Li*

## Part I. Cardiovascular Surgery

**W**hile referring to the history of cardiothoracic surgery in China, Shanghai Chest Hospital (SCH, Fig. 1) should not be forgotten. Over 50 years it is one of the best hospitals in the field of cardiothoracic surgery in China, at which over 2,000 cardiothoracic operations are performed annually.

The hospital's predecessor was Hongren Hospital, which was established in 1880 by Protestant Episcopal Church. In 1957, the hospital was converted into the SCH by Shanghai Municipal Health Bureau, following the proposal of late Professor Kai-Shi Gu to set up

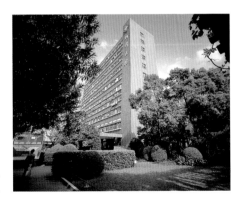

*Fig. 1. Shanghai Chest Hospital.*

a specialty hospital for the treatment of thoracic diseases. Three out of 4 pioneering cardiothoracic surgeons (Fig. 2) in China namely Drs. Jia-Si Huang, Xi-Chun Lan, and Kai-Shi Gu (except Dr. Ying-Kai Wu), had been assigned as the president of the hospital and Surgeon-in-Chief in cardiothoracic surgery successively. It is not surprising that after designation by the Chinese Ministry of Public Health as the national training base for cardiothoracic surgery in 1957, the SCH soon became the Mecca for those who need training in this specialty as well as for those who suffered from various heart and lung diseases around the country.

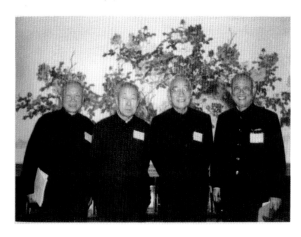

*Fig. 2A. Drs. Kai-Shi Gu, Ying-Kai Wu, Jia-Si Huang, and Xi-Chun Lan (from left to right).*

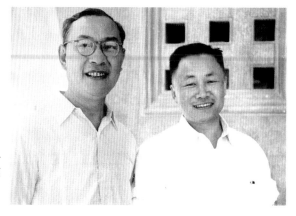

*Fig. 2B. Drs. Jia-Si Huang and Kai-Shi Gu (right) in 1955.*

## *The First Chinese Made Heart-Lung Machine*

When the SCH was established, few hospitals in China could provide closed heart operations, let alone the open-heart surgical procedure. Over the same period, surgeons in the USA and other developed countries had started to repair the intracardiac lesions using the newly invented heart-lung machine. The so-called "cardiopulmonary bypass" (CPB) technique has been popularized by Gibbon (the closure of atrial septal defect in 1953), Kirklin (correction of tetralogy of Fallot in 1955), and Cooley (repair of aorto-pulmonary window in 1957).

Though the heart-lung machines had already been commercially available in the West, it was still impossible for the Chinese surgeons to purchase one due to the deteriorative Sino-US relations and embargo policies implemented by the USA and other Western countries in 1950s.

With his ambition to establish the Chinese open-heart surgical program, Dr. Kai-Shi Gu, the vice president and Chief of the Division of Cardiothoracic Surgery of the SCH decided to make the machine. Upon visiting the Shanghai Medical Instruments Factory in June 1956, Gu expressed his desire to an engineer, Zheng-Qiu Deng (who eventually became Gu's close friend). With limited information collected from the available foreign journals, a heart-lung machine had been produced after one year's endeavor. The machine consisted of a roller pump and a bubble oxygenator (Fig. 3), which appears simple and rough by today's standard. But it was the first such device made completely by Chinese. Before clinical application, a 1-year animal experiment had been conducted to prove the efficacy and the safety of the machine.

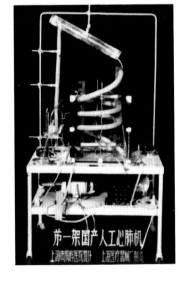

Fig. 3. *The first Chinese made heart-lung machine.*

The historic moment came on June 12, 1958, when Gu performed the first open-heart operation with the Chinese made heart-lung machine. The patient was a 12-year-old girl who suffered from the right ventricle outflow tract obstruction. The heart-lung machine worked for 12 minutes and 30 seconds. Many surgeons and cardiologists were invited to witness this breakthrough. A delegation from Argentina also showed their strong interests during a visit to the SCH in August 1958 (Fig. 4).

## The Synthetic Vascular Grafts

In 1952, Voorhees et al. developed Vinyon-N cloth tubes to replace the diseased arterial segments. Inspired by this success, Gu began to focus on the development of synthetic vascular graft. He used Kapron to produce a seamless plastic arterial graft. From August 1957 through February 1960, 17 aortic aneurysm repair operations with the seamless plastic arterial graft were performed by Gu and his team at the SCH.

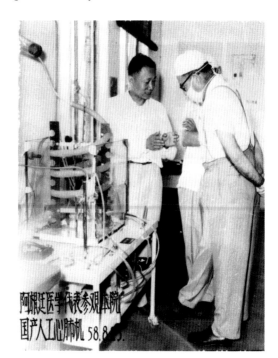

*Fig. 4. Visitors from Argentina at the SCH in 1958.*

had been performed at the SCH. The procedure had been proved to be an effective and low cost therapy for a selected group of patients with mitral stenosis.

From 1972 to 1976, SCH participated in a research project which was led by the Changhai Hospital group to develop a tilting disk mechanical mitral prosthesis. On December 11, 1978, the first clinical implantation of this new prosthesis was performed at the Changhai Hospital by Yong-Zhi Cai. One week later, Zhi Pan performed a similar case. From then on, various valvular interventions had been accomplished at the Shanghai Chest Hospital. By 2003, more than 4,000 valvular operations had been performed at this institution with an overall perioperative mortality less than 5%.

## Congenital Cardiac Surgery

### 1. Patent ductus arteriosus (PDA)

In July 1961, the successful application of a domestic-made surgical stapler for the closure of a PDA was first reported by Gu. This new surgical instrument was resulted from the collaboration between SCH and Shanghai Medical instruments Factory.

Pan and colleagues reviewed a total of 2,133 PDA closure at the SCH from November 1957 through November 1985. The perioperative mortality of the operation was 0.4% (5 deaths due to massive hemorrhage). After 1964, over 98% of the procedures were accomplished with the surgical stapler and no death was reported since January 1970 in a consecutive series of 1,838 PDA closures.

### 2. Tetralogy of Fallot (TOF)

From July 1966 through April 1975, a total of 56 cases of complete correction of TOF had been performed at the SCH. The perioperative mortality of this group of patients was 12.5%, which was one of the best surgical results at that particular period in China. The surgical result of TOF repair was further improved in 1982 by using bovine pericardium Dacron patch with mono-cusp to enlarge the right ventricular outflow tract.

## Ischemic Heart Diseases

In January 1980, the first successful CABG case in Shanghai was performed by Pan at the SCH. Pan and colleagues set up some important protocols covering indications for surgery, preoperative management, intraoperative anaesthesia and monitoring, myocardial protection, surgical techniques, and postoperative care. Meanwhile another important research, the operative transluminal coronary angioplasty (OTCA), was also in progress at the SCH. Using CABG combined with OTCA technique, Pan performed 5 successful cases. By November 1990, 98 CABG cases had been performed at the SCH. The concomitant procedures included resection of ventricular aneurysm, mitral valve replacement, closed mitral commissurotomy, coronary endarterectomy and OTCA. The perioperative mortality in this group of patients decreased from 11.3% in 1980 to 4.8% in 1990.

# Part II. Thoracic Surgery

## 1950s–1960s

Pulmonary tuberculosis was one of the most devastating and life-threatening diseases in China then. In 1954, Kai-Shi Gu first introduced the Plmbage procedure for surgical management of cavitary tuberculosis. The costal periosteum and the intercostal muscles were dissected off the ribs to create an extrapleural space. Small plastic balls were used to fill the space so as to compress the underlying lung, causing the cavities to collapse. The procedure was much less mutilating than extensive thoracoplasty, and more effective than the more primitive way of managing cavitary diseases through pneumothorax. It gained Gu international fame as the procedure was later introduced into the former USSR.

Since the late 1940s, Gu and Jia-Si Huang had started to perform pulmonary segmentectomy and lobectomy for tuberculosis and other benign lesions of the lung. In 1958, Gu performed the first pneumonectomy for lung cancer at the SCH. The patient's recovered uneventfully.

Tracheal surgery had long been considered as a forbidden area in China, except a mere tracheostomy for releasing airway obstruction. In 1959, Kai-Shi Gu resected a 5-cm trachea for a patient with tracheal tumor and successfully anastomosed both ends together to reconstruct the airway. It was not until 1961 that Grillo proposed the length of tracheal resection should not beyond 4–6 cm if the airway were to be reconstructed through end-to-end anastomosis.

For surgical treatment of esophageal cancer, the most popular method of esophagectomy in China was partial resection of the esophagus and intrathoracic anastomosis through left thoracotomy. However a right side approach, namely a modified McKeown procedure, was first proposed at the SCH. In comparison with a left thoracotomy, there are three advantages via the right side approach: (1) Resection of tumors located in the upper thoracic esophagus above the level of the carina becomes much easier, and less risky for trachea laceration or thoracic duct damage while dissecting the upper thoracic esophagus under direct vision. (2) By making the anastomosis higher up in the neck, the length of esophagus resected is greater than using the intrathoracic anastomosis method. Given the high incidence of multiple originations of esophageal squamous carcinoma and frequent submucosal metastasis, a subtotal esophagectomy would assure a more radical resection of the tumor. In addition, leakage from a cervical anastomosis is often not life threatening as opposed to an intrathoracic leak. (3) Modification was made so that two teams of surgeons could work simultaneously on the chest (through an antero-lateral thoracotomy) and on the abdomen. Hence the duration of operation as well as that of anesthesia could be greatly reduced, making the procedure less traumatic to the patients.

## 1970s–2000s

The Department of Thoracic Surgery at the SCH started to gain international fame over this period under the leadership of Shan-Fang Wu (Fig. 7), Ou-Lin Huang (Fig. 8), Yun-Zhong Zhou, and Wen-Hu Chen (Fig. 9).

Early in the 1970s, Shan-Fang Wu started a clinical study on extended indication of surgery for lung cancer. The subjects included patients aged over 70 years and patients with impaired respiratory function, with small cell lung cancer, or stage III diseases, or tumor invading into the carina, and with pleural dissemination. After retrospectively reviewing 3,120 lung cancer patients operated on over a 25-year period, Wu suggested:

(1) Age itself should not be a contraindication to lung cancer surgery. With careful case selection and meticulous perioperative management, the surgical risk in patients aged over 70 years is acceptable with a 30-day mortality as low as 2.9%. And the long-term result is quite satisfactory with a 5-year survival rate as high as 28.2%.

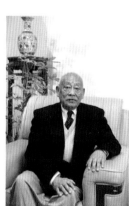

Fig. 8. Dr. Ou-Lin Huang.

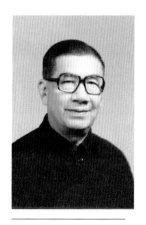

Fig. 7. Dr. Shan-Fang Wu.

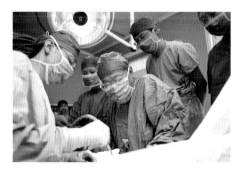

Fig. 9. Dr. Wen-Hu Chen.

(2) Pulmonary resection could still be indicated in patients with impaired pulmonary function after stringent respiratory preparation. For COPD patients, a RV/TLC>60% or AV Shunt>20% is more sensitive than routine spirometry (FVC and FEV1) in predicting postoperative complications.

(3) The 5-year survival rate after surgery for stage $T_1N_0M_0$ and $T_2N_0M_0$ small cell lung cancer was 66.7% and 37%, respectively. Contrary to the traditional opinion that small cell lung cancer was not a surgical indication, Wu proposed that surgery could play an important role in the management of early stage small cell lung cancer. Such an observation has been supported by Mountain and Shields.

(4) While stage III lung cancer was considered a contraindication to surgery then, the results from the SCH showed that the 5-year survival after resection could reach over 30% in these patients. After stratification, the 5-year survival rates for $T_3N_0M_0$ and $T_3N_1M_0$ were as high as 49.1% and 37.2%, respectively. The long-term result of $N_2$ patients remained dismal, with the 5-year survival of $T_3N_2M_0$ being only 14.4%. All these contributed to the evidence which later led to the down-staging of $T_3N_0M_0$ diseases from stage IIIa to IIb in the 1997 UICC classification of lung cancer.

(5) Included in the series were 29 cases involving 7 different methods of carinal resection and reconstruction, making it one of the earliest reports of carinal resection for lung cancer.

(6) Extrapleural pneumonectomy combined with cryotherapy was effective in the control of refractory effusion caused by pleural dissemination and hence helped to improve the quality of life of the patients. However, it did not prolong survival.

Based on the above findings, Wu made his *"Two Maximizations"* proposal, namely the maximization of resection for lung cancer and the maximization of functional preservation, which is still held true for lung cancer surgery today.

Ou-Lin Huang is known as the "Father of Tracheal Surgery in China" owing to his outstanding contributions in the area. In 1978 Huan resected a segment of 9.5 cm (almost the whole length of the trachea) in a patient with adenoid cystic carcinoma. To reconstruct the airway Huang ingeniously sacrificed the right lung and then anastomosed the reversed right main bronchus and the right intermediate bronchus to a cervical "Broncheostomy." The patient was relieved from airway obstruction and fared well after surgery. He died of diffused left lung metastasis 11 months later. Upon autopsy, the anastomosis between the right and left main bronchus was still intact, and although completely fibrotic because of lack of blood supply, the interposed airway was still patent. More than 10 procedures concerning the major airway were first introduced into China by Huang. These included local resection of tracheal tumor and repair with a muscle flap (1976), lateral wall resection and repairing of the main bronchus (1976), right sleeve pneumonectomy (1976), long segment tracheal resection and reconstruction with artificial tracheal substitute (1978), tracheal and carinal resection and reconstruction (1980), right upper lobectomy together with carinal resection and reconstruction with tracheo-right intermediate bronchial anastomosis (1983), left sleeve pneumonectomy (1984), and tracheal and carinal resection and reconstruction with Y-shaped artificial substitute (1987). Before he passed away in 2005, Huang successfully performed more than 300 resections of tracheal tumors at the SCH. This led the hospital taking a leading position in the field of tracheal surgery in China.

Huang also helped to make the modified McKean esophagectomy a standard procedure for thoracic esophageal cancer at the SCH. When Orringer proposed transhiatal esophagectomy as a less invasive procedure than the transthoracic approach, Huang also started performing transhiatal resection using inversion extraction in patients in poor performance status. He acquired fairly good results and was the first to successfully use free jejunum interposition to replace the cervical esophagus after segmental resection for benign esophageal stricture. With his support and through years of effort by his successor, Wen-Hu Chen, the Department of Thoracic Surgery at the SCH is now equipped with esophagascopy, esophageal ultrasound (EUS), and manometry. It is worth mentioning that the SCH was the first institute in China to use EUS to evaluate the progressiveness of cancers before intervention. With EUS, cervical ultrasonography and other examinations in its armamentarium, clinical trials on systemic lymph node dissection, induction therapy, and concomitant chemoradiation of esophageal cancer could finally be carried out in a more scientific manner with an accurate clinical staging. The management strategy of this once ominous disease has been changed to a multimodality approach. And the long-term results have been markedly improved.

The SCH has long been outstanding in surgical techniques in the management of large mediastinal masses. For example, it has accumulated over 1,000 cases of thymic epithelial tumors (TET) over 40 years. Based on the results of a large retrospective study and detailed clinical-pathological analysis, Chen and his colleagues concluded the heterogeneity of TETs in histological manifestation, clinical and biological behavior, and response to treatment. They proposed that since the long term outcome of TETs is related to the WHO histological classification as well as the clinical staging, these tumors should thus be treated accordingly. Clinical studies on minimal invasive diagnostic techniques for histological classification and the effectiveness of induction therapy are already underway. Due to its experience in this relatively rare disease, the SCH was invited to participate in preparing the new WHO histological classification of TETs in 2005.

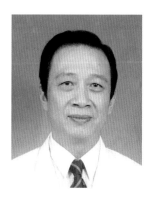

Ying-Ze Li

# The Development of Thoracic Surgery at Peking Union Medical College

*Le-Tian Xu, Qi Miao*

After the "Opium War" a number of foreign missionary groups gradually set up several hospitals as well as medical schools in China. Among them was the Union Medical College, founded by the London Missionary Society in 1906. When the China Medical Board (CMB) of the Rockefeller Foundation was launched in 1914, the Union Medical College had 90 in-patient beds, 14 foreign doctors and a total of 95 medical students. Recognizing such a "creditable beginning" the CMB purchased the Union Medical College and established the Peking Union Medical College (PUMC).

In September 1917 the cornerstone for the first new structure of PUMC (the anatomy building) was laid (Fig. 1) and the first 8 students were enrolled in the Premedical School. The formal dedication ceremony took place on September 19, 1921. Over the next two decades PUMC became "not only the leading medical center in Asia but one of the world's outstanding medical schools" [1].

Committed from the beginning to excellence, the faculty of PUMC was mainly drawn from the United States and the United Kingdom. In its early phase PUMC had 350 in-patient beds and 125 of them were for surgery (distributed mainly in three wards).

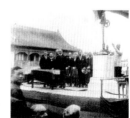

Fig. 1.

The first Chairman of the Department of Surgery between 1921 and 1927 was Adrian S. Taylor, who graduated in medicine from the University of Virginia in 1905. After ten years working experience in China he was awarded the first CMB fellowship for postgraduate study in 1915. Taylor elected to go back to Harvard to review the cutting edge of knowledge in medicine. His record at Harvard was so impressive that the CMB extended the fellowship, allowing Taylor to train at the Johns Hopkins Hospital under William Stewart Halsted, MD, the father of modern American surgery. Taylor's sterling qualities gained Halsted's respect and friendship, and they maintained an illuminating correspondence after Taylor's return to China in the fall of 1920 [1]. Taylor found the equipment at PUMC was "almost ideal" and the caliber of the surgical program satisfactory. He particularly praised the manual skills of the young Chinese assistants (Fig. 2). Taylor organized the Department with general surgery and various surgical subspecialties as Divisions (groups). All the heads of the different Divisions then were from the

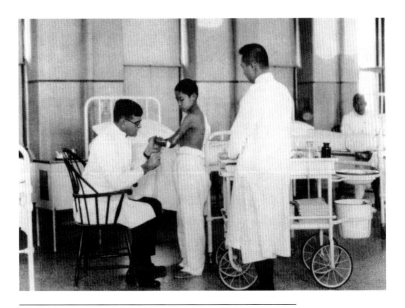

*Fig. 2. Adrian S. Taylor (left) treating a young patient with burns.*

USA, including Dr. Chester M. van Allen from the University of Chicago who was the chief of thoracic surgery between 1931 and 1935.

The second Chairman of the Department of Surgery (1928–1930) was Dr. Max M. Zinninger. He was succeeded by Dr. Harold H. Loucks (1931–1941 and 1948–1950, as PUMC was closed during World War II through December 1941 to November 1947).

Loucks graduated from Western Reserve University in the USA and came to China in 1922. He worked through residency and was promoted to the teaching ranks in surgery at PUMC. Although his primary interest was in abdominal surgery, Loucks also made his name in thoracic surgery (please refer to p. 30 of this book). Dr. Ying-Kai Wu (Fig. 3) worked under Loucks between 1933 and 1941, followed by two years advanced training in thoracic surgery at the Barnes Hospital, Washington University in St. Louis, USA.

In the 1920s and the 1930s PUMC saw some pioneering surgical accomplishments in China. These various achievements included gastrectomy, cholecystectomy, thyroidectomy, excision of intracranial meningioma, division of sensory root of trigeminal nerve, and removal of an islet cell adenoma of the pancreas. In the field

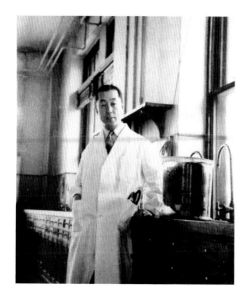

*Fig. 3. Dr. Y. K. Wu.*

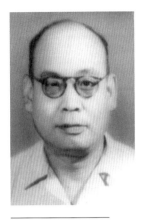

*Fig. 4. Dr. T. T. Wang.*

of thoracic surgery, the first successful left lower lobectomy for a 22-year-old female patient with bronchiectasis was performed by Dr. T. T. Wang (Fig. 4) using the tourniquet method in 1937; the first successful esophagectomy with intrathoracic esophago-gastrostomy for carcinoma for a 39-year-old male patient in 1940 by Dr. Y. K. Wu; and the first successful left pneumonectomy for lung cancer in a 49-year-old male patient in 1941 by Dr. C. C. Chang (who graduated from PUMC in 1931, Fig. 5) using individual ligation of hilum vessels and bronchus [2].

That PUMC was strikingly successful in training the leaders of medicine in China is attested by the fact that when it closed in December 1941, fewer than ten of its graduates were in private practice. Virtually all of the alumni were teaching medicine, leading hospital medical services, or in governmental positions in public health. In 1949 six of the national medical schools of China were under the leadership of PUMC graduates, and six others were headed by individuals who had received part of their training at PUMC [1].

During his second working term (1948–1950), Loucks was also appointed the Director of PUMC. Eventually, PUMC was "nationalized" in January 1951. After the departure of Loucks, Ying-Kai Wu was appointed as the Chairman of the Department of Surgery.

In April 1956 Wu moved to Heishanhu Hospital (also known as the No. 309 People's Liberation Army Hospital, the first dedicated chest hospital in China) together with all the staff members of the Division of Thoracic Surgery from PUMC. Over the next

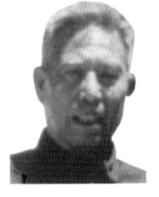

*Fig. 5. Dr. C. C. Chang.*

5 years, therefore, no thoracic surgical services were available in PUMC. Dr. Hsien-Chiu Tseng, who graduated from PUMC in 1940, was Chairman of the Department of Surgery from 1956 to1985. Dr. Le-Tian Xu, who graduated from Beijing Medical University in 1950, was the subsequent Chairman (from 1985 to 1987).

After the establishment of the People's Republic of China, PUMC and its teaching hospital were taken over by the Government in 1951. The PUMC (now named the Union Medical College of China) was made a division of the Chinese Academy of Medical Sciences in late 1957. The hospital was then named the Capital Hospital and was established as a separate institution. However it reverted to PUMC Hospital in 1985 (please refer to p. 6 of this book).

In 1972 the Division of Thoracic Surgery was officially re-established at PUMC and Le-Tian Xu was appointed as the head of the Division. Thus within the Department of Surgery there were five Divisions, namely General Surgery, Orthopedics, Urology, Neurosurgery, and Thoracic Surgery—later called Cardiothoracic Surgery.

In 1995, in the new hospital building, the Division of Cardiothoracic Surgery first had an independent ward with 40 beds, including a dedicated intensive care unit. In 2004 the thoracic surgical team was separated from the cardiac surgical unit, the latter being led by some acknowledged cardiac surgeons in China including Drs. Xiao-Cheng Liu and Xiao-Dong Zhu, who worked at PUMC in the late 1990s and the early 2000s.

Under the leadership and influence of many distinguished pioneer surgeons such as Drs. Y. K. Wu and C. S. Huang, younger generations of thoracic surgeons at PUMC progressed rapidly. They benefited from its valuable traditions in patient care. Attention to detail has always been emphasized. The balance between strict surgical training and meticulous scientific research has been regarded as a necessary basis for the young surgeons in their professional career [3–6]. Over the past five decades, the Division of Cardiothoracic Surgery at PUMC has enjoyed an extraordinary reputation in China in all areas of clinical practice, medical education, and scientific research.

Carcinoma of the esophagus and lung cancer have been the two most common diseases dealt with at the thoracic unit. For the former, we often perform infra- or supra-aortic esophago-gastrostomy. The overall surgical mortality is less than 1%. We also do total gastrectomy with esophago-jejunostomy, Roux-en-Y, for advanced lesion of the cardiac portion, and cervical esophago-gastrostomy for supra-aortic lesion of the esophagus. The five year survival rate in 850 patients reported in 1985 was 22%, 10 year survival in 368 patients was 9%, and 20 year survival in 34 patients was 7% [7]. For lung cancer patients we conduct postoperative comprehensive chemo- or radio-therapy following their lung resection procedures whenever feasible. The five year survival rate in these patients was above 30%.

In 1987 we reported 50 surgical cases of intraluminal tracheo-bronchial tumor with thorough analysis of pathological histology [8]. We summarized our experiences in resection of pulmonary metastatic choreocarcinoma in 43 drug-resistant patients [9]. We also reviewed the long term survival data in patients after thymectomy for myasthenia gravis or tumor [10]. Eight patients with Cushing syndrome due to intrathoracic tumor had good results after surgery and their diagnoses were confirmed by blood test (N-POMC) [11].

The history of cardiac surgery at PUMC can be traced back to the 1960s, when experimental investigations on mechanical assistance with extracorporeal circulation for open heart surgery were carried out. In 1972 we performed the first open heart operation under direct vision (closure of a VSD) at PUMC. In recent years our 30-day mortality in hundreds of patient after CABG was less than 1%. We have an increasing number of cases of combined CABG with valvular or other major surgical procedures such as interventions for lung cancer, gastric cancer, peripheral arterial thrombosis, myoma of uterus etc. We are also taking care of more and more elderly patients nowadays.

For over two decades in the first part of last century, PUMC and Tsinghua University were the two principal intellectual bridges between China and the West (i.e. the United States). With the recent agreement on merging these two influential Chinese universities, it is logical to expect that the new institution will play an even more important role in health care, education and scientific research, both nationally and internationally.

# References

1.  Bowers JZ (1972) Western medicine in a Chinese palace: Peking Union Medical College, 1917–1951. The Josiah Macy Jr. Foundation, Philadelphia.
2.  Wu YK The Department of Surgery at the Peking Union Medical College: 1921–1941 and 1948–1956. (unpublished manuscript in English).
3.  Tseng HC, Xu LT, et al. (1984) Current surgical interests in China. Surgery 95: 165.
4.  Xu LT (1987) In memory of Professor Huang Jiasi (Chia-Ssu Huang) with great affection. *Chin Med J* 100:513–516.
5.  (1988) A briefing of the Peking Union Medical College Hospital. *Proc CAMS & PUMC* 3:64–365 (in Chinese).
6.  Dai YH (1988) Medical education at Peking Union Medical College. *Med Edu* 22:261–264.
7.  Xu LT, et al. (1983) Surgical treatment of carcinoma and cardiac portion of the stomach in 850 patients. *Ann Thorac Surg* 35:542–547.
8.  Xu LT, et al. (1987) Clinical and pathological characteristics in patients with tracheobronchial tumor: report of 50 patients. *Ann Thorac Surg* 43:472–476.
9.  Xu LT, et al. (1985) Resection of pulmonary metastatic choreocarcinoma in 43 drug-resistant patients. *Ann Thorac Surg* 39:257–259.
10. Xu LT, et al. (1990) Analysis of 124 thymectomies for myasthenia gravis or thymoma. *Endoc Surg* 7:361–364.
11. Zhang ZY, Xu LT, et al. (1993) Diagnosis and surgical treatment in 8 patients with cushing syndrome due to intrathoracic tumor. *Chin J Thorac Cardiovasc Surg* 9:329–331 (in Chinese).

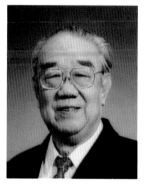

Le-Tian Xu

# The Development of Esophageal Surgery in China

*Guo-Jun Huang*

T he history of esophageal surgery in China is primarily the history of esophageal resection for carcinoma. Carcinoma accounts for the bulk of surgical esophageal disease, and often requires urgent intervention. In common with most other developed countries, esophageal surgery was first undertaken in China approximately 60 years ago. Although surgery on the intra-abdominal portion of the esophagus was already established by this time, surgery on the thoracic esophagus required the introduction of endotracheal intubation and positive pressure ventilation before it could be performed safely.

Prior to the 1930s most reports of esophageal surgery were limited to esophageal exteriorion or esophageal tube surgery, such as that reported by Torek in 1913 [1]. Early attempts at surgical resection for carcinoma at the Peking Union Medical College by Taylor and colleagues in the 1920s uniformly ended in failure. This institution's first successful case of thoracic esophago-gastrostomy for carcinoma was eventually undertaken by Ying-Kai Wu (Fig. 1) on April 26, 1940 [2], only two years after the pioneering surgery reported by Marshall [3] and Adams [4]. The 58-year-old male patient had a tumor involving the distal intra-thoracic esophagus, that was resected via a left trans-thoracic approach, with a supra-diaphragmatic anastomosis (Fig. 2). The patient recovered well after surgery, and left the hospital

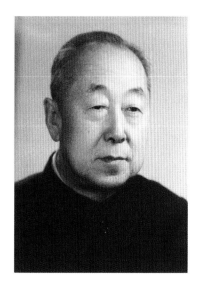

*Fig. 1. Ying-Kai Wu (1910–2003).*

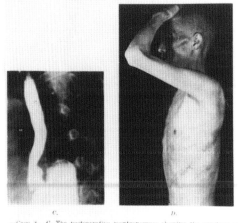

*Fig. 2. A photograph of the first successful case of surgical resection for esophageal carcinoma with thoracic gastro-esophageal anastomosis. Left: Contrast swallow radiography demonstrating a smooth gastro-esophageal anastomosis. Right: the patient's left thoracotomy scar.*

after three weeks. This successful result was a turning point for esophageal surgery in China, which began in earnest in the Peking Union Medical College Hospital and several other hospitals in the late 1940s. A clinical esophageal carcinoma research group had already been established in Peking Union Medical College Hospital in 1939, and was the fore-runner of dedicated esophageal research in China.

At the time of his pioneering surgery, Ying-Kai Wu was only 30 years old, but already established as an independent surgeon at the Department of Surgery, PUMC. Between 1940 and 1941, he and H. H. Loucks, the chief surgeon, undertook a further 11 cases of esophageal resection. Four cases had tumors located in the mid-thoracic esophagus, five involved the distal esophagus, and two cases involved the gastric cardia. Three deaths were reported (27%), all secondary to intra-thoracic complications (pneumothorax, pneumonia, mediastinitis). Only two patients survived more than a year from surgery. One patient survived eight years, an impressive result even by today's standards. This case also received radiotherapy after surgery, and might therefore be considered one of the first cases of combination therapy for esophageal carcinoma.

Between 1941 and 1943, Ying-Kai Wu was trained at Barnes Hospital, St. Louis, Missouri, under the supervision of the renowned thoracic surgeon Evarts A. Graham. Graham had already performed the world's first successful pneumonectomy for carcinoma of the

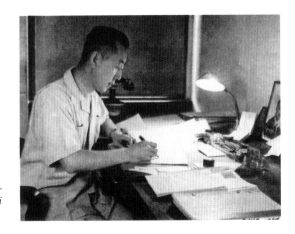

*Fig. 3. A picture of Ying-Kai Wu in the early 1940s.*

lung, but had never performed a successful resection for esophageal carcinoma. Once he became aware of Ying-Kai Wu's experience of esophageal surgery, Graham invited him to present his results to a local surgical society. His report was subsequently published in the *Journal of Thoracic Surgery* in 1942 [5], and represents our department's earliest internationally published clinical report of esophageal carcinoma surgery.

From 1946 to 1960, Wu and colleagues performed almost a thousand surgical resections for esophageal carcinoma at a number of surgical institutions. These included Tianjin Central Hospital, Peking Union Medical College Hospital, the Chinese People's Liberation Army Thoracic Hospital and the China Academy of Medical Science Fuwai Hospital. Several other hospitals in China also started to undertake esophageal surgery for both carcinoma and benign disease. During the same period of time the mortality rate of esophageal resection for carcinoma decreased from over 25% in the earlier years to approximately 10%.

It had been noted that esophageal carcinoma was predominately found in the Shanxi, Henan, Hebei, and Shandong provinces of Northern China. Studies of the epidemiology and etiology of this condition were urgently needed. These were initiated by Ying-Kai Wu in April 1959, at the "Four Provinces (Shandong, Shanxi, Henan and Hebei) and One City (Beijing)" Scientific Research on Prevention of Esophageal Carcinoma Meeting, at Fuwai Hospital in Beijing. Wen-Xian Yang, Qiong Shen and Fang-Yuan Liu from Henan Medical School, Guang-Heng Li from the Shanxi Medical School of Oncology, Yu-De Zhang from the Fourth Hospital of Hebei Medical School, Xian-Ting Cao from the Affiliated Hospital of Shandong Medical School, and Ying-Kai Wu, Guo-Jun Huang, Yu-Qing Liu and Xia Wu from Fuwai Hospital all actively participated in the conference. They subsequently decided to initiate a comprehensive survey of esophageal carcinoma in their own high-risk regions. In August 1959, the First "Four Provinces One City" Symposium on Scientific Research on Esophageal Carcinoma Prevention was held in Taiyuan, Shanxi (Fig. 4). A few months later a comprehensive population survey was conducted in Yangquan District in Shanxi, and Linxian

District in Henan. The incidence of esophageal carcinoma in adults over the age of 30 was 30.6 per 100,000 in the former, and 67.3 per 100,000 in the latter. The establishment of these regular symposia enabled the dissemination of experience of esophageal surgery throughout China.

In May 1964 the Third Symposium on Scientific Research on Esophageal Carcinoma Prevention was held in Anyang, Henan (Fig. 5). The incidence and mortality rates for esophageal carcinoma

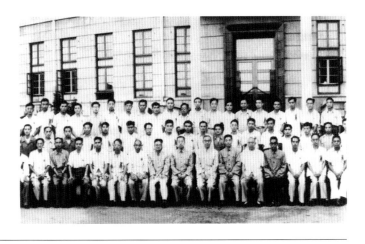

*Fig. 4. A group picture (partial) of the First "Four Provinces One City" Symposium on Scientific Research on Esophageal Carcinoma Prevention held in Taiyuan, Shanxi, in August 1959.*

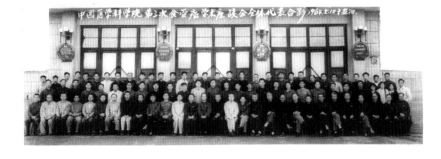

*Fig. 5. A group picture of the Third Academic Symposium on Esophageal Carcinoma held in May 1964 in Anyang, Henan.*

throughout China were reported, among which, Linxian of Henan, Yangquan of Shanxi, and Feicheng of Shandong had the highest risk figures.

The 1960s heralded a new era of esophageal surgery in China, as specialist thoracic surgical and oncology units were established. An esophageal surgical unit was established at Linxian County Hospital in Henan in 1964, initially under the supervision of Guo-Jun Huang of Fuwai Hospital, then subsequently under the guidance of Ling-Fang Shao (Fig. 6). Over the next few years local units were restructured and consolidated. Eventually, under the supervision of Director Bing Li, research into every aspect of the epidemiology, etiology, diagnosis, investigation and treatment of esophageal carcinoma was conducted at Linxian and its local hospitals. This solid research base, allied with the high local incidence of esophageal carcinoma enabled this unit to sub-specialize to such a degree that it eventually undertook only surgery for this disease, and in 1984 it was renamed the Linxian Esophageal Carcinoma Hospital (Fig. 7).

The surgical management of benign esophageal diseases developed in parallel with that of carcinoma. Congenital esophageal atresia is an uncommon and challenging condition that remains a surgical challenge even today. Nevertheless, early in 1964, Shao-Chuan Pan and Ya-Xiong She had both published reports of successful surgery for this disease [7, 8].

The surgical management of achalasia was another challenge for pioneering esophageal surgeons. Xian-Jiu Ceng and Ying-Kai Wu described the technique of surgical cardioplasty for this disease in 1949 [9]. The subsequent recognition of significant post-surgical reflux esophagitis eventually led to this technique being abandoned, with a move towards Hellers myotomy (esophageal muscularis externa incision) combined with an anti-reflux procedure as the surgical gold standard. Esophageal surgeons in China continued to contribute extensively to published literature on advances in the management of the spectrum of benign esophageal disease throughout the 1960s [10–15].

It has already been described how the high incidence of esophageal carcinoma had been a prime motivator to the

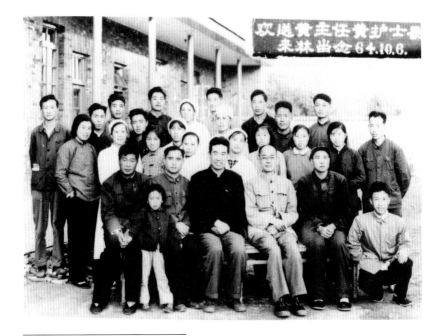

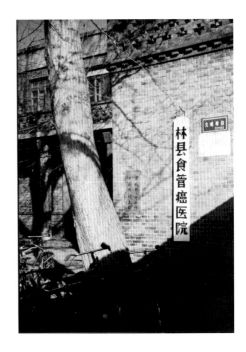

*Fig. 6. Group photograph of the leaders of Linxian County Hospital in Henan, including Guo-Jun Huang (front row, third from right) and County Committee Secretary Gui Yang (front row, 4th from right) taken in 1964.*

*Fig. 7. Linxian Esophageal Carcinoma Hospital (taken in 1984).*

development of surgery in China. Conditions associated with gastro-esophageal reflux e.g. reflux esophagitis, Barretts esophagus and benign stricture, by contrast, are uncommon in China and the East, and have therefore attracted little research attention in the past [16, 17]. However, reflux-associated conditions are increasing in incidence in Western countries, and attracting much research interest, particularly since the association between Barretts esophagus and adenocarcinoma has been recognized.

Leiomyoma is the most common benign esophageal tumor in China. In 1950 Ling-Fang Shao, Ying-Kai Wu and colleagues published an early report on the diagnosis and surgical therapy of esophageal leiomyoma [18]. In 1991 Guo-Jun Huang and colleagues published their surgical results for a cohort of 100 patients, which at the time was the largest reported case series [19]. They subsequently reported their surgical technique in 1994 [20]. Continued research into esophageal leiomyoma in China has recently yielded an unexpected result: the application of new diagnostic techniques had demonstrated that several tumors previously identified as leiomyomas were re-classified as gastrointestinal stromal tumors [21]. Unlike leiomyomas, gastrointestinal stromal tumours have a potential for malignant change. The concerns that this discovery raised were a further impetus to the establishment of a benign esophageal diseases study group in the Chinese Academy of Medicine in the 1990s.

The extensive screening of esophageal carcinoma in adults in high-risk areas was difficult to initiate, but has yielded exciting results. The poor prognosis of esophageal carcinoma is in part a reflection of the fact that it usually presents late. The use of esophageal balloon cytology in this survey identified significant numbers of cases with early esophageal and cardiac carcinoma [22, 23]. In 1981 Ling-Fang Shao and his colleagues reported the results of surgical treatment in 253 cases of stage I esophageal carcinoma. Mortality after surgery was 2.8%; 5-year survival was 89.9%; and 10-year survival was 60% [25]. These outstanding results surpassed any previously reported series. The benefit of resection for early stage disease was emphasized by the results reported by Pei [26]. He followed-up 23 cases of stage

I esophageal carcinoma which were not resected. The average survival was only 43.6 months.

The further development of esophageal surgery was impeded during the Cultural Revolution. Clinical and basic scientific research almost came to a halt. Not until the mid 1970s did the situation start to recover. In the 1980s the increase in international co-operation and communication, the introduction of modern facilities and the development of new technology enabled esophageal surgery in China to re-establish its pioneering progress and disseminate its experience. In 1983 the English version of the book *Esophageal and Cardiac Carcinoma* edited by Guo-Jun Huang and Ying-Kai Wu, was published [27]. This book summarized the experiences and achievements in basic research and clinical practice on every aspect of esophageal and cardiac carcinoma in China, and introduced the pioneering results of this group to the world for the first time, attracting international recognition and praise.

Further refinements in the surgical treatment of esophageal carcinoma have been developed in China. The choice of surgical approach is principally determined by the location of the tumor. Originally a left postero-lateral thoracotomy was the approach of choice, as this gave good access to the distal thoracic esophagus. From 1962 to 1964, Shao-Qian Sun, Xia Wu, Xun-Sheng Lin and colleagues studied 100 esophageal carcinoma resection specimens. They found evidence of residual tumor involving the resection margins in 15% of cases. Separate discrete foci of neoplastic change within the esophageal mucosa at some distance from the primary tumor site were also identified, giving rise to the concept of a field change [28]. These findings helped explain the relatively high incidence of local recurrence after surgery, and it became apparent that the extent of esophageal resection and lymph node clearance needed to be increased, if better results were to be achieved. There has accordingly been a shift towards more radical surgery, often utilizing a cervical anastomosis (Figs. 8 and 9). Alternative surgical routes that avoided thoracotomy were proposed for tumors that involved the cervical or intra-abdominal esophagus [29, 30].

Although early stage cancers accounted for an increased

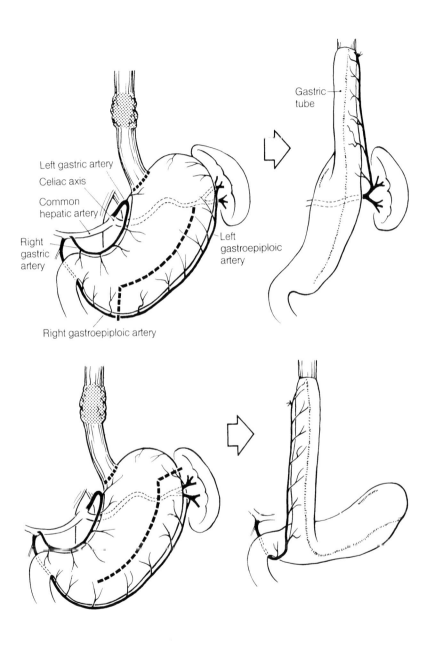

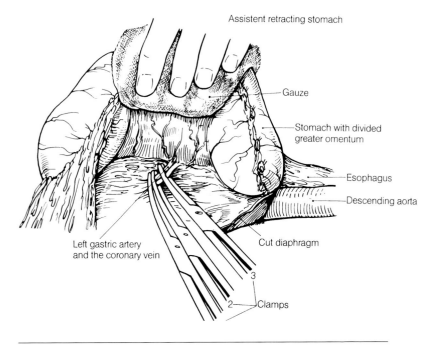

*Fig. 9. Figure from [27]: Surgical techniques. Reproduced with permission from Springer Verlag.*

proportion of tumors in most series from high-risk areas of China, the majority of cases were still presenting relatively late. It was recognized that the local extent of tumor progression (T stage), the presence of lymph node metastases (N Stage) and completeness of resection were all factors that critically influenced long-term survival [31]. However, although the extent of local resection influenced local and distant relapse in those with early stage disease, increasing the extent of resection in those with more advanced tumors seemed to increase the risk of post-operative complications, without offering a survival advantage. The concept of cancer as a systemic disease was introduced, and adjuvant therapies were introduced into clinical practice.

There is a relatively long history of combination therapy for esophageal carcinoma in China, which includes the use of traditional

Chinese medicine. However, the lack of scientifically rigorous trial data has made effectiveness difficult to evaluate. The potential benefits of additional radiotherapy were first recognized several years ago. In 1962, Guo-Jun Huang and colleagues had reported their results utilizing radiotherapy prior to surgical treatment in 113 cases of esophageal carcinoma [32]. They remained at the forefront of pioneering research into combination therapy, and subsequently published the results of larger randomized studies of combined surgery and radiotherapy [33–35]. More recently the timing of radiotherapy has shifted. Min Zhu and colleagues reported an improvement in five-year survival from 41.7% with surgery alone, to 74.2% with the addition of adjuvant radiotherapy, although other small series have not always supported their conclusions [37]. The benefits of neo-adjuvant chemotherapy are now also established, and there has been a shift away from adjuvant radiotherapy except in cases of incomplete resection.

The choice of conduit and the optimal method of anastomosis are also subjects that have provoked much debate and research. The stomach is the most commonly-used and convenient conduit, although jejunum and colon are alternative options in selected patients. In Guo-Jun Huang's large reported series of 3,335 cases of esophagectomy, stomach was used to replace the resected esophagus in more than 98% of patients [38]. The quality of anastomosis is also critical to a good outcome in esophageal surgery. Anastomotic leak is a dreaded complication, and is associated with a high mortality rate if it occurs within the chest. In the pioneering days of esophageal surgery post-operative mortality approached 10%. The mortality associated with anastomotic leak was nearer to 60%, and accounted for more than a third of the total post-operative deaths [39]. The incidence of anastomotic leaks remained approximately 4% for the next two decades, but has now started to reduce further [40–42]. Several different anastomotic techniques have been promoted over the years [43–51]. The introduction of mechanical stapling devices into China in the 1980s has potentially made anastomotic failure a rarity. However, cost implications and other factors limits their use and most anastomoses are still performed by hand. The improvements in surgical technique, allied with better anesthetic and perioperative management, have had a significant impact on surgical mortality following esophagectomy, which has also fallen, and is now approaching 3% in most units in China [52].

The long-term outcome following esophagectomy in large-volume units in high-risk regions of China compares favorably with reported series from elsewhere, but remains unsatisfactory in terms of patient survival. In the 1970s, 5-year survival following esophagectomy approached 25% [53, 54]. In the 1980s and 1990s the reported figures in some hospitals approached 30% or better [55]. Poor outcome is predominantly a reflection of the fact that many patients still present late. For example, in a report published by Guo-Jun Huang and his colleagues in 1985, only 3% of the 1874 patients presented with stage I disease. Stage II patients accounted for 16.8%, whereas stage III and stage IV cases accounted for 70.5% and 9.7% respectively. Overall 5-year survival was less than 30% [56]. It is clear that strategies that enable earlier diagnosis and better pre-operative staging are vital if any impact on survival is to be achieved.

Video-assisted thoracoscopic surgery (VATS) has already had a huge impact on the practice of non-esophageal thoracic surgery. It enables the surgeon to undertake most thoracic surgical procedures without the need for thoracotomy, which has significant potential benefits for both the patient and the surgical unit. Our unit began to use VATS in the 1990s, primarily to facilitate lymph node sampling and improve tumor staging. The resection of esophageal diverticula, the removal of leiomyomata, and Hellers myotomy have all been successfully performed via a VATS approach. Combined laparoscopic and thoracoscopic techniques have been used for the surgical management of reflux disease in China, but the role of VATS as a method of esophageal resection is still being evaluated.

Another area of increasing interest relates to the use of video-assisted esophagoscopy and mucosal staining to facilitate the identification of very early stage esophageal mucosal carcinoma, particularly in high-risk regions. Endoluminal esophageal mucosal resection is now a recognized treatment for superficial mucosal carcinoma, once the extent of disease and lymph node status has been defined. Accurate staging is vital, as extension into the submucosal layers is associated with a significant incidence of lymph node metastases [57–65].

The current standard of esophageal surgery in China today is world class [66]. When we look back at the development of esophageal surgery, we cannot forget the contributions of those pioneering surgeons and their non-surgical colleagues. We must also acknowledge and accept that limited exchange of information at critical times may have obscured important contributions that have not been specifically mentioned. The author therefore sincerely asks for understanding and forgiveness from colleagues if there is any inadequacy in this review.

At the beginning of the 21st century we are confident of the future of esophageal in our country. As some of the pioneers leave us, nevertheless we are also pleased to find new blood entering the esophageal surgical team. They are stepping forward into the new era with dignity, easing the suffering of esophageal carcinoma patients, and working together to promote esophageal surgery in China to ever greater heights.

## Acknowledgement

The editors are very grateful to Dr. Juliet E. King, FRCS, for her conscientious editorial assistance.

## References

1. Torek F (1913) The first successful case of resection of the thoracic portion of the esophagus for carcinoma. Surg Gynecol Obstet 16:614.
2. Wu YK and Loucks HH (1941) Surgical treatment of carcinoma of the esophagus. Chin Med J 60: 1.
3. Marshall, SR (1938) Carcinoma of the esophagus. Surg Clin North Am 18:643.
4. Adams WE, Phemister DB (1938) Carcinoma of the lower esophagus: Report of a successful resection and esophagogastrostomy. J Thorac Surg 7:621–632.
5. Wu YK, Loucks HH (1942) Resection of the esophagus for carcinoma. J Thorac Surg 11:516.
6. Wu YK (1997) Seventy years in medical field. Beijing: China Scientific Technology Press, 60–61.

7. Pan SC et al (1964) Five examples of esophageal atresia, clinical experience and effectiveness. J Pediatrics 13:445.

8. She YX (1964) Surgery therapy of congenital esophageal atresia. Sci J China 12: 377.

9. Tseng HC, Wu YK (1949) Cardioplasty for achalasia of the esophagus. Chin Med J, 67:596–602.

10. Liu SG et al. (1961) Surgery therapy of cardiospasm. J Chin Surg 7:591.

11. Yan Zhikun et al. (1964) "Barium Bladder" dilation therapy for cardiospasm. J Chin Surg 10:47.

12. Sun YQ and Zhu DL (1965) Therapy of esophago-cardiac achalasia with diaphragm cardia plastic surgery. J Chin Surg 13:718.

13. Du XQ et al. (1965) Therapy of esophago-cardiospasm with diaphragm cardia plastic surgery. J Tianjin Med 5:400.

14. Cao XT et al. (1966) An anti-reflux therapy for esophageal achalasia. J Chin Surg 3:159.

15. Huang GJ et al. (1996) Evaluation of mucosa muscularus resection surgery for cardiospasm. J Chin Surg 6:586.

16. Wang QZ et al. (1993) Diagnosis and surgical treatment of gastroesophageal anti-reflux. J Chin Surg 31:232–235.

17. Wang QZ (1958) Anti-reflux in Gastro-esophagus. Tianjin: Tianjin Scientific Press, 1994.

18. Shao LF, Wu YK et al. (1958) Esophageal leiomyoma. J Chin Surg 6: 979–982.

19. Huang GJ et al. (1991) Surgery for leiomyoma of the esophagus—experience in 100 patients. J Dis Esophagus 4:43–46.

20. Huang GJ (1994) Extramucosal enucleation of leiomyoma of the esophagus. In: Jamieson GG, Debas HT. (eds) Surgery of the upper gastrointestinal tract. 5th ed. Chapman & Hall Medical, 237–243.

21. Wang QZ, Wang XL, Li BQ et al. (2004) Surgical treatment of esophageal leiomyoma and differentiation from stromal tumors. J Chin Cardiovasc 20:178–179.

22. Shen Q, Qiu ZL, Zhao HZ (1963) Preliminary report of esophageal cell biology. J Chin Etiology 1:19–23.

23. Shen Q (1990) Diagnosis of esophageal carcinoma and cardiac carcinoma and early discovery. Ref: Huang GJ, Wu YK. Esophageal carcinoma and cardiac carcinoma. Shanghai: Shanghai Scientific Technology Press, 114–115.

24. Huang GJ and Wu YK (1965) Early-stage esophageal carcinoma and several clinical phenomena. J Chin Surg 13:435–437.

25. Shao LF, Huang GJ, Zhang DW, et al. (1981) Detection and surgical treatment of early esophageal carcinoma. Proceedings of the Beijing symposium of cardiothoracic surgery. Beijing: China Academic Publishers, 168–171.

26. Pei YH, Zhang YD et al. (1982) Random observation on natural progress of early-stage esophageal carcinoma. Therapy on Carcinoma 9:75.

27. Huang GJ, Wu YK (eds) (1984) Carcinoma of the Esophagus and Gastric Cardia. Springer Verlag Berlin Heidelberg New York Tokyo.

28. Sun SQ and Wu X (1965) Pathology of esophageal carcinoma. In: Wu YK and Huang GJ, Esophageal Carcinoma and Cardiac Carcinoma. Shanghai: Shanghai Scientific Technology Press.

29. Wu TQ and Jiang XM (1979) Non-open chest esophageal therapy for cardiac carcinoma. J Chin Surg 59:358.

30. Huang GJ, Zhang DW, Lin H et al. (1979) Non-open chest esophageal therapy for early-stage esophageal carcinoma. J Chin Oncology1:245–248.

31. Huang GJ (1989) Prognostic significance of lymph node metastasis in surgical resection of esophageal carcinoma. Proc IV World Congress of ISDE.

32. Huang GJ, Wang JZ, Liu YQ and Wu X (1962) General therapy on pre-surgical radiotherapy on esophageal carcinoma on 113 cases. J Chin Surg 12: 770–774.

33. Huang GJ, Gu XZ et al. (1980) General therapy on pre-surgical radiotherapy on esophageal carcinoma on 113 cases. J Chin Oncology 2:15–18.

34. Huang GJ, Wang LJ, et al. (1989) Combined preoperative irradiation and surgery versus surgery alone for carcinoma of the esophagus: A prospective randomized study in 360 patients. Proc IV World Congress of ISDE.

35. Zhang ZX, Huang GJ, Zhang DW et al. (1992) Evaluation of pre-operative radiotherapy for esophageal carcinoma—analysis of 1012 cases. J Chin Radio Oncology 1:169–171.

36. Zhu M, Chen GW, Wang YX et al. (1998) Pre-surgical radiotherapy for esophageal carcinoma. J Chin Radio Oncology 7:46–48.

37. Yang ZY (1997) Recent development of surgical treatment and radiotherapy on esophageal carcinoma, cardiac carcinoma. J Chin Radiotherapy Oncology 6:75–76.

38. Huang GJ (2000) Replacement of the esophagus with the stomach. In: Shields TW, LoCicero J III, Ponn RB, Eds. General Thoracic Surgery, 5th ed. Lippincott Williams & Wilkins, 1723–1732.

39. Huang GJ (1963) Esophagogastric anastomosis imperfection after surgical resection on esophageal carcinoma and cardiac carcinoma. J Chin Surg 11:859.

40. Zhang YD, Du XQ, Zhang W et al. (1982) Esophageal carcinoma and cardiac carcinoma: experience of 4,310 surgical cases. J Chin Oncology 4:1–4.

41. Shao LF, Li ZC et al. (1982) Esophageal carcinoma and cardiac carcinoma with 3,155 surgical treatment cases. J Chin Surg 20:19–22.

42. Huang GJ, Zhang DW et al. (1982) Effectiveness and existing problems in the surgical treatment of esophageal carcinoma. Chin. French Review on Acad. Discussion, Kunming, 35.

# The Surgical Treatment of Pulmonary Tuberculosis in China

*Yu-Ling Xin, Xiao-Jia Chen*

Tuberculosis has long been a very serious life-threatening infectious disease in human beings. When we had no specific chemotherapeutic or antibiotic medicines for tuberculosis, symptomatic treatment such as rest, nutrition, fresh air and sunshine were the only effective measures. The discovery of the Tubercle Bacillus (Koch R., 1882) and the production of streptomycin (Waksman, S. A., 1950), isoniazid (1950), para-amino-salicylate sodium (1946), rifampicin etc. improved the treatment of tuberculosis and established the scientific basis for the surgical procedure for pulmonary tuberculosis.

## Surgical Treatment of Pulmonary Tuberculosis in the Early Years

Before the major surgical procedures used for pulmonary tuberculosis were developed, lung-collapse treatments such as artificial pneumo-thorax, artificial pneumoperitonium, intrapleural adhesion dissection and phrenic nerve compression operations were routine methods in the anti-tuberculosis clinics.

The purpose of the lung-collapse procedure was to decrease the respiratory movement and blood circulation in the local collapsed lung. Desaturation of oxygen does not favor the growth of tubercle bacilli, yet it is beneficial for the lung tissue at the pathogenic focus to have a rest and repair process. In the 1930s Dr. Da-Tong Wang (Peking Union Medical College) and others in China had used the above mentioned procedures in all of the anti-tuberculosis clinics. But after quite a long period of wide clinical practice these procedures were discarded gradually due to the complications of diffused pleural adhesion, pleural thickening and damaged pulmonary function etc.

In 1885 Dr. Cerenville (Switzerland) tried to perform a major permanent lung collapse operation—thoracoplasty—to treat pulmonary tuberculosis. He performed a partial resection of the ribs to collapse the thoracic wall, but with a high morbidity and mortality rate. In 1907 Drs. C. Braur and Fredrich tried to resect 5–9 ribs in one stage of an operation. They had a 30% mortality rate due to mediastinal flutter and paradoxical respiratory movement. In 1925 Dr. Alexander improved the technique, performing one operation in 2–3 stages, fixing the anterial costal end of the resected ribs and separating the apical pleura instead of resecting the first to third ribs etc. These procedures decreased markedly the operative complications and mortality rate, and also improved the post-operative results. These procedures were used as the most common operation for the surgical treatment of pulmonary tuberculosis in Europe and North America at that time. Later on Drs. Shade and Heller designed more radical procedures than traditional thoracoplasty for patient with tuberculous emphysema and broncho-pleural fistula.

In the early 1930s Dr. Da-Tong Wang in Peking Union Medical College, and Dr.Yong-Qi Dong in Shanghai Red Cross Hospital practiced thoracoplasty successfully.

In 1950 Drs. Woods and Lucas first successfully separated the parietal pleura accompanied by intercostal muscles and costal periostium and filled up the extrapleural intrathoracic space with tens of plastic balls to compress the diseased lung lobe. These procedures avoided the permanent deformity of the thorax, scoliosis of the spine and compensational emphysema of the counter-side lung which occurred after thoracoplasty. But there was some incidence of secondary infection, displacement of the plastic balls and broncho-pleural fistula.

When surgeons had not yet perfected the technique to dispose the lung hilum, when the anesthesiologists did not yet have the intratracheol technique, and when there was not yet antituberculous chemotherapy and antibiotics, many surgeons had already started to try pulmonary resection for tuberculosis, with high complications and mortality (Blokd, 1881). But there were still many surgeons who had successful cases (Tuffier 1891, Friedlander 1934, Eloesser and O'Brien 1935, Rienhoff 1936). In 1945 Overholt reported 200 cases of pulmonary resection for tuberculous patient with 5.5% mortality. After that pulmonary resection instead of thoracoplasty became the most common choice for tuberculosis cases.

# The Development of Surgical Treatment of Pulmonary Tuberculosis after the Establishment of the People's Republic of China

The Central Government of the People's Republic of China paid much attention to the problem of prevention and treatment of tuberculosis for the country's people. Anti-tuberculosis organizations and hospitals specializing in tuberculosis were established throughout the country. Both resection and collapse procedures were developed in the surgical treatment of pulmonary tuberculosis. In 1955 at the Department of Thoracic Surgery, Peking Institute of Tuberculosis, Dr. Yu-Ling Xin reported on extra-pleural pneumothorax, extra-pleural oil-thorax and filling up the extra-parietal space (intrathoracic) with sponge material to treat pulmonary tuberculosis (cavity type) in 150 cases. The postoperative effective rate was 80–90%. He also reported on 183 patients with serious type pulmonary tuberculosis who had undergone thoracoplasty. In 1954 Dr. Kai-Shi Gu reported 53 cases of plastic ball filling operations with good results in the early postoperative period. In 1962 Ling-Fang Shao, Ying-Kai Wu and Xiao-

Mai Huang reported 15 patients undergoing thoracoplasty with fixation of the anterial costal end. These patients had very good postoperative results and avoided postoperative paradoxical respiratory movement. In 1945 Chia-Ssu Huang (Jia-Si Huang) started to perform pulmonary resection for tuberculosis in several of Shanghai's hospitals and reported 200 cases with a 94% effectiveness rate at the 28th Congress of International Thoracic Association. After that pulmonary resection for tuberculosis was widely used in many hospitals in the major cities of China. Segmental resection and bilateral pulmonary resection were also at one stage used in Peking and Shanghai (Kai-Shi Gu and Yu-Ling Xin).

After 1956, under the direction of the Ministry of Health, a special techniques course for thoracic surgery was taught by the Peking Institute of Tuberculosis. More than 200 surgeons from different provinces of China became highly qualified through these courses. When they returned to their own province's hospital, they started to establish their own sections of Thoracic Surgery and started to use the new techniques they had learned in the practice of pulmonary resection for tuberculosis.

Dr. Yu-Ling Xin designed an extra-mucosal closure suture to prevent bronchial fistula after lobectomy on the basis of large amounts of animal experiments. In the first series of 200 tuberculous patients undergoing pulmonary lobectomy using the extra-mucosal closure suture, there was no cases of bronchial fistula. During the same period there was a 1.5% occurrence rate of fistula in 200 tuberculous patients after traditional closure suture of the bronchus (whole layer closure suture), and a 5% occurrence rate of bronchial fistula in 100 tuberculous patients after mechanical instrument closure suture. During a 20 year period (1961–1981) they accumulated 4,200 tuberculous patients of pulmonary lobectomy by extra-mucosal closure suture; the bronchial fistula rate was only 0.4% (17 cases/ 4200 patients ). In this period pulmonary resection for tuberculosis (chiefly lobectomy and also segmental resection, wedge shaped resection and pneumonectomy) was widely used throughout the country. In some complicated cases modified thoracoplasty, incision and drainage of tuberculous cavity, closure of the bronchus after division, and ligation of the pulmonary artery of certain lobes were also practiced.

## Current Status of Surgical Treatment of Pulmonary Tuberculosis in China

In the late 1970s as a whole, anti-tuberculosis work in our country achieved great advances.

1. The modern standard antituberculous program was carried out throughout the country;
2. Systematic immunization with B.C.G was started for new born babies;

Effective new anti-tuberculosis medicines were produced in many big cities. All of this work much decreased the number of patients indicated for surgery. But recently the drug-resistant tubercle bacilli, variation in tubercle bacilli, the recurrence of old lesions and the acquired immune deficiency problem etc. have been discovered. Up until now the statistics confirm that the old disease of human tuberculosis is still one of the major killers in our country. A lot of preventative and clinical work should be carried out and many problems should be investigated further. The surgical treatment of pulmonary tuberculosis is still one of the effective procedures in some special cases such as: 1) Thick wall tuberculous cavity with positive antifast stain sputum after conservative treatment; 2) Tuberculous bronchiectasis complicated with persistant hemoptysis; 3) Pulmonary tuberculoma; 4) Pulmonary atelactasis by the compression of enlarged hilum lymph nodes; 5) Pulmonary tuberculosis with secondary infection and destructed lung lesion; 6) Fungus infection (fungus ball formation) in the tuberculous cavity due to anti-tuberculous medication for a long duration; 7) Thick wall tuberculous emphysema or complicated with broncho-pleural fistula etc.

In China recently there has been great progress in the field of basic medicine (bacteriology, immunology etc), biomedical engineering and video-assisted thorochoscopic techniques. All of these new techniques and new ideas provide our thoracic surgeons

with many possibilities for improving clinical practices and patients'
prognosis in the treatment of pulmonary tuberculosis. It means that
our thoracic surgeons have new chances and face big challenges in
the new era.

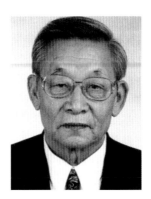

Yu-Ling Xin

# Open Heart Operation under Acupuncture Anesthesia

*Yi-Shan Wang*

Since the first case of open-heart operation with extra corporeal circulation under acupuncture anesthesia performed on April 19, 1972, we have operated on 265 cases (1990 statistics) of various congenital and acquired heart diseases with good results provided that patients were well selected and mediasternotomy was employed.

Various acupuncture points on the ear, chest, and both upper and lower extremities on the proper meridian leading to the chest were chosen for controlling chest pain and arrhythmia. These points were used for the first three years. Later ear points were eliminated, because puncturing into both ears caused severe local pain and the patient usually found this unacceptable. Since then we have routinely used bilateral "Neiguan" and "Lieque" on the upper extremities and bilateral "Yu men" at the middle subclavicular region on the frontal chest wall. These combinations of acupuncture points were proven very effective for mediasternotomy.

Following are the specific requirements for choosing patients for extracorporeal circulation under acupuncture anesthesia.

1. Because general anesthesia is not used, the patient is mentally clear. They usually cannot stand too long a period of restriction of the whole body on the operating table, especially in the case

of young children. So acupuncture anesthesia for open-heart operations is indicated for operations which are simple with rather a short operation time (no longer than one and half hours).

2. The patients should be over 14 years of age, as at that age they are able to cooperate well.
3. It must be the first cardiac operation on the patient.
4. The respiratory function of patients should be normal and the hemodynamic function stable with few rhythmic problems.
5. The patient's neuropsychic state should be stable.

Acupuncture points are distributed widely throughout the whole body area. Old traditional extensive knowledge and experience give us guidelines for choosing the proper points for puncture which enable us to inhibit pain in the frontal area of the chest for mediasternotomy. But these points for the inhibition of pain and sensation in this area do not cover the whole area, so we need to apply several specific operative techniques and procedures in compensation.

Mediastinotomy incision for open-heart operations under acupuncture anesthesia possesses the advantage that there is less muscular attachment in comparison to that for lateral thoracotomy and abdominal incisions. There is less tensile stress and painful effects produced during stretching the wound and the muscles around it. The pain usually produced during the operative procedure mainly occurs during the incision of the skin, electrocauterization, finger dissection of xiphold process and tissue behind the manubrium, sawing the sternum, spreading or pulling together the split sternum parts, and closing the wound at the termination of the operation. If supplementary medicine such as a light dose of sedatives and analgesic drugs are added, and if specific maneuvers such as gentle, accurate, stable and speedy operative handling are strictly executed, the majority of patients can endure this operation uneventfully, even in the case of younger children (Fig. 1)

The pain produced during operative procedure mainly occurs as noted above. Thus before cutting through the sternum we routinely administer a local infiltration of 1:200,000 adrenalin-saline solution to the incision line to reduce bleeding so that the need for application of electrocauterization and the pain caused by it is much lessened.

During open sternum or dissection of substernal tissue, pleura may be torn. The ruptured hole should be closed right away by suture. If necessary a drainage tube for suction is inserted through the intercostal space in order to keep the lung expanded.

Assisted respiration by a mask is usually not necessary except for a brief interval during extensive tearing of mediastinal pleura or discontinuation of the bypass. Preoperative training of slow abdominal respiration instead of chest respiration for a period of about one week or longer, until patient can do this naturally, is a very important requirement. During dissection of deep tissues under the sternum or manipulation of the heart and great vessels or intracardiac structures patient has no sensation, even if deep hypothermia and electrical defibrillation is applied to the heart. Usually normothermia or light hypothermia is applied. The stress reaction of the heart to manual stimulation is small. Occurrence of

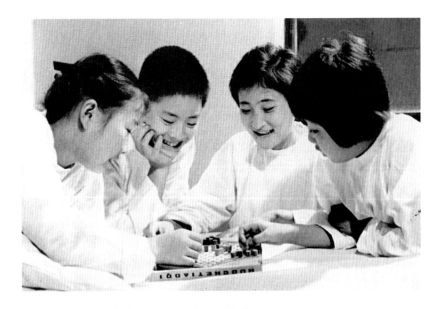

*Fig. 1. 1 boy, 3 girls, 14–15 years old, all endured the operation very well, ready to be discharged from hospital.*

arrhythmia is much less than with a conventional general anesthesia with moderate hypothermia. Compression to the heart and great vessels should be avoided; even elevation of cardiac apex should be limited, lest low cardiac output and hypotension may lead to loss of consciousness of the patient or cause nausea and vomiting. Body temperature by blood cooling should not be lower than 33°C lest the patient suffers shivering. It is important to maintain the mean arterial blood pressure above 50 mmHg. Below this level the patient usually loses consciousness. Recently we performed a case of ventricular septal defect repair, two cases of atrial septal defect and one case mitral valve plastic with good results by carefully following the above mentioned guide lines, and by using specific manipulation and operative techniques.

## Advantages

The majority of patients were kept consciousness introperatively and immediately postoperatively. If their blood pressure was normal they could drink water and sit up in bed (Fig. 2). General recovery of function of the whole body usually occurs within a few days. The patients were usually discharged within one week. Because an intratracheal tube was not used, there were no respiratory complications postoperatively. The patients' general condition was very good.

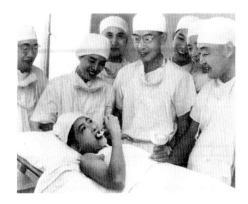

*Fig. 2. Rigth after operation, she can drink water on operation table.*

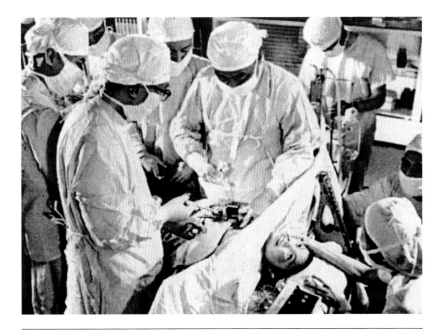

*Fig. 3. First open heart operation. Heart was widely opened, she was mentally clear, eyes wildly opened.*

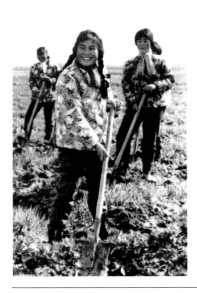

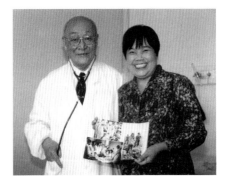

*Fig. 5. 49 years old, follow up check health, very healthy.*

*Fig. 4. Not long after operation, she could join field work.*

The first open heart operation was performed on a girl aged fifteen to repair tetralogy of Fallot on April, 19, 1972. The mediasternum was widely opened. She was mentally clear. Both of her eyes were wide open (Fig. 3). Her postoperative recovery was smooth. Not very long after the operation she joined in work in her father's field without problem (Fig. 4). We followed up state of health recently. She appeared very healthy. She is now 49 years old (Fig. 5) and owns a small shop. Her daughter is about 23 years old.

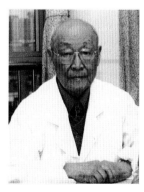

Yi-Shan Wang

# The Evolution of Cardiology in China

*Tsung O. Cheng*

L ike most specialties of medicine today, the current practice of cardiology in China owes much to the wisdom, knowledge and accomplishment of earlier generations. It is often surprising how far back one must look to find the real beginning of cardiology in China. The milestones in the evolution of cardiology in China are many and varied, and to attempt to annotate all of them would be an almost impossible task indeed. In this chapter, however, I will discuss a random but fascinating selection of major discoveries over many centuries and decades by many important people that together have contributed to the current state of cardiology in China [1].

## CARDIOLOGY IN ANCIENT CHINA

Although Hippocrates was generally recognized as the Father of Cardiology in the Western world [2, 3], Huang Di, or the Yellow Emperor of China (2695–2589 BC), was the Father of Cardiology in China [3]. Huang Di, also an ancient Chinese physician, sometimes has been called the Hippocrates of China [3]. But Huang Di was born more than 2,200 years before Hippocrates (460–c 375 BC) [2]. Therefore, it would seem more appropriate to call Hippocrates the Huang Di of Greece than to call Huang Di the Hippocrates of China. The fact that Hippocrates was referred to homophonically as Ch'i Po or Qi Bo (岐伯), the most important interlocutor of Huang Di in *Huang Di Neijin* (The Yellow Emperor's Canon of Internal Medicine), did not contradict in any way this point of view [3]. As was commonly understood, some of the writings in *Hippocratic Corpus* were evidently composed much later than the bulk of the Corpus, obviously by Hippocrates' followers. So was the case with *Huang Di Neijin*.

Although there was no specific reference to coronary artery disease in the *Huang Di Neijin*, coronary artery disease existed in China as far back as one century BC [4]. Severe occlusive coronary atherosclerotic disease was found in a 50-year-old ancient Chinese lady who died over 2,100 years ago and whose body was excavated in China in 1972 (Fig. 1) [4]. The woman was overweight and had a severely occluded left anterior descending coronary artery which was responsible for her sudden death from an acute myocardial infarction an hour or so after eating. Packets of herbal medicines

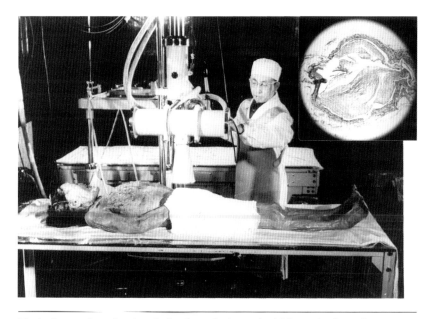

*Fig. 1. Severe atherosclerotic occlusive disease in the proximal left anterior descending coronary artery (inset) of a 50-year-old Chinese lady who died of acute myocardial infarction over 2,100 years ago.*

containing cinnamon, magnolia bark, and peppercorns found in the tomb (Fig. 2) suggest that the woman probably had angina pectoris. According to Han medical canons, these were prescribed for coronary heart disease just as they still are by Chinese traditional doctors today [4]. Incidentally, she must have Type A personality, because 138 musk melon seeds were found in her stomach. She must gulp down the melon in a great haste [5].

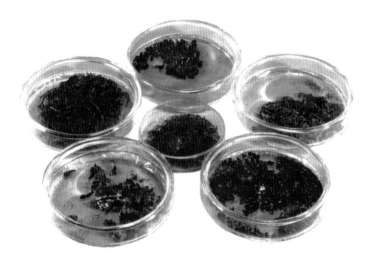

Fig. 2. *The unearthed herbs that were buried in the ancient lady's tomb, such as magnolia, orchid, fragrant reed, Chinese prickly ash, cassia bark, wild ginger, etc., suggesting that the lady probably had angina pectoris. (Courtesy of Hunan Provincial Museum).*

Whereas Hippocrates' countless classics have become obsolete in the West, the *Huang Di Neijin* still holds the prestige of antiquity and scientific interest. This is a medical attitude which cannot be disregarded, especially since it has survived all the political revolutions in China. It gives Chinese medicine its timeless, monolithic aspect in which, however, each generation has left its mark, usually discernible on careful examination [3].

Chinese physicians were skilled in feeling the pulse before the dawn of Hippocratic medicine [6]. In *Huang Di Neijin* the art of feeling the pulse was well described. The importance of feeling the pulse in diagnosing various diseases has been passed down until the present time (Fig. 3). In Chinese traditional medicine, each organ has its

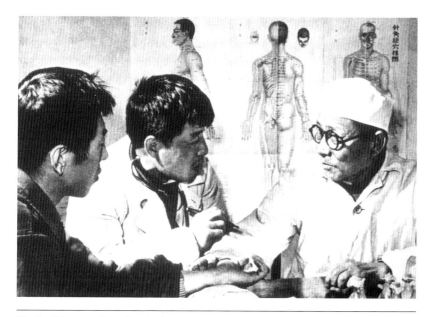

*Fig. 3. Chinese traditional medical doctor palpating the patient's radial pulse while his student watched and learned.*

proper pulse and 28 kinds of pulses have been described [7, p 32]. Among those that are of importance in the evaluation and management of cardiovascular diseases are:

(1) 細脉，微脉，伏脉 (fine pulse, filiform pulse, and hidden pulse). Fine pulse is felt as a thin thread and found in severe mitral stenosis, tricuspid stenosis, constrictive pericarditis and pericardial effusion. Filiform pulse is felt as almost imperceptible below the fingers and found in cardiogenic shock. Hidden pulse is hidden (or sunken) and is encountered in aortitis.

(2) 洪脉 (flooding pulse). This corresponds to the bounding pulse in Western medical terminology.

(3) 芤脉，革脉 (hollow pulse and leather pulse). Hollow pulse, "like the stalk of a spring onion," is seen in conditions associated with peripheral vasodilatation and decreased peripheral vascular resistance. Leather pulse, "like tapping the skin of a drum," corresponds to the water-hammer pulse in aortic valve regurgitation.

(4) 遲脉 (slow pulse). Slow pulse means three or less pulse throbbings at wrist per each respiration, normal being four. It is seen in sinus bradycardia and various degrees of heart block.

(5) 促脉，結脉，代脉 (hasty pulse, knotted pulse, and intermittent pulse with long pauses). They represent various tachyarrhythmias and bradyarrhythmias.

The art of feeling the pulse was so advanced in ancient China that the court physician, summoned to examine the ailing queen but not allowed to either see or touch the queen, could feel the pulse of the patient by tying a thin thread around her wrist and feeling her pulse at the other end of the thread in next room (Fig. 4). This technique was probably the beginning of modern-day plethysmography.

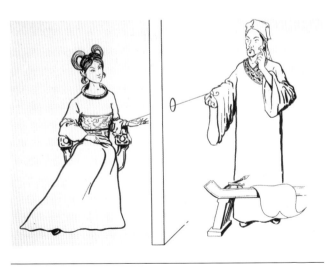

*Fig. 4. Court physician in the next room feeling the ailing queen's radial pulse by means of a thread tied around the queen's wrist.*

The Chinese traditional medical doctors are experienced not only in feeling the pulse but also in examining the tongue (Fig. 5). Because tongue is considered to be the window to the heart, it is examined very thoroughly if the patient is suspected of suffering from any heart disease. Many diagnoses could be made by mere inspection of patient's tongue (Fig. 6) [8].

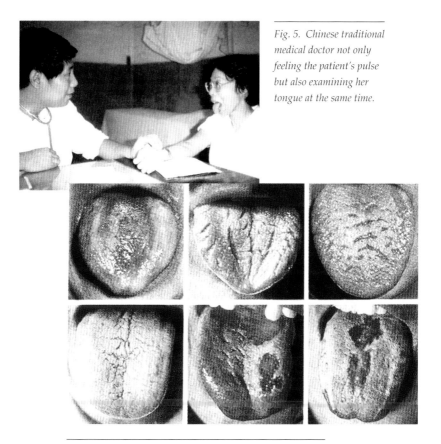

*Fig. 5. Chinese traditional medical doctor not only feeling the patient's pulse but also examining her tongue at the same time.*

*Fig. 6. Tongue appearances in various cardiovascular diseases.*
*Top: left, normal coated tongue of a cigarette smoker with nicotine staining; middle, normal fissured tongue ("scrotal tongue"); right, transverse fissuring of tongue in Down's syndrome. Bottom: left, combined horizontal, vertical, and diagonal fissuring of the tongue in a patient with cardiac arrhythmias; middle, geographical tongue in a patient with coronary artery disease and cerebral artery spasm; right, chicken heart tongue in a patient with coronary artery disease.*

In recent times, the phenomenon of decreased heart rate variability as a predictor of sudden death in a variety of disease states has received increasing attention [9]. From the plethora of publications in the cardiological literature, one would have thought that this is a new discovery. Actually the observation that decreased heart rate variability as a predictor of sudden cardiac death has been known in China for 17 centuries. The Chinese physician Shu-He Wang (265–317 AD) wrote, in *The Pulse Classic*, "If the pattern of the heart beat becomes as regular as the tapping of a woodpecker or the dripping of rain from the roof, the patient will be dead in four days." [10].

The positive correlation between sodium intake and blood pressure has been confirmed both experimentally and epidemiologically for many years, both outside and inside China (Fig. 7) [11]. But the role of salt in hypertension was recognized in China a long, long time ago when the Yellow Emperor in *Huang Di Neijin* said "… if too much salt is used for food, the pulse hardens …" [12].

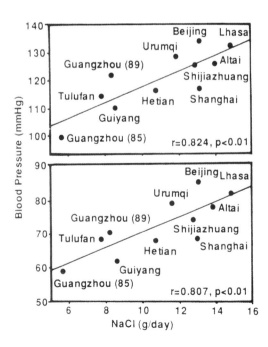

*Fig. 7. Close relation between daily urinary sodium excretion (x-axis) and systolic (top) and diastolic (bottom) blood pressure (y-axis) in China. The numbers in parentheses after the city of Guangzhou denote the different years, i.e., 1985 and 1989, during which period there was a large increase in the fast food restaurants in the city.*

# C. L. TUNG, FATHER OF MODERN CARDIOLOGY IN CHINA

Dr. Paul Dudley White, born in 1886, was graduated from Harvard in 1911 and the world's leading authority on heart and heart diseases as well as America's most influential academic cardiologist [13]. He was often called the Father of Modern Cardiology. He was my mentor. I was greatly influenced by him to always practice and "teach any and all about the heart, to investigate some of the unsolved problems associated with the heart, and to write as long as the words flowed from my pen." [14]

There is a Paul D. White in every country around the world. The Paul D. White of China is Dr. Chen-Lang Tung from Shanghai. I was

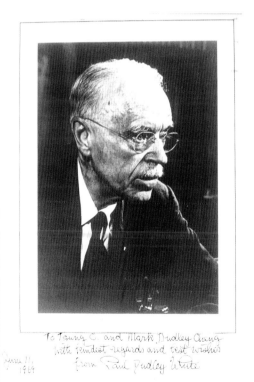

To Tsung C. and Mark Dudley Chung
with kindest regards and best wishes
from Paul Dudley White
June 11
1969

*Fig. 8. Paul Dudley White, MD, Boston.*

fortunate to have both White as my mentor (Fig. 8) and Tung as my long-time idol (Fig. 9).

Tung was born in 1899—13 years after White—and received his MD degree from the University of Michigan Medical School, Ann Arbor, Michigan in 1924 (Fig. 10). Upon graduation he returned to China to be on the faculty of the Peking Union Medical College (PUMC), the extraordinary accomplishment of the Rockefeller Foundation in China (Fig. 11). Because of his special interest in cardiology he was sent by PUMC back to the University of Michigan in 1930 for another year of postgraduate training under Frank N. Wilson, the world leader in electrocardiography [15, p 18] and the inventor of the unipolar precordial leads in ECG [15, p 122]. Ten years later, Tung was sent by PUMC to the United States again for further training in such renowned institutions as the Mayo Clinic. But he always returned to his motherland to serve his own people. As one of the great promoters of rational medicine in China, a country beleaguered and shrouded by several major turmoils including the Cultural Revolution during which medicine was in shambles, medical schools were closed, many physicians were exiled to the countryside, and contact with any foreigners was a punishable crime, he helped keep the gates open to Western medical advances and infused many young colleagues in China with a sense of mission and connection with the world at large.

Like White, Tung carried out several pioneering studies and published many important articles, too many to name them all here. Many of his publications revolutionized the care of patients with cardiovascular diseases not only in China but worldwide. His first landmark publication was on myxedema heart disease in 1931 when he was with Wilson in Michigan. Until then, the association of hypothyroidism and heart disease was either unknown or controversial; but he demonstrated that patients with myxedema could have cardiomegaly on chest X-rays due to pericardial effusion and low voltage of P, QRS and T complexes on EKG, all of which disappeared following thyroid replacement therapy [16]. Another landmark publication was on chronic cardiac adaptation to chronic repetitive exercise. Tung's interest was aroused in 1930 when he in

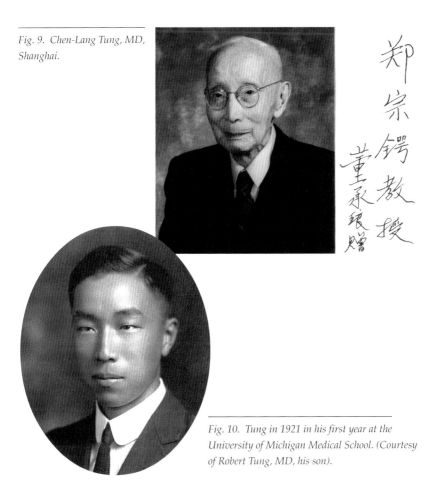

*Fig. 9. Chen-Lang Tung, MD, Shanghai.*

*Fig. 10. Tung in 1921 in his first year at the University of Michigan Medical School. (Courtesy of Robert Tung, MD, his son).*

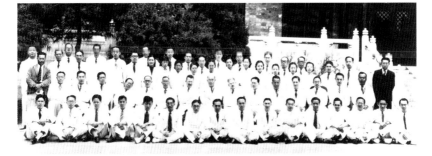

*Fig. 11. Tung at PUMC in 1941. He is the 6th sitting person from left. Dr. I. Snapper, chairman of the department of medicine at PUMC, is the second person to his left.*

the course of a routine physical examination found a markedly enlarged heart in an otherwise healthy ricksha puller, employed in one of the departments of the PUMC. This finding led to the study of 46 healthy ricksha pullers, nearly half of whom showed definite cardiac enlargement, which he reported in 1934 [17]. Until then, cardiac enlargement was considered to be a pathognomonic sign of heart disease. Tung, therefore, was the first to differentiate between physiological and pathological cardiac enlargement. His landmark article anteceded the much later publications on the subject [18–21] by seven decades. Tung was also among the first to point out in 1930 that digitalis was a double-edged sword; whereas digitalis in therapeutic doses was effective in slowing the ventricular rate in atrial fibrillation, it in toxic doses might induce transient atrial fibrillation [22]. Another important observation first made and published in 1941 by Tung was the value of EKG in differentiating cardiac enlargement due to heart failure from that due to pericardial effusion; QT interval on EKG was prolonged in cardiac failure but normal in pericardial effusion [23]. Before the advent of echocardiography in making the diagnosis of pericardial effusion, this simple EKG sign not only was of diagnostic significance but also had important therapeutic implications; whereas pericardiocentesis was indicated in pericardial effusion, pericardiocentesis in a dilated heart without pericardial effusion might yield disastrous results.

All of these landmark articles were published in the *American Heart Journal* which was the official scientific publication of the American Heart Association at the time. Later on, Tung had the honor of being appointed in 1980 by George E. Burch, editor-in-chief of the journal, to its international editorial board (Fig. 12).

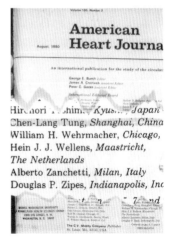

*Fig. 12. Tung appointed to the international editorial board of the* American Heart Journal *in 1980.*

According to Tung, his most significant contribution to the cardiologic literature was on the heart in severe anemia which was published in the *Chinese Medical Journal* in 1937 [24]. He demonstrated that severe anemia could cause cardiomegaly, heart failure and heart murmurs in both systole and diastole, all of which disappeared after correction of the anemia. This publication of Tung made such a great impression on White that, although in the first edition of his textbook on heart disease in 1931 and second edition in 1937 White refuted the idea that anemia could induce heart failure, he reversed his opinion by citing Tung's article in his 3rd edition in 1944 and again in his 4th edition in 1951 (Fig. 13).

To me, the most significant article published by Tung was the one in 1958 in the *Chinese Medical Journal* [25] (Fig. 14). In that article, he attributed the low prevalence of coronary artery disease in China to the low serum cholesterol content. His observation of close association of cholesterol and atherosclerosis anteceded by at least a decade the report by the Framingham Study [26]. Tung subsequently validated and updated this association in a chapter in my book *The International Textbook of Cardiology* (Fig. 15) [7, pp 10–14].

Like White's authoritative textbook *Heart Disease*, Tung's textbook entitled *Practical Cardiology* was the first such book published in China and considered by many to be the "Bible" in heart diseases (Fig. 16A). Unlike White who did not revise his textbook after its fourth edition in 1951—nearly a quarter of a century before he died in 1973, Tung continued to update his book and completed his greatly expanded third edition just before he died on November 21, 1992 at the age of 93, and the book was published posthumously in 1993 (Fig. 16B).

In 1988 Tung emigrated to the United States to be with his son Robert who is also a cardiologist. I continued to maintain close contacts with Tung after his arrival in the United States (Fig. 17). As an appreciated capstone to Tung's long and distinguished career, the American College of Cardiology in 1991 bestowed upon him an Honorary Fellowship (Fig. 18A). I had the distinct honor of acting as his marshal at the convocation (Fig. 18B). That year Tung was one of three recipients of the American College of Cardiology Honorary Fellowship awards; the other two were Inge Edler from Sweden who

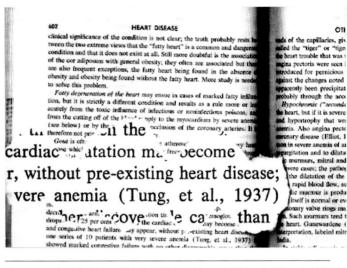

*Fig. 13. In the 4th edition of his book* Heart Disease, *White cited Tung's 1937 article on anemia causing heart failure. White refuted this association in the 1st and 2nd editions of his book.*

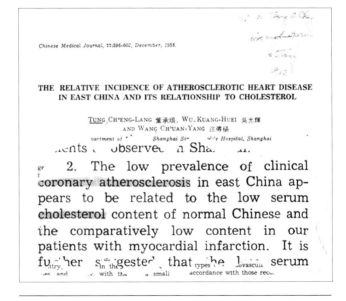

*Fig. 14. Tung's landmark article on the association of cholesterol and coronary artery disease published in 1958.*

# 2 The Changing Incidence of Heart Disease in Modern China

*Cheng Lang Tung, MD and Tsung O. Cheng, MD*

10   AVAILABLE CRUDE AND CAUSE-SPECIFIC
        MORTALITY DATA
10   AVAILABLE HOSPITAL ADMISSION DATA
11   CHANGING PROPORTION OF VARIOUS ETIOLOGIC
        TYPES
11   VARIOUS ETIOLOGIC TYPES IN OTHER PARTS OF
        CHINA

12   REGIONAL DIFFERENCES
12   CHANGES IN CERTAIN ENVIRONMENTAL FACTORS
13   RHEUMATIC HEART DISEASE
13   OTHER ETIOLOGIC FORMS OF HEART DISEASE
13   REFERENCES

Changes in the average life expectancy in modern China bear a close relation to the incidence of heart disease in the population at large. The average life span has nearly doubled in the last 30 years. In old China the average life span was 35 to 40 years according to various estimates, whereas in 1981 it was 67.88 years (66.43 years for males

and 111.14 to 151.79 in rural areas), the latter figur accounting for over 17% of all causes of death, a r markable increase in the mortality rate from heart disea of about 90%. However, an investigation conducted certain Chinese cities for a more recent period apparent disclosed cerebrovascular disease as the number tv

(A)

(B)

## Foreword

When Dr. Cheng asked me if I would write a short foreword for his book *The International Textbook of Cardiology*, memories came flooding back to me of our wonderful early trips to China and the Soviet Union, to the many other countries we visited, and to the many friends we made there. A whole portrait gallery of those who came here to Boston to study and work and visit is imprinted on my mind. What a rich inheritance!

I am well aware of the distinguished position Dr. Cheng holds among his colleagues, of the tremendous number of outstanding contributions he has made in the field of cardiology. It is indeed an honor to write a short foreword to his book. There is another reason that is more personal and that delights me. Dr. Cheng has a son, Mark Dudley Cheng, named after Paul, born in 1957 in Boston when Dr. Cheng was at the Massa-husetts General Hospital working with Dr. White. In 1972 Dr. Cheng visited the People's epublic of China, the first China-born physician from the United States to have that rivilege. In 1973 he went again to China, this time taking his son, Mark Dudley.

For many years Dr. Cheng thought, as most physicians do now, that the science and practice of medicine have a special role to play in bringing the people of the world together. Physicians have "no axe to grind," their sole purpose being to work and study together to help solve the multiplicity of problems that face them for the betterment of all people.

This book, edited by Dr. Cheng, would have been of enormous interest to Dr. White because it draws from the scientific studies done by Dr. Cheng and by other men and women from all parts of the world.

I thank Dr. Cheng for giving me the opportunity to feel again the excitement and value of this great work.

Ina Reid White
(Mrs. Paul Dudley White)

(C)

*Fig. 15. Tung's chapter (A), validating the close association between cholesterol and coronary artery disease, in my book* The International Textbook of Cardiology *(B) for which Mrs. Paul Dudley White wrote a Foreword (C).*

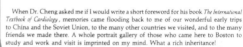

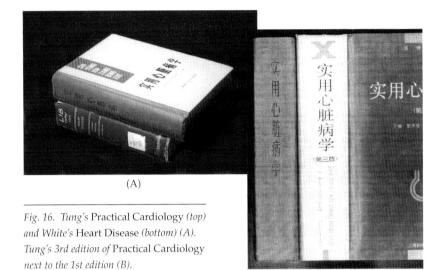

(A)

*Fig. 16. Tung's* Practical Cardiology *(top) and White's* Heart Disease *(bottom) (A). Tung's 3rd edition of* Practical Cardiology *next to the 1st edition (B).*

(B)

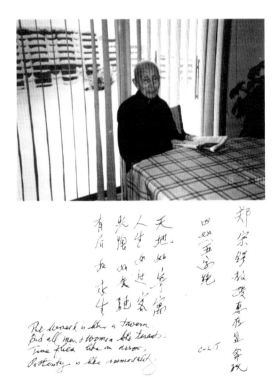

*Fig. 17. Tung in the United States in 1990.*

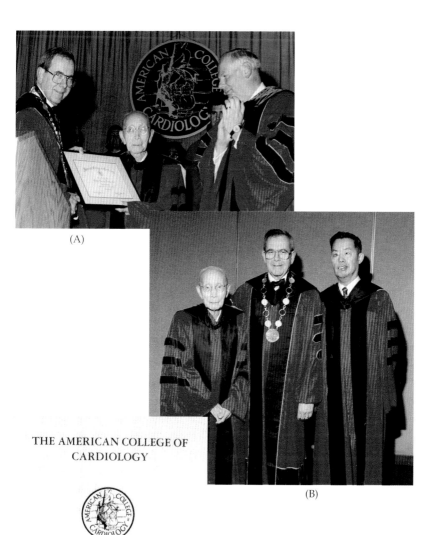

(B)

THE AMERICAN COLLEGE OF
CARDIOLOGY

FORTIETH ANNUAL
CONVOCATION

...ration of Honorary Fellowship Awards
Recipient, Earl E. Bakken
Marshal, Dwight E. Harken, M.D., F.A.C.C.

Recipient, Inge Edler, M.D.
Marshal, William L. Winters, Jr., M.D., F.A.C.C.

Recipient, Chen-Lang Tung, M.D.
Marshal, Tsung O. Cheng, M.D., F.A.C.C.

(C)

*Fig. 18. Tung receiving his American College of Cardiology Honorary Fellowship in 1991 (A), with me as his marshal (B), the other two recipients of the award being Edler and Bakken (C).*

219

introduced echocardiography and Earl E. Bakken who founded Medtronic, world's premier manufacturer of pacemakers and other medical devices (Fig. 18C).

Tung's remarkable career, spanning more than six decades, has been truly phenomenal and enormously productive in terms of countless doctors trained or influenced by him, thousands of patients treated by him, many important concepts of disease process that revolutionize the practice of medicine and cardiology, and numerous landmark contributions to the cardiological literature.

# ELECTROCARDIOLOGY

## *ELECTROCARDIOGRAPHY*

The invention of electrocardiograph by Dutch physiologist Willem Einthoven in 1902 represented a major advance in the methods available for the diagnosis of heart disease [27]. Although Tung was the first physician in China to report ECG changes in myxedema [16], digitoxicity [22] and pericardial effusion [23] between 1930s and 1940s using the imported Cambridge ECG machine, the first clinical use of a China-made moving string galvanometric ECG machine took place at PUMC in early 1950s under the direction of Shi-Zhen Liu (Fig. 19) [20, p 34] and Wan Huang (Fig. 20) [28, p 34]. Huang, who

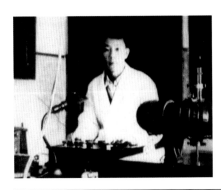

*Fig. 19. China's first moving string galvanometric ECG machine put into use under the direction of Shi-Zhen Liu (Courtesy of Rui-Long Sun).*

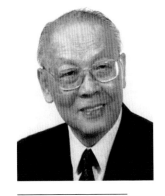

*Fig. 20. Wan Huang, MD (Courtesy of Rui-Long Sun).*

received training at Michael Reese Hospital in Chicago under Louis Katz, Richard Langendorf and Alfred Pick, America's three giants in ECG, started courses in ECG on a national level in early 1950s [28, p 20]. Huang wrote China's first ECG book in 1956 (Fig. 21A); the book is now in its 5th edition published in 1998 (Fig. 21B) and considered by many to be China's most authoritative textbook on ECG.

The first use of unipolar ECG in diagnosing acute myocardial infarction was by Hao-Zhu Chen in 1954 [29] (Fig. 22) who also reported the first use of intracardiac ECG in 1969 [28, p 32]. In 1982 Chen edited the magnum opus the *Chinese Encyclopedia of Cardiology* (Fig. 23).

Stress ECG started in China in early 1950s with Master's two-step test which was replaced by multi-stage treadmill exercise test

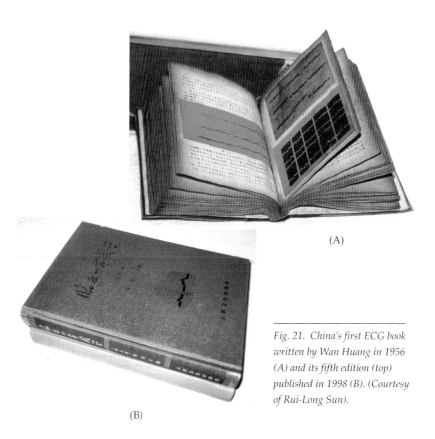

(A)

(B)

Fig. 21. *China's first ECG book written by Wan Huang in 1956 (A) and its fifth edition (top) published in 1998 (B). (Courtesy of Rui-Long Sun).*

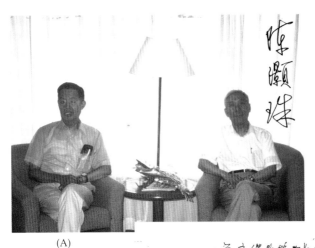

(A)

*Figure 22. Hao-Zhu Chen (A) and his 1954 article reporting the first use in China of unipolar ECG leads in diagnosing acute myocardial infarction (B).*

(B)

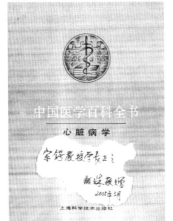

*Fig. 23* Chinese Encyclopedia of Cardiology, *edited by Hao-Zhu Chen.*

(C)

using modified Bruce protocol in the 1970s. The postprandial stress test which was quite popular in 1950s and 1960s had been abandoned. Persantine stress test is nowadays used quite often [Rui-Long Sun, personal communication, February 15, 2005].

In commemoration of the centennial of invention of ECG, Ji-Hong Guo in 2002 wrote the book, entitled *History of Electrocardiology in China*, in which he elegantly reviewed the evolution of electrocardiology in China by individuals as well as provinces (Fig. 24) [28]. The book contains many historic photographs, some of which are reproduced in this chapter with his gracious permission. As the Chinese saying goes, one picture is better than a thousand words.

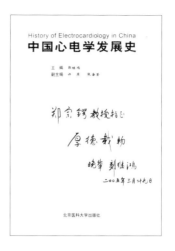

*Fig. 24.* History of Electrocardiology in China, *by Ji-Hong Guo*

Vectorcardiography was started in China in 1950s using the Grishman system and continued in 1960s using the Frank system [Rui-Long Sun, personal communication, February 15, 2005]. The first clinical application in China of vectorcardiography took place in 1961 by Yu Gao [28, p 112]. The first book on VCG was published in 1976 and written by Bing-Xian He of Xinjiang Medical College (Fig. 25).

Holter monitoring or ambulatory ECG was started by Fu-Sheng Gu in 1971 with the assistance of Bernard Lown in Boston [28, p 80]. She was also the first cardiologist in China to advocate the use of leads V7 and V8 in diagnosing acute myocardial infarction [28, p 80]. Ventricular late potential, heart rate variability and QT dispersion which were in vogue in the 1980s gradually lost their appeal in recent years [Rui-Long Sun, personal communication, February 15, 2005]. Torsade de pointes was first reported in China by Lan-Sheng Gong in 1974 [28, p 88]. Hypokalemia causing serious arrhythmias was first reported by Shou-Chi Tao in 1956 [28, p 8]. The

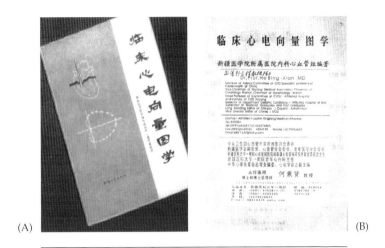

(A)                                                                                          (B)

*Fig. 25. China's first book on vectorcardiography (A) written by Bing-Xian He (B). (Courtesy of Bing-Xian He).*

first report of Osborn wave in hypothermia was made in 1959 by Yi-Ming Tang [28, p 119].

## Electrophysiology and Ablation of Arrhythmias

Esophageal electrodes are used to perform electrophysiological studies in many hospitals in China, because this procedure is easy to perform and is popular in hospitals where there is no catheterization laboratory. Its first use was reported by Wen-Ping Jiang in 1979 [28, p 44]. A programmable stimulator manufactured in China is used for transesophageal electrophysiological studies. It has almost the same functions as the Medtronic 5,325 programmable stimulator and other allied stimulators, except that the output strength has a range of 7–45 volts and the pulse width has a range of 2–10 ms [30].

In China, the first recording of His bundle electrogram was reported by Rui-Long Sun in 1974 [28, p 38] and of sinus node electrogram by Ji-Hong Guo in 1980 [28, p 46]. The first catheter ablation procedures for Wolf-Parkinson-White syndrome were performed in China using direct-current shocks in 1986 [Rui-Long

Sun, personal communication, February 15, 2005], but this energy source has now been supplanted by radio-frequency energy.

China performed its first successful catheter ablation for atrial fibrillation in January, 1996 [31]. Between January, 1996 and April, 2005, 2,580 catheter ablation procedures from 48 centers were carried out, and 152 reports have been published. Several strategies were used, including right atrial compartmentalization in 233 patients, left atrial compartmentalization in 129 patients, ablation of the triggering focus in 993 patients, and pulmonary vein electrical disconnection in 1,225 patients. Paroxysmal atrial fibrillation was the indicated arrhythmia in 90% of the patients, and persistent and permanent atrial fibrillation in 10% of the patients. As to the source of energy used, 2,460 patients received radiofrequency current ablation; 6, cryotherapy ablation; 104, ultrasound ablation; and 6, microwave ablation. Of almost all the patients completing the procedure, 60% became asymptomatic without drugs after the first procedure over 3–6 months follow-up, 70%–75% after the second procedure (20%–30% of patients received the second procedure), 85%–90% after the third procedure (10% of patients received the third procedure and 2%–3% more than three procedures). The total incidence of complications was 1%–3% [31]. Therefore, the Chinese experience is on a par with that of the rest of the world reported recently [32]. China has also published the guidelines for the management of all types of supraventricular tachyarrhythmias which are thorough and up-to-date [33]. The recent publication by Tang and associates from Fuwai Hospital [34] of a review article on the anatomic and electrophysiologic characteristics of the coronary sinus is very timely, because of the latter's involvement in several types of arrhythmias from both the diagnostic and therapeutic points of view.

## Pacemaker, Cardioverter and Defibrillator

The first successful use of a Chinese-made temporary pacemaker was reported in a patient in Shanghai in 1963 [28, p 62]. Transvenous pacing was started in China in early 1970s [35]. During my 1973 visit to China I saw several models of cardioverters (Fig. 26A), defibrillators (Fig. 26B) and cardiac pacemakers (Figs. 26C,D,E), all made in China, being widely used throughout China. China's first implantable pacemaker was introduced by Zu-Xiang Fang in 1974 [28, p 88]. Qinming is China's biggest manufacturer of implantable pacemakers [28, p 62]. For Brugada syndrome the current therapy is ICD implantation [36].

## Phonocardiography and Ballistocardiography

The first book on cardiac auscultation and phonocardiography was published in China in 1962 (Fig. 27A), although phonocardiograms of various cardiovascular diseases had been published as early as 1955 (Fig. 27B). Intracardiac phonocardiography was first introduced in China in 1965 by Hao-Zhu Chen (Fig. 27C).

Ballistocardiography was invented by William Dock in the United States [37] who published a book on ballistocardiography in 1953 [38]. Because of scarcity of any Chinese literature on this subject, Guo-Rui Yu published a book on ballistocardiography in 1961 based mainly on Dock's work (Fig. 28A). Actually, the construction and application of ballistocardiograph were first described by De-Wen Guo in 1958 [Fig. 28B) [39].

## Publications

Besides Huang's ECG book (Fig. 21), He's VCG book (Fig. 25) and Yu's BCG book (Fig. 28A), several other major textbooks on electrocardiology have been published in China over the years (Fig. 29). Among these, the book by Zhen-Wu Xie on ECG in the Chinese population published in 2002 is a significant contribution [Rui Long Sun, personal communication, February 15, 2005]. It serves as a valuable reference for evaluation of normal and abnormal patterns among the Chinese individuals, taking into consideration the ethnic differences unique for the Chinese. Xie also published in 1980 China's first book on ECG in normal children [28, p 60]. As far as I am aware, I do not know of any similar books published in any other countries around the world.

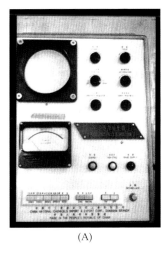

(A)

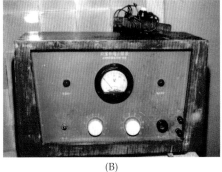

(B)

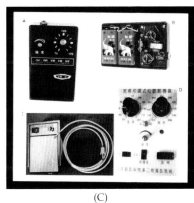

(C)

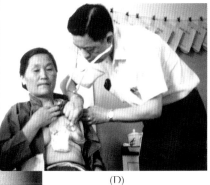

(D)

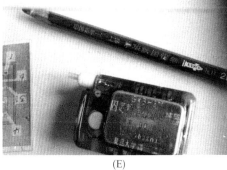

(E)

Fig. 26. Early Chinese models of synchronized cardioverter (A), Shanghai made defibrillator (B), Nanking made transvenous temporary pacemakers (C,D), and implantable permanent pacemaker made by Shanghai's Fudan University (E).

227

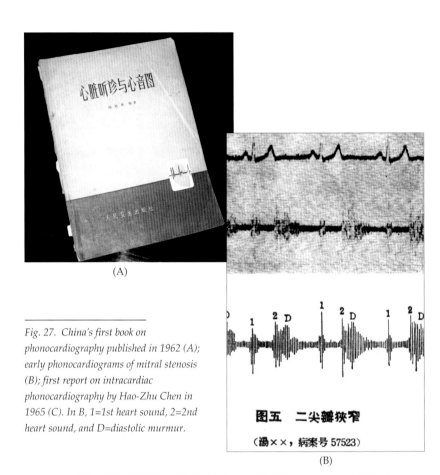

Fig. 27. *China's first book on phonocardiography published in 1962 (A); early phonocardiograms of mitral stenosis (B); first report on intracardiac phonocardiography by Hao-Zhu Chen in 1965 (C). In B, 1=1st heart sound, 2=2nd heart sound, and D=diastolic murmur.*

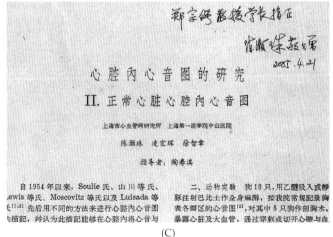

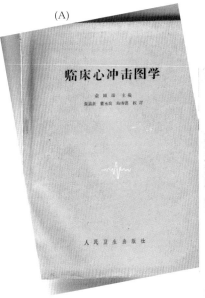

(A)

(B)

*Fig. 28. China's first book on ballistocardiography (A) and first article on ballistocardiography (B) (Both courtesy of De-Wen Guo).*

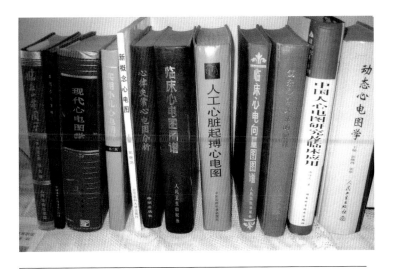

*Fig. 29. Chinese books published on electrocardiology. (Courtesy of Rui-Long Sun).*

Several journals have also been published. Fourteen years after the publication in 1968 in the United States of the *Journal of Electrocardiology*, the *Chinese Journal of Electrocardiology* (*Xindianxue Zazhi*) was published in 1982.

# ECHOCARDIOGRAPHY

## Early Innovations

Although Edler [40] from Sweden was the first to use ultrasound to examine the heart and published with Hertz the first paper in 1954, China began to use cardiac ultrasound in very early years too [41]. Despite his initial efforts in using ultrasound to examine the heart, Edler really did not anticipate this technique to flourish, was primarily concerned with its application in mitral stenosis, never became involved with any of the newer echocardiographic techniques, e.g., detection of pericardial effusion, evaluation of left ventricular function, etc., and retired in 1976 [41].

However, in the late 1950s, investigators in both Shanghai and Wuhan were already making and using ultrasonic devices to examine the hearts of their patients. In 1958, researches on ultrasound were very popular in all industries throughout China. Shi An successfully used the converted flaw detector of Shanghai Shipbuilding Yard to examine the human body. Xin-Fang Wang, China's pioneer and foremost authority in echocardiography (Fig. 30), began to study

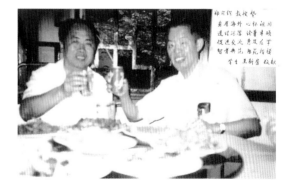

*Fig. 30. Xin-Fang Wang, China's pioneer in echocardiography (left) with me in Wuhan.*

sonography in 1961 and devoted himself to echocardiography since 1963 [Xin-Fang Wang, personal communication, February 23, 2005].

Shanghai Sixth People's Hospital started initially in 1958 with an A-mode ultrasound device and then in 1962 developed the B-mode and an M-mode recorder to study patients with mitral stenosis (Fig. 31). Wang duplicated the findings of Edler with regard to mitral stenosis [42, 43]. In addition, his group clarified the mechanisms of various points, peaks and segments of the echocardiograms in mitral stenosis and was the first in the world to show that the opening snap coincides with the E-peak (Fig. 32).

Zhi-Zhang Xu (formerly spelled Chih-Chang Hsu) in Shanghai (Fig. 33) reported in 1961 the first use of A-mode echocardiography in detecting pericardial effusion and guiding pericardiocentesis [44–46], 4 years before such application was reported in the English literature by Feigenbaum in the USA in 1965 [47]. Wang was also the first to use fetal echocardiography in 1964 [48] (Fig. 34), 8 years before such application was reported in the English literature by Winsberg in 1972 [49].

Contrast echocardiography is now a well-recognized technique, useful in studying various cardiovascular disorders. However, in early days it did not enjoy the widespread use due to lack of a safe inexpensive agent that can reliably produce dense, sustained contrast effects with either M-mode or 2D echocardiography. Wang and associates in 1979 [50] reported that microbubbles were formed when hydrogen peroxide reacted with leukocyte peroxidase and catalase to form water and oxygen, and suggested that hydrogen peroxide would be an ideal echocardiographic contrast agent [50–52]. This contrast agent has been applied to medical ultrasonography all over the world. Wang's publications in 1978–1979 anteceded the article of Gaffney et al. [53] by 4 years. Xu [54] from Shanghai in 1981 and Hua [55] from Wuxi in 1982 later reported the use of carbon dioxide as an echocardiographic contrast agent. Roelandt's group from the Netherlands [56] published their work the same year in 1981.

Simple continuous-wave Doppler equipment was developed in Shanghai in 1964 [57]. It was used to detect the moving structures and blood vessels. Pulsed spectral Doppler and color Doppler flow

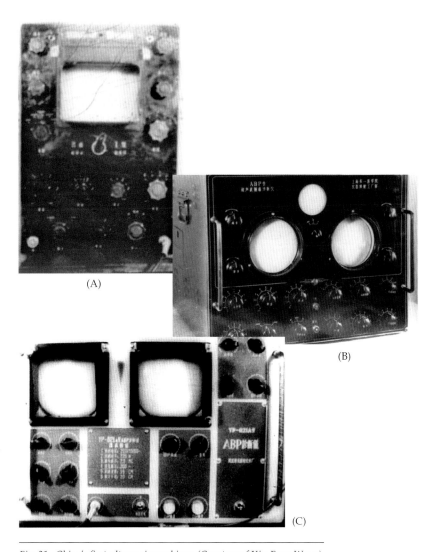

*Fig. 31. China's first ultrasonic machines. (Courtesy of Xin-Fang Wang).*
*(A) The earliest ultrasonic diagnostic device, the A-mode, made in Jiangnan Shipyard in*
*Shanghai and used to diagnose liver abscess, pleural effusion, pericardial effusion and pregnancy*
*by An S and Wang XF in 1961–1963.*
*(B) ABP ultrasonic diagnostic device made in Shanghai First Medical College capable of display*
*of the M-mode curves (with slow scan circuit) to diagnose mitral stenosis by Xu ZZ in 1963.*
*(C) ABP ultrasonic diagnostic device made in Wuhan Wireless Element Factory capable of*
*simultaneous display of the M-mode curves with ECG and phonocardiogram (with slow scan*
*circuit) to diagnose mitral stenosis and pregnancy by Wang XF in 1963.*

(A)

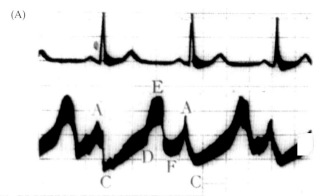

阙下鱼河陷消失，呈一平段，即所谓缓慢样改变。迅与此所入之狭啮（E 啮、A 啮）相现象
不同。此种改变为二尖瓣狭窄之特征，国内外作者均以此征作为诊断二尖瓣狭窄之重要依
（图7—7）。

(B)

图 7-7　二尖瓣狭窄患者之瓣叶曲线
直接描记快录得，纸速 25 毫米/秒。图中见舒张期曲线下降

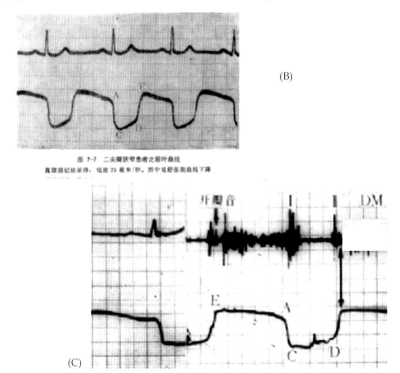

(C)

*Fig. 32. China's early echocardiograms in a normal subject (A) in contrast to patients with mitral stenosis (B,C) with world's first demonstration of coincidence of the E-peak (double-headed arrow in C) with the opening snap (arrow in C) followed by the diastolic murmur (DM in C). (All courtesy of Xing-Fang Wang).*

**Table 1.   Major Cardiac Procedures Done in Modern China**

|  | 1973–1995 | Up to 2002 | Up to 2004 |
|---|---|---|---|
| Coronary Arteriography | 10,000 | 180,000 | 380,000 |
| PTCA | 2,000 | 75,000 | 155,000 |
| CABG | 1,000 | 20,000 | 38,000 |
| Heart Transplantation | 7 | 150 | 200 |
| Coronary Stenting | 30 | 73,300 | 153,300 |
| Brachytherapy | 0 | 200 | 240 |
| Percut Balloon Mitral Valvuloplasty | 5,543 | 20,000 | 22,000 |
| Radiofrequency Ablation, PSVT | 10,000 | 70,000 | 90,000 |
| Radiofrequency Ablation, PVT | 40 | 3,000 | 5,000 |
| Perc Transluminal Septal Myoc Ablation | 0 | 400 | 700 |

Modified from Ref 1 and courtesy of Prof R. L. Gao, Cardiovascular Institute, Beijing Fuwai Hospital. PTCA, percutaneous transluminal coronary angioplasty; CABG, coronary artery bypass grafting; Percut, percutaneous; PSVT, paroxysmal supraventricular tachycardia; PVT, paroxysmal ventricular tachycardia; Perc, percutaneous; Myoc, myocardial.

Percutaneous transluminal coronary angioplasty (PTCA) was first performed in Xi'an, China in 1984. Percutaneous coronary intervention (PCI) grew rapidly in China at an annual rate of increment of around 40% [87, 88] until 2003 when the rate of increment reached nearly 70% (Fig. 41). The success rate also improved rapidly. For instance, in 2001, 16,345 procedures were performed with a success rate of 97% [87, 88]. This, of course, is a rather small number as compared with the United States where, in 1999, 601,000 procedures were performed [89]. Similar to the trend in the Western world, the Chinese cardiologists have also become more aggressive in the management of acute coronary syndromes. According to a recent report of a study, which is a part of the international multicenter registry, selective coronary arteriography was carried out in 35% of these patients, in half of whom (17%) PTCA was performed; thrombolytic therapy was carried out in only 3% of the patients and

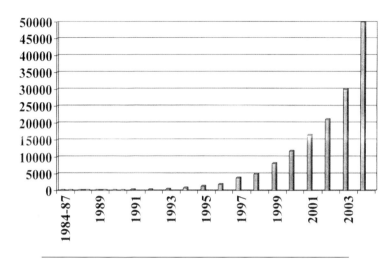

Fig. 41. *Percutaneous coronary interventions performed in China between 1984 and 2004. (Courtesy of R. L. Gao).*

coronary artery bypass grafting in 4% [90]. Coronary stenting has also rapidly expanded in number; according to the Third National Coronary Intervention Registry, published at the end of 2002, over a 3-year period from 1999 to 2001, stents were implanted in 81% (43,304 of 53,695) of PCIs with a success rate of 99% [88]. In 2005, almost 100% of the patients undergoing PCI received stents, averaging 1.4 stents per patient [Gao RL, personal communication, April 12, 2005].

The number of PCIs has now surpassed that of percutaneous balloon mitral valvuloplasty which, after the initial report in 1987 [91] (Fig. 42), used to be the most frequently performed interventional cardiologic procedure in China [92–98]. This reversal in trend reflects the change in the etiologies of heart disease in modern China over the past two decades, namely, an increase in coronary artery disease and a decline in rheumatic heart disease (Table 2).

Frequent symposia on interventional cardiology are held regularly at both national and local levels to keep the cardiologists abreast of the latest development in interventional cardiology. These meetings are usually supported by foreign pharmaceutical companies or/and device manufacturers which also take care of the travel expenses of Chinese cardiologists going overseas to attend

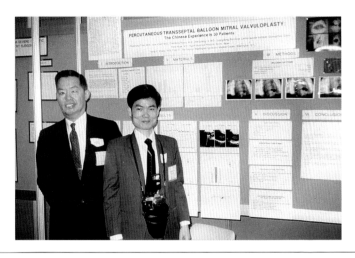

*Fig. 42. First poster presentation from China of percutaneous balloon mitral valvuloplasty at the American College of Cardiology annual meetings in 1987 (C. R. Chen standing on left side of me).*

### Table 2.   Changing Patterns of Heart Disease in China, 1948 to 1999

| Etiologic Types | 1948–57 | 1958–68 | 1969–79 | 1980–89 | 1990–99 |
|---|---|---|---|---|---|
| (Cardiac/total adms | 10% | 16% | 21% | 23% | 24%) |
| Coronary | 6% | 16% | 26% | 27% | 39% |
| Rheumatic | 50% | 44% | 30% | 24% | 10% |
| Hypertensive | 18% | 7% | 3% | 5% | 7% |
| Syphilitic | 9% | 3% | 1% | 0.2% | 0.1% |
| Pulmonary | 7% | 10% | 8% | 2% | 2% |
| Congenital | 2% | 12% | 17% | 13% | 2% |
| Myocarditis | 1% | 1% | 7% | 11% | 8% |
| Cardiomyopathy | 0.05% | 0.16% | 2% | 3% | 5% |
| Pericarditis | 2% | 2% | 2% | 2% | 1% |
| Thyroid | 2% | 1% | 0.24% | 1% | 0.2% |
| Mitral valve prolapse | – | – | – | 0.1% | 0.5% |
| Others | 2% | 3% | 3% | 10% | 25% |

Modified from Chen H et al. (2003) Chin J Intern Med 42:829–832.
adms = admissions to the hospitals

international cardiologic meetings. Unlike the United States where such practices are now forbidden, many Chinese cardiologists who otherwise would not be able to afford such international trips on their meager salaries[2] are able to attend these cardiologic meetings in both Europe and North America. Upon returning to China from such meetings, they promptly report the highlights of such meetings in the national or local medical journals in China. Such practices serve to educate the rest of the cardiologists in China who otherwise would not have an opportunity to keep abreast of the recent advances in cardiology due either to lack of financial means to go overseas or to unfamiliarity with the English language.

# NUCLEAR CARDIOLOGY

Nuclear cardiology is one of the newest subdivisions of cardiology around the world, including China. A PubMed/Medline search on June 16, 2005 yielded 752 references, 145 of which were from the United States, 56 from Europe, 7 from Asia, and none from China.

### Nuclear Medicine

Nuclear medicine had an early, though humble, beginning in China. The year 1956 witnessed the birth of nuclear medicine in China, when the first course, Biomedical Applications of Isotopes, was offered by the Peking Union Medical College [99]. This course was preceded by a training course in nuclear instruments in which trainees learned to construct the radiation detection devices required for performing experiments using radioisotopes. In 1958, several courses in clinical nuclear medicine paved the way for the first generation of nuclear medicine physicians in China. In 1996, several approaches to the teaching of nuclear medicine were adopted in China [100]: (1) Nuclear medicine is taught as part of the clinical curriculum in most medical schools. (2) Three medical schools provide undergraduate training

---

[2] Despite frequent gifts from their grateful patients which may range from a chicken from a farmer to a Mercedes-Benz automobile from a well-to-do businessman.

in nuclear medicine. (3) Four medical schools train nuclear medicine specialists at graduate level. (4) Eight medical schools are authorized to provide a postgraduate programme in nuclear medicine leading to an MS degree. Among them, four are also permitted to offer Ph.D. degrees. (5) No less than 20 medical schools offer a course in isotope techniques and their biomedical applications for graduate students in various fields of medicine. (6) Many departments of nuclear medicine in medical schools offer short-term training courses or continuing education workshops on specific topics in nuclear medicine (Fig. 43). (7) Some schools of pharmacy offer radiopharmacy courses. (8) Members of hospital staff undergo in-service training in computer science, foreign languages, radiology, etc. (9) Graduate students and more senior scientists or physicians are sent abroad to pursue advanced training. (10) Foreign students from developing countries are admitted to nuclear medicine centers in China for further training, (11) Foreign guest speakers are invited to China to demonstrate (Fig. 44) or participate in symposia (Fig. 45). At present,

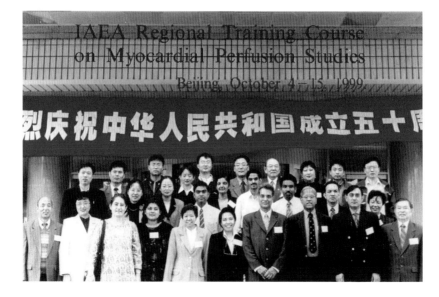

*Fig. 43. Regional training course on myocardial perfusion studies in Beijing in 1999. (Courtesy Z. W. He).*

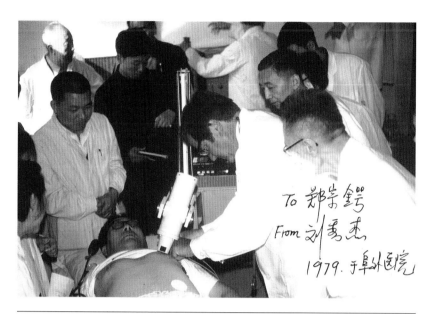

To 郑崇锷
From 刘秀杰
1979. 于阜外医院

Fig. 44. First demonstration in China of Nuclear Stethoscope at Fuwai Hospital by Henry Wagner of Johns Hopkins University in 1979. At the head of the patient is Xiu-Jie Liu and behind him is Y. K. Wu.

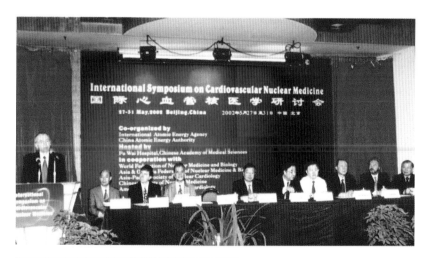

Fig. 45. International Symposium on cardiovascular nuclear medicine in Beijing in 2002. (Courtesy of Z. X. He).

there are 32 medical schools offering an undergraduate course in nuclear medicine; and 12 and 44 schools are authorized to train M.D. and M.S. in nuclear medicine, respectively [Wang SC, personal communication, May 18, 2005].

Some of the major historical events in the development of nuclear medicine in China include [99]: (1) operation of the first reactor, producing 33 radioactive isotopes in 1958; (2) first linear scanner built in 1960; (3) setting up an organization for the control of radiopharmaceuticals in 1961; (4) distribution of the first batch of cyclotron-produced isotopes in 1963; (5) development and use of the first radioimmunoassay procedure in 1963; (6) production of tritium in 1964; (7) production of 99.8% enriched heavy water in 1965; (8) supply of $^{99}$mTc and $^{113}$mIn generators in 1972; (9) first gamma camera imported in 1972 and first homemade gamma camera installed in 1977; (10) founding of Chinese Society of Nuclear Medicine in 1980; (11) publication of the *Chinese Journal of Nuclear Medicine* in 1981; (12) first single photon emission computed tomograph (SPECT) imported in 1983. At present, there are in China 856 nuclear medicine departments with 5,600 staff members [Wang SC, personal communication, May 18, 2005] and 600 nuclear cardiology departments [He ZX, personal communication, May 26, 2005].

Gamma cameras were first manufactured in Beijing in the late 1970s by a factory affiliated with the Ministry of Aviation and Space Technology [101]. The cameras thus produced now hold a dominant position in the domestic market and account for more than half of the total in use. The emergence of software for image analysis designed by the Tsinghua University, to be used in combination with the gamma cameras, has further improved the vitality of nuclear medicine imaging.

Following its import in 1983 [101], the number of SPECT in China has grown rapidly at an average rate of 20%–25% each year. At present there are 500 SPECTs in China [He ZX, personal communication, May 26, 2005]. According to the regulation set up by the Ministry of Health, class A hospitals in China must all be equipped with a SPECT and thus be able to perform high-quality diagnostic studies with isotopic tracers [101].

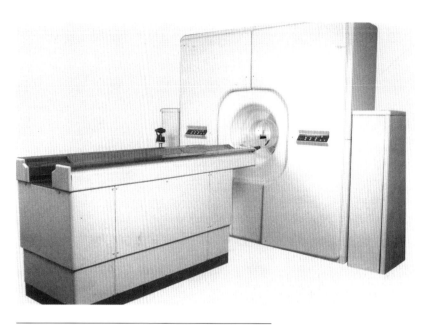

*Fig. 46. China's first PET scanner. (Courtesy of S. C. Wang).*

Positron emission tomography (PET) is most valuable in the diagnosis of coronary artery disease and cerebral disorders. In 1986 China made its first PET scanner (Fig. 46). At present, there are 15 PET centers in Beijing, Shanghai and Guangzhou [He ZX, personal communication, May 26, 2005], marking a big step forward from old-fashioned nuclear medicine to molecular nuclear medicine with this cutting-edge diagnostic technique.

## Nuclear Cardiology

Nuclear cardiology started relatively early in China [102, 103]. The first study with the Nuclear Stethoscope, a handy device for monitoring cardiac function, was performed at the Fuwai Hospital on September 25, 1979 (Fig. 44) [7, p 137]. Nuclear cardiology progressed quickly due to the introduction of SPECT and the availability of a great number of new cardiac imaging agents. The dopamine stress test, which was started in China in 1993 [He ZX, personal communication, May 26, 2005], has been widely used in detecting coronary artery disease when physical exercise cannot be carried out. By the quantification of the left ventricular ejection fraction, cardiac circular shortening fraction and change in wall thickness during gated cardiac perfusion imaging, it is possible to measure cardiac contractile function, which is very useful in predicting myocardial viability.

Detection of myocardial viability in severe ischemia or myocardial infarction is also investigated by various methods such as [$^{99}$mTc] MIBI tomography, Tl$^{201}$ delay and reinjection imaging, [$^{18}$F] FDG PET metabolic imaging, and Tl$^{201}$ myocardial imaging by intervention with nitrates. These procedures are very valuable in differentiating viable myocardium from scar tissue in rendering decisions on the therapeutic strategy for patients with coronary artery disease, predicting the outcome of coronary artery bypass surgery or PTCA, and postoperative follow-up. The special merit of cardiac radionuclide scintigraphy lies in its noninvasiveness and its ability to detect whether the coronary artery is restenosed.

Metabolic cardiac imaging, in addition to myocardial perfusion imaging, is essential in the assessment of myocardial viability. For this purpose, [$^{18}$F] FDG PET imaging proved to be a sensitive and specific method. It is the "gold standard" for identifying whether patients will likely benefit from myocardial revascularization procedures. Clinical investigation of hypertrophic cardiomyopathy using $^{123}$I-BMIPP (beta-methyl-iodophenyl pentadecanoic acid) has also been performed since free fatty acid is the main energy source of the myocardium. Cardiac imaging using $^{123}$I-MIBG (metaiodobenzylguanidine), which was initially developed for the diagnosis of pheochromocytoma, has become a valuable tool in assessing cardiac sympathetic activity in diabetes, hypertension, ischemic and nonischemic cardiomyopathy and congestive heart failure.

Radionuclide ventriculography is a useful noninvasive approach for evaluating valvular heart disease, the effect of mitral valve replacement or repair, surgical indications of congenital heart disease

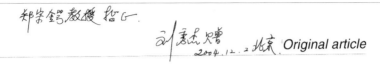

Original article

# Long-term prognostic value of exercise 99mTc-MIBI SPET myocardial perfusion imaging in patients after percutaneous coronary intervention

Xiaoli Zhang, Xiujie Liu, Zuo-Xiang He, Rongfang Shi, Minfu Yang, Runlin Gao, Jilin Chen, Yuejin Yang, Wei Fang

Cardiovascular Institute and Fu Wai Hospital, PUMC & CAMS, Beijing, China

Received: 17 June 2003 / Accepted: 25 October 2003 / Published online: 22 January 2004
© Springer-Verlag 2004

**Abstract.** The purpose of this study was to evaluate the long-term prognostic value of exercise technetium-99m methoxyisobutylisonitrile ($^{99m}$Tc-MIBI) single-photon emission tomography (SPET) imaging in patients after percutaneous coronary intervention (PCI). Three hundred and eighteen consecutive post-PCI patients who underwent exercise and rest $^{99m}$Tc-MIBI SPET myocardial perfusion imaging (MPI) were followed up for 38±27 months. Patients with early revascularisation (<3 months after MPI) were excluded. A semiquantitative visual according to whether patients were symptomatic or asymptomatic (*P*>0.05). However, the annual soft event rate in patients with irreversible defects and symptoms was 5.0%, which was higher than that of 0.6% in asymptomatic patients ($\chi^2$=6.11, *P*<0.05). Multivariate Cox analysis showed that SSS was the best independent predictor for hard cardiac events ($\chi^2$=12.70; *P*<0.001) and SDS was the strongest independent predictor for soft cardiac events ($\chi^2$=11.72; *P*<0.001). Post-PCI patients who have normal exercise $^{99m}$Tc-MIBI SPET MPI have a

*Fig. 47. A recent paper from Fuwai Hospital on the largest series of patients to undergo $^{99m}$Tc-MIBI for evaluation of prognosis following percutaneous coronary interventions published in the* European Journal of Nuclear Medicine and Molecular Imaging *(2004;31:655–662).*

such as tetralogy of Fallot and the therapeutic effectiveness of surgery. It is also used in monitoring drugs which are toxic to the myocardium, such as adriamycin.

During the 7th World Congress of Nuclear Medicine and Biology, China ranked sixth in the total number of papers accepted for presentation [101]. Many important contributions to the world literature have emanated from China, including the largest series of patients (n=318) to undergo $^{99m}$Tc-MIBI for evaluation of prognosis following PCI (Fig. 47). Therefore, nuclear medicine, including nuclear cardiology, in China has a very promising future indeed.

## PULMONARY EMBOLISM

Pulmonary embolism used to be thought to be rare in China [104] and among the Chinese in other parts of the world [105–110]. But this is no longer the case [1, 111–113]. My good colleague in Shenyang and a renowned cardiologist, Shao-Zhou Pan, died in 1980 of massive pulmonary embolism after hip fracture following a fall. In 1991 Xian-Sheng Cheng and associates from Fuwai Hospital reported the incidence of autopsy proven pulmonary embolism to be 11%, of which 76% were confirmed to have pulmonary infarction with an antemortem diagnosis made in only 13% [114, 115].

In a recent analysis of 37 documents of Chinese-language case studies involving misdiagnoses of pulmonary embolism published from January 1980 to June 2001 and identified by searching the Chinese Biomedical Literature Database [116], 310 patients with misdiagnosed pulmonary embolism were identified. The five commonest misdiagnoses were coronary artery disease in 20%, pneumonia in 14%, primary pulmonary hypertension in 10%, cardiomyopathy in 7%, and pleurisy in 6% [116]. China is launching a campaign to increase the awareness of this disease and its management, as evidenced by several recent publications in major Chinese medical journals [116–119] and three recent monographs published in China (Fig. 48).

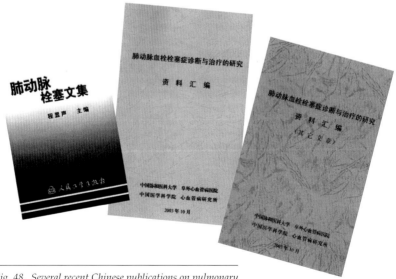

*Fig. 48. Several recent Chinese publications on pulmonary embolism. (Courtesy of X. S. Cheng, Fuwai Hospital).*

There are several explanations for underdiagnosing or misdiagnosing pulmonary embolism in China:

(1) Traditional teaching by such authorities as Snapper, who was highly regarded in old China as one of the most astute diagnosticians, was that pulmonary embolism was rare in China. He did not even mention it in his book *Chinese Lessons to Western Medicine* [120].

(2) Even as recent as 1970s, pulmonary embolism was thought to be rare in China [104]. The rarity of pulmonary embolism was even more remarkable when one considered the widespread use of birth control pills among the Chinese women of child-bearing age [104]. Perhaps the use of acupuncture anesthesia, which permitted early ambulation after major surgery, accounted for the low incidence of postoperative pulmonary embolism in China [1]. Because acupuncture anesthesia is seldom employed in modern China, this protective factor is no longer operative.

(3) More accurate in vivo diagnosis of pulmonary embolism is now possible because of improved diagnostic techniques.

## PREVENTIVE CARDIOLOGY

Preventive cardiology is another relatively new subdivision of cardiology, although the Yellow Emperor of China advocated it thousands of years ago (Fig. 49). It is well known that the occurrence of coronary artery disease is closely related to a society's economic development [121]. Coronary artery disease, which used to be rare in China, has increased considerably in prevalence over the past several decades [1] (Table 2). The cause is multifactorial: longevity [1], change in dietary habit [1], obesity [1], cigarette smoking [1], and increased mechanization [122]. With the exception of more people in China living to an older age [1], all the rest are preventable risk factors.

Modern Chinese love the atherogenic fast food and devour them at an ever faster rate. The huge success of world's two of the best known fast-food giants, McDonald's and Kentucky Fried Chicken, is the result of a change of Chinese life styles which are becoming

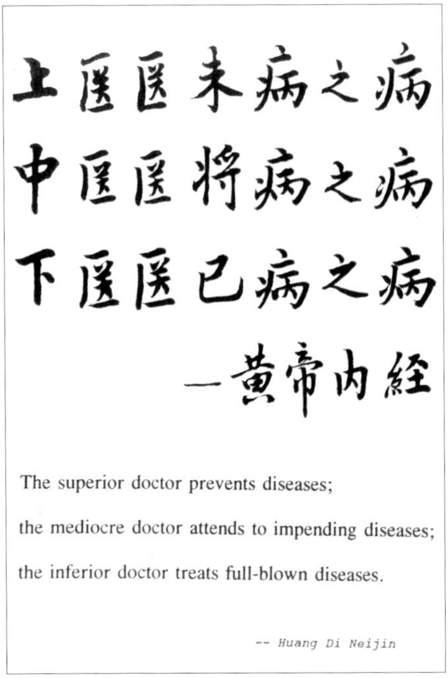

上醫醫未病之病
中醫醫將病之病
下醫醫已病之病
　—黃帝內經

The superior doctor prevents diseases;

the mediocre doctor attends to impending diseases;

the inferior doctor treats full-blown diseases.

-- Huang Di Neijin

*Fig. 49. A Chinese saying from* Huang Di Neijing *with English translation (Chinese calligraphy by Mme Qi-Yun Ge, wife of the late Chinese Ambassador to US Xu Han).*

more geared to speed, convenience and variety. As a consequence of the recent change in the dietary habits in China, the normal plasma cholesterol values in modern China have shown a steady increase. In 2003, the upper limit of normal was 6.0 mmol/L or 232 mg/dL and the mean value was 5.06 mmol/L or 196 mg/dL [123]. These "normal" values, which were very similar to those reported recently from another study of 1,211 retirees in Beijing [124] and the Chinese MONICA project involving 5 million Chinese from 16 provinces [125] were considerably higher than the normal values in China published in 1958 (155 mg/dL) [7, p 12], in 1981 (191 mg/dL) [7, p 12], and in 1997 (200 mg/dL) [126]. In a country known traditionally for its low plasma cholesterol values and low incidence of coronary artery disease, this upward adjustment of the so-called "normal" values in modern China represents an alarming trend that deserves special attention. This trend is bound to get worse, because of the long "incubation period" between exposure to this major risk factor and its maximum effects on morbidity and mortality from coronary artery disease [127].

China used to be known for her slender people. I never saw a fat person in China till recent years (Fig. 50). Now China is fighting obesity, especially childhood obesity which is as high as 28% [128],

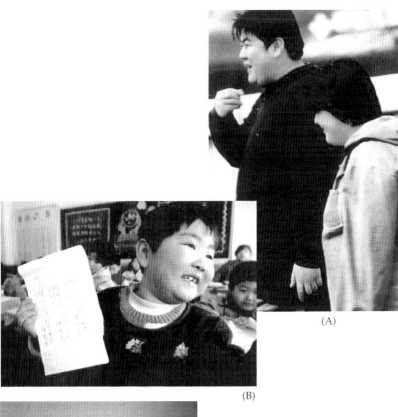

(A)

(B)

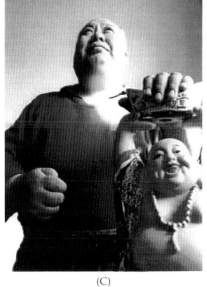

*Fig. 50. Obesity is prevalent in China among not only adults (A) but also children (D). Obese people in China are often compared to Buddha (C) and represent prosperity. (Courtesy of* Beijing Review).

(C)

as the rest of the world [129]. Excessive caloric intake from fast food [130] and insufficient exercise from increasing availabiltiy of, and increased reliance on, automobiles [122] and popularization of television result in weight gain. The effect of television viewing on pediatric obesity has recently been documented: each hourly increment of TV viewing is associated with 1% to 2% increase in the prevalence of obesity in urban China [131].

The prevalence of obesity continues its upward trend in China as the rest of the world. By the end of 2000, the obesity rate of male students in Beijing reached 15%, doubling that of 1990 and approaching that of developed countries [128]. Traditionally, a fat child in China meant a healthy child, one who was likely to survive the rigors of undernourishment and infections. This misconception still prevails today in many parts of China which unfortunately is a participant in an international epidemic of childhood obesity [132, 133]. The situation is made worse by China's one-child policy [134]. China is strict in allowing only one child per family. There is a saying in China: "2-4-8 (pronounced as 'er', 'si' and 'ba', respectively), you get fat." With only one child in the family, the doting parents (2 in number), grandparents (4 in number) and great grandparents (8 in number) pamper the "little emperor" by overfeeding him. Furthermore, food that used to be distributed among his siblings is now devoured by just one person. Fat children grow up to be fat adults. Overweight in China (BMI $\geq$ 25) has shown a progressive increase in both men and women over the past two decades [135]. It is estimated that overweight is present in 50–60% of northern Chinese and 20% of the total Chinese population [135]. Obesity (BMI $\geq$ 30) is present in 10% of the population in northern China and 5% in southern China; the total number of obese people in China is now estimated to be 30 to 40 million [135].

The Chinese have a lower baseline BMI to begin with (baseline value = 21 [136], mean = 18.5–23.9 [137]), and it takes less increment to reach an obese level, so that BMI of 24–27.9 is considered as overweight and $\geq$ 28 as obese [137]. It takes smaller increments to increase the risk of hypertension, coronary artery disease and type 2 diabetes in the Chinese population [136, 138, 139]. China is in the midst of an obesity epidemic [140]. Obesity in China has reached such a serious stage that the Chinese government has started a national campaign against it [141]. Among the encouraging signs that I noticed is that, contrary to his two predecessors Tse-Tung Mao and Ze-Min Jiang, the current Chinese president Jin-Tao Hu is not a bit paunchy (Fig. 51). At my last visit with Y. K. Wu in 2002 (Fig. 52), he handed me several brochures describing the major risk factors for coronary artery disease in China and methods of prevention (Fig. 53). He repeatedly reminded me of the importance of preventive measures that need to be taken against the rising incidence of coronary artery disease in modern China.

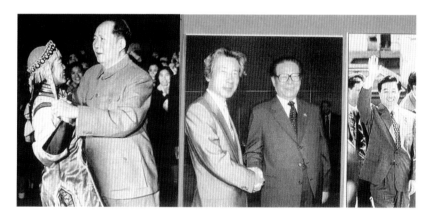

*Fig. 51. Paunchy Tse-Tung Mao (left) and Ze-Min Jiang (middle) in contrast to trim Jin-Tao Hu (right).*

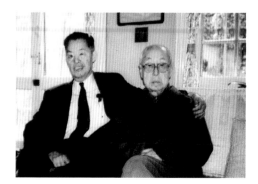

*Fig. 52. Visiting Y. K. Wu at his home in October 2002.*

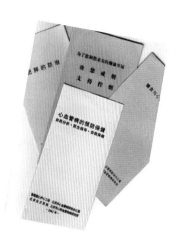

Fig. 53. *Several brochures on preventive cardiology given to me by Y. K. Wu at our last gathering in October 2002.*

# GENE AND GENOMIC RESEARCH

Medical genetic research in China started in the late 1950s [142]. Molecular genetic research started in China in the 1990s [142]. As the Human Genome Project was initiated in the United States at the beginning of the 1990s, China also launched a national human genome project as part of its contribution to international efforts to sequence the human genome [143].

Though a late comer, China has contributed much to the field of human genome research through international collaborations and strong government support. According to one official from the National Science Foundation of China, "The Chinese account for over one-fifth of the world's population, and the country has 56 ethnic groups. As a result, no databank of human genetic information can be said to be complete without a detailed study of the Chinese human genome" [143]. The project has important practical implications, as the Chinese with her powerful sequencing capacity and capability in the genome project are expected to contribute vital information that may lead to the early diagnosis and treatment of more than 5,000 hereditary diseases [143].

In 1998, China's scientific leaders overcame skepticism from some members of the Human Genome Project to become the only developing country to take a role in sequencing the human genome by contributing 1% of the published sequence—an achievement that is of huge symbolic importance [144]. Chinese researchers are now setting up programmes in everything from stem-cell research, through large-scale efforts to determine protein structures, to population studies to hunt for human disease genes [144]. There is even talk of trying to clone the endangered giant panda [144]. The whole governmental budget for genome research and other relevant projects, mainly devoted to research running costs, is about 200 million US dollars for the years 2001–2005 [145]. Dozens of research centers and laboratories have been established nationwide [145].

In the field of cardiology, China has made much progress in research work on the molecular etiology and gene therapy of hypertension, coronary artery disease and myocardial infarction.

## Hypertension

Hypertension is a common late-onset disease that exhibits complex genetic heterogeneity. Several genome-wide scans recently accomplished in ethnic Chinese populations revealed a number of candidate loci possibly contributing to essential hypertension, and appeared to be replicable in 2q14-q23 and 5q32 [146, 147]. Zhu and associates [148, 149] reported linkage to the chromosome 2q14-q23 region for essential hypertension in a south China population. Several genes located in that region are considered to be relevant to the regulation of blood pressure and the development of essential hypertension. These genes include several G-proteins and G protein-coupled receptors, a voltage-gated sodium channel protein and the gamma subunit of the sodium/potassium ATPase [150]. Another region, 5q32, harboring the $\beta_2$-adrenergic receptor gene, has been reported to be linked to essential hypertension in Hans Chinese residing in Taiwan [151]. To repeat these results and perform quantitative linkage analysis, Gu's group [152] genotyped members of 148 hypertensive families containing 328 affected sib pairs, and grouped families from Beijing and Jiangsu province with five highly informative microsatellite markers (D2S151, D2S142, D5S2090,

D5S413 and D5S2013). Their results provided no evidence to support a significant linkage of 2q14-q23 or 5q32 with essential hypertension or blood pressure quantitative traits in the ethnic Chinese, and indicate the etiologic diversity and complexity of hypertension.

Another study reported recently by Gu's group [153, 154], which involved linkage analysis in 148 Chinese hypertensive families, showed that a region of chromosome 8 flanking the lipoprotein lipase gene might contribute to the individual blood pressure variations in Chinese. Using the linkage model in variance component analysis of the computer program SOLAR (Sequential Oligogenic Linkage Analysis Routines), a region of linkage with systolic blood pressure to a 10.6 cM on chromosome 8 (8p22) was identified by markers D8S1145, D8S261 and D8S282 with a maximum two-point logarithm of odds (LOD) score of 2.03 near the marker D8S261. In the qualitative trait linkage analysis, evidence for linkage between the marker D8S1145 and essential hypertension was found (p=0.029); transmission/disequilibrium test (TDT/S-TDT) also supported a significant linkage disequilibrium with essential hypertenion of the allele 3 of D8S261 (chi2=8.643, p<0.01).

## Coronary Artery Disease and Myocardial Infarction

Genetic studies of coronary artery disease (CAD) and myocardial infarction (MI) are lagging behind other cardiovascular disorders, because CAD or MI is a complex disease, caused by many genetic factors, environmental factors and interactions among these factors [155]. Among many risk factors, family history is one of the most significant independent risk factors for CAD/MI [155]. Over the past few years several studies have focused on the role of hemostatic markers that reflect the inherited or acquired propensity to CAD/MI, and several genetic mutations affecting coagulation proteins have been suggested as prothrombotic risk factors [156, 157]. Thrombomodulin (TM) is the anticoagulant endothelial cell membrane-bound protein cofactor in the thrombin-mediated activation of protein C [158]. However, conflicting data have been reported recently regarding the possible contribution of the TM–33G/A polymorphism to CAD [159–165]. In view of these contradictory findings and the smaller sample sizes of the previous reports, Gu's group [158] investigated this polymorphism in 808 patients with angiographically verified CAD or a history of an acute MI and 813 age- and sex-matched controls. Their results failed to support a significant association of the TM –33G/A polymorphism with CAD or MI in their population [158].

### Traditional Chinese Medicine

On the long list of organisms that should be sequenced, the Beijing Genomics Institute has already started investigations into proteomics and drug discovery, including a project to isolate the active compounds in the herbs used in traditional Chinese medicine [166]. There are many Chinese herbs that are widely used in this country, especially for treatment of coronary artery disease and congestive heart failure [167]. Unfortunately, they tend to interact unfavorably with commonly prescribed Western cardiac drugs, including warfarin [168–177], digoxin [172, 178–181] and hypoglycemic agents [182]. Therefore, the isolation of the active compounds in these herbs will facilitate the understanding of the pharmacodynamics of these herbs and thus avoid their inadvertent adverse interactions with the Western medications [167, 169].

## INTERNATIONAL EXCHANGES AND COLLABORATION

Former US president Nixon's historic visit to China to meet Chairman Mao in February 1972 (Fig. 54) was a turning point in world history, not only for its geopolitical significance but also in the medical world including cardiology. Due to nearly a quarter of a century of isolation from the rest of the world, medicine, especially cardiology, in China was little known to the outside world. Nixon's 1972 visit led to opening of China to the West. At the Great Wall, Nixon said, "As we look at this Great Wall, we do not want any walls of any kind between people."

After the initial excitement over acupuncture anesthesia for closed (Fig. 55A) and open (Fig. 55B) heart surgery, the Western cardiologists began to realize that cardiology in China is more than using acupuncture needles (Fig. 55C) to induce analgesia for cardiac surgery [183–187] and to treat angina pectoris [188, 189]. Unbeknownst to the outside world, China has made many important advances in cardiology, e.g. echocardiography (vide supra), traditional medicine [35, 104, 167, 190], cardiopulmonary resuscitation [35, 104, 190] and synthesis of insulin (Fig. 56) [104].

## Paul White Visiting China in 1971

Although Nixon was widely known as the first VIP from the United States to set foot on the Chinese mainland since the founding of the People's Republic of China in 1949, much less well known was the

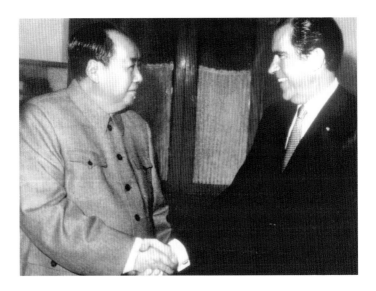

*Fig. 54. Historic visit to China in February 1972 by US President Richard Nixon to meet Chairman Mao.*

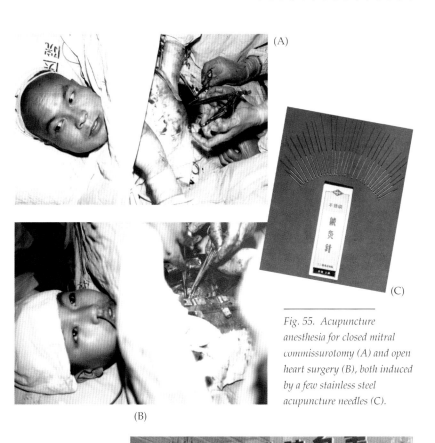

(A)

(C)

Fig. 55. Acupuncture anesthesia for closed mitral commissurotomy (A) and open heart surgery (B), both induced by a few stainless steel acupuncture needles (C).

(B)

Fig. 56. Scheme for China's synthesis of bovine insulin and the crystals of the synthetic insulin depicted in detail at the Shanghai Industrial Exhibition which I visited in 1972.

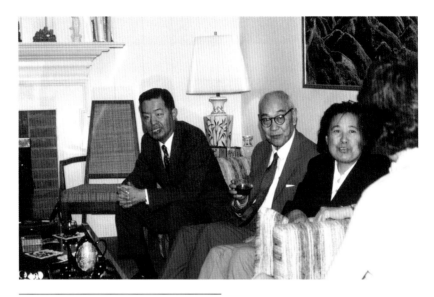

*Fig. 57. Jia-Si Huang visiting my home in 1979.*

fact that Paul D. White's visit preceded Nixon's by 5 months. White's China visit actually could have taken place much earlier. In 1962 at the VIII International Cancer Congress in Moscow, White was invited to visit China by Jia-Si Huang, president of the Chinese Academy of Medical Sciences, but the invitation was cancelled owing to the "reactionary attitude of the U.S. government toward new China" [13]. This incident was later confirmed to me by Huang during his visit to my home in 1979 (Fig. 57). But White was not daunted by this rejection; from 1962 on, he sought advices and efforts involving many of his contacts and friends including me [35]. His long sought journey to China finally came in the Fall of 1971.

White's visit was a huge success. He and his wife along with another cardiologist E. G. Dimond and his wife, a public health expert Victor Sidel and his wife, and an otologist Samuel Rosen and his wife, were warmly welcomed upon arrival in Beijing (Fig. 58). It might be of interest at this juncture to mention a small incident at the Beijing airport where Mrs. White was curious about the large red Chinese characters all over the place and asked Y. K. Wu, one member of the

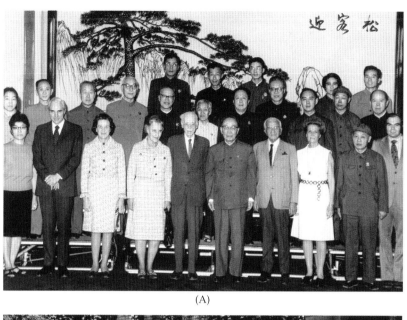

(A)

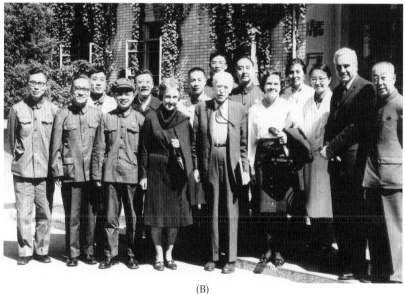

(B)

Fig. 58. *Paul D. White visiting China in 1971 and being received by Mo-Ruo Guo at the People's Great Hall (A) and Y. K. Wu at Fuwai Hospital (B). In A, Dr. White and Mrs. White stood on the right side of Guo; in B, Mrs. White and Dr. White were 4th and 5th from left in the front. (Courtesy of Ji-Hong Guo).*

welcoming party, whether they were meant to welcome the visiting American guests. Wu said, "Sorry, they mean 'Down with American Imperialists'" [191]. Mrs. White was shocked, "Oh, my God!", she exclaimed. However, it was Wu's honesty and frankness that greatly impressed the American visitors.

White visited several hospitals and medical schools and saw a few patients with various types of heart disease including CAD. As a matter of fact, there was an erroneous announcement over the BBC that White's visit to China was to treat Chairman Mao's heart disease [13]. White was so impressed by his visit that soon upon his return to the United States he urged me to "return to visit your motherland to see for yourself the medical progress that new China has made." I do not think there is any doubt that White's pioneering visit to China played a major role in what followed afterwards. There were further medical visits and exchanges between the United States and China that followed the historic visit of White in 1971. As White always said, medicine knows no international boundary and is the world's best goodwill ambassador [35]. It was White's inspiration that started many of my return visits to China. I chose as the title of the American College of Cardiology's Second Annual Paul D. White Lecture in 1973 "Cardiology in the People's Republic of China" [35].

## Chinese Medical Association Delegation Visiting the US in 1972

The first official medical delegation from China to visit the United States following White's historic visit to China came in the Fall of 1972. The four American physicians who visited China a year earlier along with the National Academy of Sciences Institute of Medicine and the American Medical Association were the official hosts; I was asked to be the special liaison between the two sides.

The leader of the Chinese medical delegation was Wei-Ran Wu, a surgeon, and the deputy leader was Chiao-Chih Lin, an obstetrician. The delegation was comprised of two cardiologists (Yen-San Li, an echocardiographer from the same medical school in Wuhan as Xin-Fang Wang; Jia-Yu Xu, an expert in nuclear medicine from Shanghai and also my classmate in medical school), a surgeon (Guan-Han Zhou, from Beijing, versed in operating under acupuncture anesthesia) and a researcher in acupuncture anesthesia (Shu-Hsun Zhang from Chinese Academy of Medical Sciences in Beijing) and others.

The visit was a major event, as evidenced by the fact that on the first day the delegation was greeted at the White House by president Nixon (Fig. 59). On the other hand, the visit was so unprecedented that, because of a quarter of a century of separation between the United States and China and because both sides were still unsure of each other, the Chinese delegation throughout the 18-day, 4,000-mile journey across the United States was closely shepherded for security reasons by many US Secret Service agents. The latter even paid a visit to my house and checked out the neighborhood a couple of days before some members of the Chinese delegation came to a reception at my home I held in their honor.

On their Boston tour, they received their highest praise from Eugene Braunwald, professor of medicine at Harvard and chairman of medicine at Peter Bent Brigham Hospital. "We discussed Freis' study of hypertension among Veterans Administration patients," he said, referring to the cooperative study in the 1960s that won Freis a

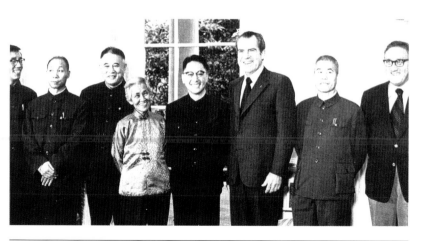

*Fig. 59. First Chinese Medical Association delegation visiting the US in 1972, led by Wei-Ran Wu, Chairman of Surgery at Beijing Hospital (5th left) and received by US President Nixon at the White House.*

Lasker Award and established the value of drug therapy in essential hypertension. "They understood the value of a large, randomized controlled study like that. They immediately grasped what we were doing in our coronary and dialysis units. In the radioisotope area, they showed familiarity with what is a rather sophisticated branch of medicine. They are well read and up to date" [192].

## Michael DeBakey Visiting China in February/March 1973

The world-renowned American heart surgeon Michael E. DeBakey was invited by the Chinese Medical Association to visit China in February/March 1973 (Fig. 60). His trip like Paul White's was also delayed 10 years. According to Y. K. Wu, "We almost had him here ten years ago but something came up. We have a great deal of respect for him" [193, p v].

In his *China Diary* (Fig. 61), DeBakey summarized his experiences by saying that "My visit to China, albeit brief, was truly one of the

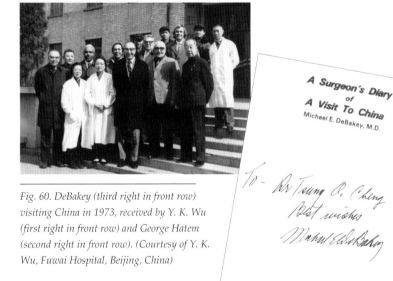

*Fig. 60. DeBakey (third right in front row) visiting China in 1973, received by Y. K. Wu (first right in front row) and George Hatem (second right in front row). (Courtesy of Y. K. Wu, Fuwai Hospital, Beijing, China)*

*Fig. 61. A Surgeon's Diary of A Visit to China by DeBakey.*

most memorable and exciting experiences I have ever had in my extensive travels to foreign lands around the world. The organization of the Chinese health care system, the way in which it was implemented within a short time despite the shattering social upheaval that occurred during the Cultural Revolution, and the extraordinary results they have achieved with limited resources are indeed a magnificent tribute to the dedication of the Chinese medical leaders and to the altruism and industry of the health workers…. I was deeply impressed with the warmth, friendliness, and forthrightness of all the people whom I met. Everywhere we went we were accorded a genuinely cordial and hospitable reception. The people were honest in their explanations to us about what they were trying to do and the progress they had made, as well as the problems they have yet to solve" [193].

DeBakey is a great man [194]. Despite hundreds and thousands of articles, book chapters and books he had written, he paid meticulous attention to details. I would never forget the superb chapter on "Diseases of the Aorta and Its Branches" [195] which he contributed to my book *The International Textbook of Cardiology* [7]. He proofed the galleys personally. When I suggested a better print be made for one of the illustrations in his chapter, he promptly dispatched one to me within 72 hours by express mail. He also generously contributed several illustrations of his new small LVAD, the DeBakey/ NASA Axial Flow Ventricular Assist Device (Fig. 62), to my

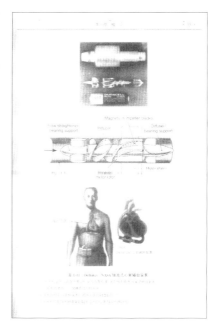

*Fig. 62. DeBakey/NASA Axial Flow Ventricular Assist Device as illustrated in my book* Congestive Heart Failure.

recent book on *Congestive Heart Failure* [196]. He was pleased to receive a copy of my book containing these illustrations which I presented to him in person recently (Fig. 63). Most recently, after reading my article on the current state of cardiology in China [1], he was greatly impressed by how advanced cardiology in China has become since his 1973 visit (Fig. 64).

## My Visit to China in June/July 1973

On the 1972 visit to the United States by the Chinese Medical Association delegation, Wei-Ran Wu expressed a great deal of interest in coronary artery bypass grafting (CABG) for coronary artery disease but told the reporters "We haven't started yet" [192]. One of the prerequisites for CABG is, of course, accurate diagnosis of the location and severity of the obstructive process in the coronary arterial system.

Following my initial private visit to China in 1972, I was officially invited by the Chinese government (Fig. 65), Chinese Medical

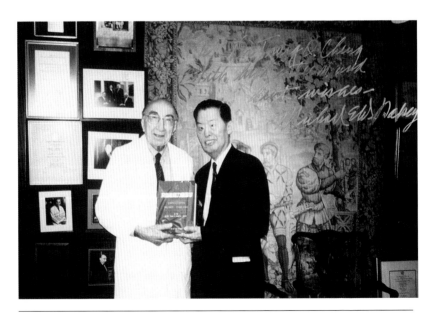

*Fig. 63. DeBakey being presented a copy of my book* Congestive Heart Failure *at his Houston office in 2003.*

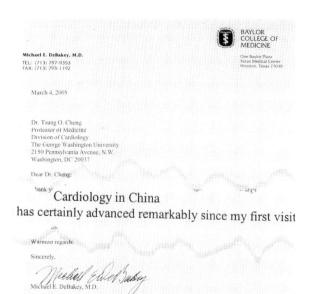

*Fig. 64. DeBakey's comment about the advances China made in cardiology as expressed in a recent letter of his to me.*

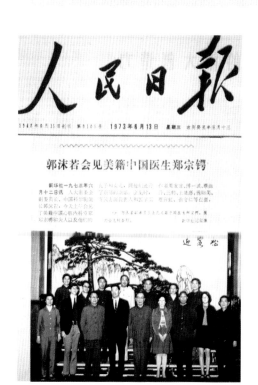

*Fig. 65. My invited visit to China in 1973 with my family as officially announced in the* People's Daily *which showed me being received by Mu-Ruo Guo at the People's Great Hall. The original photo of the meeting was superimposed on the printed newspaper clipping for better reproduction.*

Association and Chinese Academy of Medical Sciences (Fig. 66) to return to China to update the Chinese cardiologists on modern diagnostic technology including selective coronary arteriography. I performed China's first selective cine coronary arteriogram in Fuwai Hospital, Cardiovascular Institute, Chinese Academy of Medical Sciences on June 7, 1973 (Fig. 40). One year later China successfully performed its first CABG surgery in the same hospital in October 1974 [197, 198]. It was a single-vessel saphenous vein graft to the left anterior descending coronary artery in a 40-year-old male patient who survived for 8 years [Xiao-Dong Zhu, Fuwai Hospital, personal communication, August 1, 1997]. Since then, over 38,000 CABGs have

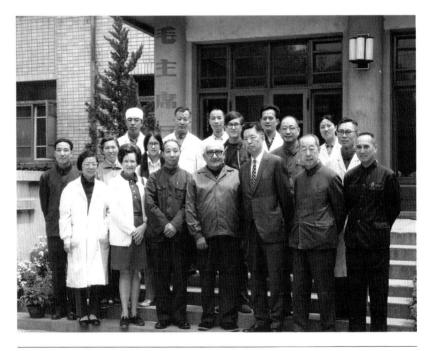

*Fig. 66. My visit to Fuwai Hospital, Cardiovascular Institute, Chinese Academy of Medical Sciences in 1973 with my wife (3rd from left in the front row), my daughter (between and behind my wife and I-cheng Fu, Secretary General of Chinese Medical Association) and my son (behind and between George Hatem and me). On the other side of me were Y. K. Wu (second from right) and Rui-Sun Tsai (first right), director and deputy director, respectively, of Fuwai Hosptal. Yu-Qing Liu, chief of radiology, stood behind and between Wu and Tsai.*

been carried out in China (Table 1). This number is, of course, very small as compared with the United States, i.e., less than 40 per million of population in China as compared with 2,000 per million population in the United States.

Hypertrophic cardiomyopathy was an unfamiliar diagnosis in China until I introduced selective cine coronary arteriography in 1973 [35]. Three of the 11 patients catheterizaed because of exertional chest pain did not have any coronary artery obstruction but had hypertrophic obstructive cardiomyopathy. The first case of angiocardiographically documented hypertrophic cardiomyopathy in China was that of a 29-year-old man with chest pain, a soft mid-to-late systolic murmur without a click, and pulsus bisferiens. His coronary arteriograms were normal. But his left ventriculograms were typical of hypertrophic cardiomyopathy (Fig. 67). This disease entity is now encountered more and more often in China [199–203]. As a matter of fact, the interventional cardiologists in China have also become quite aggressive in treating these patients with the

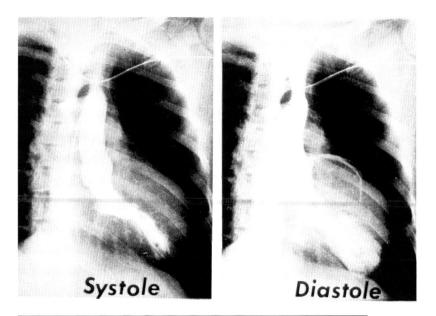

Fig. 67. *China's first case of hypertrophic cardiomyopathy showing the characteristic features on left ventriculography in systole (left) and diastole (right).*

percutaneous technique of transluminal septal myocardial ablation with one center alone reporting in early 2004 performance of such a novel procedure in 119 patients with excellent short- and long-term results [74]. At present, 700–800 such procedures have been carried out in more than 50 hospitals throughout China (Zhang WW, personal communication, May 19, 2005).

Mitral valve prolapse is another entity that was unknown in China until 1973 when I introduced selective cine coronary arteriography. Of the 11 patients with chest pain to undergo selective cine coronary arteriography, one had mitral valve prolapse. She was a young woman with typical auscultatory findings of mitral valve prolapse, namely, a midsystolic click and a late systolic murmur. In order to illustrate the various angiocardiographic features of mitral valve prolapse as well as to ensure that her coronary arteries were normal, I reluctantly agreed to perform coronary arteriography and left ventriculography on her. She had the typical angiographic features of mitral valve prolapse and as expected normal coronary arteriograms. Once my Chinese colleagues became aware of this entity which is prevalent all around the world [204], they began to carry out several epidemiological studies. They found an overall prevalence of 1.9% in schoolchildren in Guangdong [205], 4.3% in Hans in Sichuan [206] and 5.3% in Kazaks in Xinjiang [207]. They also found mitral valve prolapse to be more prevalent in women than men [205, 206]. Therefore, mitral valve prolapse is a global disease, including China [208]. As the old saying goes, one recognizes only what one looks for, one looks for only what one knows, and one then knows what more to look for. The heightened interest of cardiologists in China in mitral valve prolapse was refleced by the fact that I was invited to write a review article on the subject in the *Chinese Journal of Internal Medicine* which was published in 1988 [209] (Fig. 68). The emergence of mitral valve prolapse as a well documented entity in China is further evidenced by a recent disease prevalence study from 1948 to 1999 reported by Chen et al. [210] that, whereas mitral valve prolapse was not reported up to 1979, its prevalence was reported to be 0.1% in the 10-year period between 1980–1989 and 0.5% in the 10-year period between 1990–1999 (Table 2).

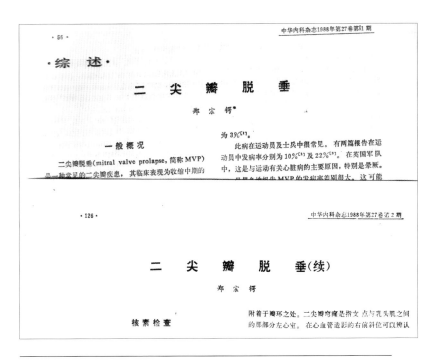

*Fig. 68. My review of mitral valve prolapse published in the* Chinese Journal of Internal Medicine *in two installments in 1988. The review was written by me in English and translated into Chinese by my classmate Yi-Jian Qian.*

## Chinese Cardiologist Delegation Visiting the USA in 1978

The first cardiologist delegation from China to visit the United States took place in November 1978 under the sponsorship of the US-China Physicians Friendship Association, of which Bernard Lown from Harvard was the president and I the treasurer. The delegation was comprised of authorities in their respective fields in China (Fig. 69). Among them were cardiologists (Ming-Hsin Huang, Jui-Lung Sun, Chih-Chiang Pien, Huan-Le Tao and Yi-Tsien Tsien), cardiac surgeons (Mei-Hsin Shih and Chi-Hua Chih), pulmonologist (Ju-Sheng Tsai) and biochemist (Ying-Shan Chang).

The first stop of the 24-day visit covering six cities across the United States was Washington, D.C. where the delegation visited the George Washington University Medical Center (Figs. 70 and 71).

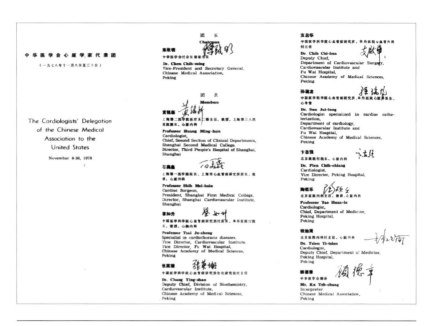

Fig. 69. Members of the Cardiologist Delegation of the Chinese Medical Association visiting the United States in 1978.

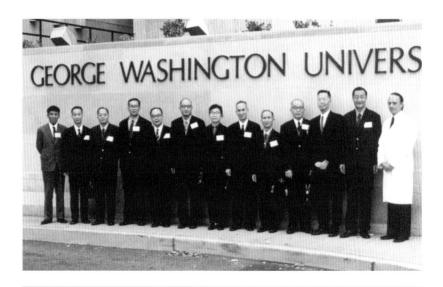

Fig. 70. The Chinese Cardiologist Delegation visiting the George Washington University Medical Center.

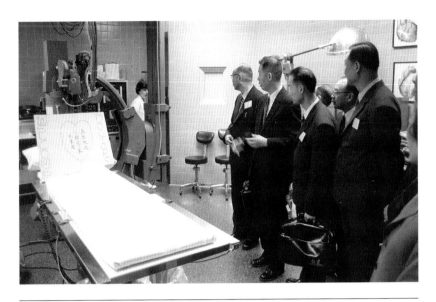

*Fig. 71. The Chinese Cardiologist Delegation visiting the cardiac catheterization laboratory, of which I was the director, of the George Washington University Medical Center.*

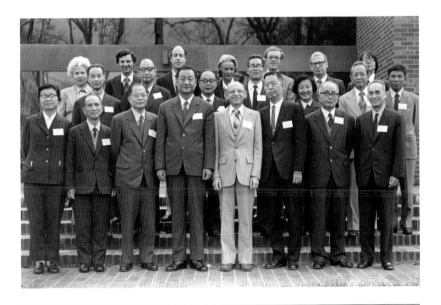

*Fig. 72. The Chinese Cardiologist Delegation visiting the American College of Cardiology and National Heart, Lung, and Blood Institute of the National Institutes of Health.*

Its members were also the guests of the American College of Cardiology at a special symposium organized in their honor in collaboration with the National Heart, Lung, and Blood Institute of the National Institutes of Health (Figs. 72 and 73). Eight members of the College presented informative talks on recent advances in their fields of expertise. A closing panel discussion permitted the Chinese visitors to question the faculty about specifics of the lectures. An evening banquet was attended by some 60 persons including Health Education & Welfare Assistant Secretary for Health Julius Richmond and Chinese Ambassador Xu Han of the Liaison Office of the People's Republic of China. From Washington, D.C. the delegation went on to Baltimore to visit the Johns Hopkins University Medical Institutions, my alma mater (Fig. 74).

In Texas, the delegates were the guests of honor at the 51st Scientific Sessions of the American Heart Association which convened in Dallas, November 13–16, 1978 (Fig. 75). One of the highlights of the meeting was a press conference during which both the Chinese and American cardiologists had a chance to compare information on medical management of heart diseases, frequency of heart attacks and life style factors that contribute to coronary heart disease. A lively discussion moderated by Elliott Rapaport, a past president of American Heart Association (Fig. 76), touched on topics ranging from cardiac surgery to herbal medications. Another highlight of the Dallas visit by the Chinese cardiologists was a pre-arranged meeting with the old China hand, Henry Kissinger (Fig. 77). From Dallas the delegation went on to Houston to meet Michael DeBakey (Fig. 78).

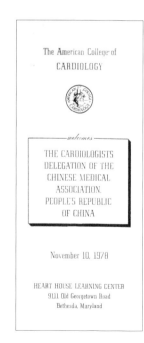

The American College of
CARDIOLOGY

*welcomes*

THE CARDIOLOGISTS
DELEGATION OF THE
CHINESE MEDICAL
ASSOCIATION,
PEOPLE'S REPUBLIC
OF CHINA

November 10, 1978

HEART HOUSE LEARNING CENTER
9111 Old Georgetown Road
Bethesda, Maryland

*Fig. 73. Special all-day symposium organized by the American College of Cardiology in honor of the Chinese Cardiologist Delegation's visit.*

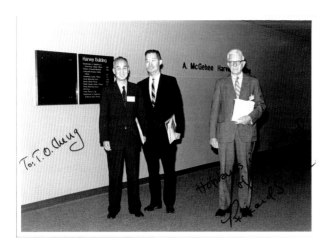

*Fig. 74. The Chinese Cardiologist Delegation visiting the Johns Hopkins University, my alma mater, upon the invitation of Dean Richard Ross.*

*Sessions of the*

# American Heart Association

**February, 1979**

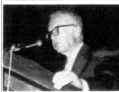

**Dr. Ross**

**Convention Reporter** is a single-purpose publication covering medical conventions and highlighting significant presentations and events for the benefit of the busy physician. This issue is devoted to the 51st Scientific Sessions of the American Heart Association, November 13,-16, 1978, in Dallas.

**Convention Reporter** is published by PW Communications, Inc., and distributed as a service by GEIGY Pharmaceuticals, Division of CIBA-GEIGY Corp., Ardsley, N.Y. The editorial content is the sole responsibility of PW Communications, Inc., 515 Madison Avenue, New York, N.Y., 10022.

## Chinese Cardiologists Detail Traditional Forms of Treatment

DALLAS — The largest selection of educational opportunities ever afforded those who treat heart disease greeted more than 15,000 scientists, physicians, nurses, exhibitors, and guests at the 51st Scientific Sessions of the American Heart Association which convened here, November 13-16, 1978.

AHA President W. Gerald Austen, MD, said the call for abstracts launched an overwhelming number of submissions — nearly 3,000 — of which 991 were presented at the convention. "These fine examples of responsible scientific investigation...illustrate both the high quality of the investigators involved and the equilibrium between basic research and clinical analysis that the Association strives to maintain," said Dr. Austen.

In addition to the scientific paper presentations, the AHA meeting encompassed postgraduate seminars, scientific exhibits, guest lecturers and the 3rd National Conference on Thrombosis and Hemostasis (see page 2).

One of the highlights of the meeting was a press conference with cardiologists hailing from the Peoples' Republic of China. A chance to compare information on medical management of heart disease, frequency of heart attacks, and

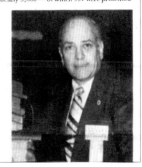

*Fig. 75. Newspaper clipping announcing the Chinese Cardiologist Delegation attending the American Heart Association Annual Scientific Meetings in Dallas.*

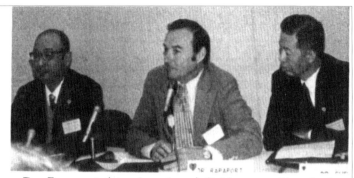

Dr. Rapaport (at microphone) fields a question during the press conference on cardiology in the Peoples' Republic of China. Tsung O. Cheng, MD, (r.), a frequent visitor to China, helped arrange this special AHA session. Dr. Cheng is professor of medicine at The George Washington University Medical Center, in Washington, D.C.

*Fig. 76, Press conference at the American Heart Association Scientific Meetings in Dallas.*

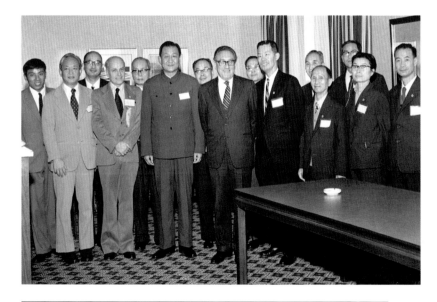

*Fig. 77. Meeting of the Chinese Cardiologist Delegation with Henry Kissinger at Dallas.*

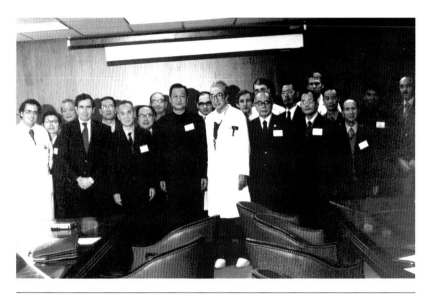

*Fig. 78. Chinese Cardiologist Delegation received by DeBakey (in white coat) in Houston.*

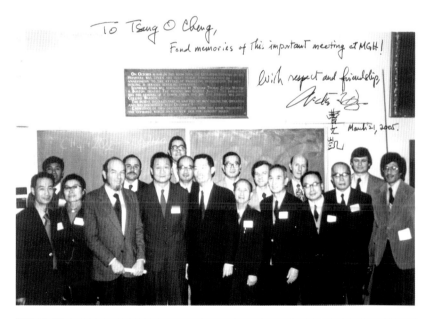

*Fig. 79. Chinese Cardiologist Delegation visiting the Massachusetts General Hospital in Boston; the photograph was taken in the historic Ether Dome (Dr. Victor Dzau at extreme right).*

In Boston, the delegation visited Harvard University Medical School and Massachusetts General Hospital where the group had a group photo taken at the historic Ether Dome (Fig. 79). Among the Harvard faculty members greeting the delegation was Victor Dzau, who was a junior faculty at Harvard then and one of the world's great medical visionaries who later became the chairman of medicine first at Stanford University and then at Brigham and Women's Hospital in Boston and most recently assumed the important post of Chancellor for Health Affairs and President and Chief Executive Officer of Health System at Duke University. The initial meeting of the Chinese delegates with Dzau at Massachusetts General Hospital left such a lasting impression on him that he has visited China quite a few times to lecture and exchange valuable information, the latest one being in November 2005 when he accepted an invitation to participate at the Great Wall International Symposium in Beijing despite his extremely busy schedule since assumption of the new executive position at Duke.

In New York City, the delegation visited the New York Hospital–Cornell Medical Center and Columbia University–Presbyterian Hospital where all the delegates were warmly welcomed by old and new friends.

Upon returning to China, the delegation made a report of what they saw and learned and their impressions of the state of cardiology in the United States that was published in 1979 in the *Chinese Journal of Internal Medicine* (Fig. 80). This report was of huge significance, because it was the first of its kind by the Chinese cardiologists reporting firsthand on the state of art in cardiology in the United States.

## American College of Physicians Teaching Delegation to China in 1979

The American College of Physicians sent its First Teaching Delegation to China in the Fall of 1979 upon the invitation of the Chinese Medical Association (Fig. 81). I was the leader of the delegation and Samuel Asper, the deputy executive vice president of the College, the deputy

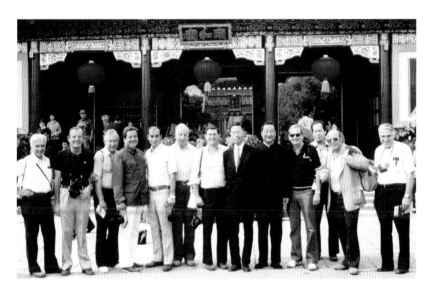

中华内科杂志1979年第18卷第2期 · 155 ·

· 国外医学动态 ·

美 国 心 血 管 内 科 的 一 些 新 进 展

中华医学会心脏病学家代表团应美中医师友好协会的邀请于1978年11月7日至30日赴美访问。曾在六个城市共十和小医学中心参观学习。美国医务界对这次访问很重视。他们接待热情，态度友好，介绍了心脏病学方面的成就，使代表团获益不少。

美国近二十年来在心脏病学的领域内进展很快，我们与之差距很大。因此必须加倍努力，迎头赶上。本刊根据代表团回国后所作的学术报告，选择在心血管内科方面进展较多的一些题目摘要介绍如下。

一、冠心病的病因及其预防的研究，近十余年来美国心脏血管疾病死亡率下降约30%，但冠心病仍居死亡原因的首位。他们认为影响冠心病死亡率的主要原因有三种，即高血压、高胆固醇血症及吸烟。其他的次要原因有糖尿病、高甘油三酯血症、缺乏运动、紧张的生活及姓族等。在美国国立心、肺、血研究所

烁照相机连续摄出⁹⁹ᵐ铥从上腔静脉经右心房、右心室、肺动脉、肺、左心房、左心室至主动脉的首次通过的图象。可以看出各房室的相对大小与解剖关系，借以瞭解心室的收缩功能。还可以推算射出比数。此法的优越性是检查时间短，只需30秒钟即能完成，适用于重笃病人及门诊病人。另一种是门电路控制的心脏血

*Fig. 80. A report of the 1978 visit by the Chinese Cardiologist Delegation published in the* Chinese Journal of Internal Medicine *the following spring.*

*Fig. 81. The First Teaching Delegation of the American College of Physicians to China in 1979. From left to right: Harry Shumacker, Edward Hook, Samuel Asper, Henry Wagner, Erza Amsterdam, Alexander Nadas, Allen Myers, Tsung O. Cheng, Chih-Ming Chen, Robert Rogers, John Salvaggio, David Bregman and Earl Wood.*

leader. Many members of the delegation were either cardiologists (Alexander Nadas from Boston Children's Hospital, Earl Wood and James Hunt from Mayo Clinic, Henry Wagner from Johns Hopkins University and Erza Amsterdam from the University of California at Davis) or cardiac surgeons (Harry Shumacker from Indiana University and David Bregman from Columbia University College of Physicians and Surgeons in New York City). Other members included a pulmonologist (Robert Rogers from the University of Oklahoma), an infectious disease specialist (Edward Hook from the University of Virginia at Charlottesville), an immunologist (John Salvaggio from Tulane University in New Orleans), and a rheumatologist (Allen Myers from Temple University in Philadelphia). F. Mason Sones from Cleveland Clinic, the father of selective cine coronary arteriography, was also to be a member of the delegation until the last minute when, much to his regret, a newly discovered eye problem forced him to withdraw (Fig. 82). However,

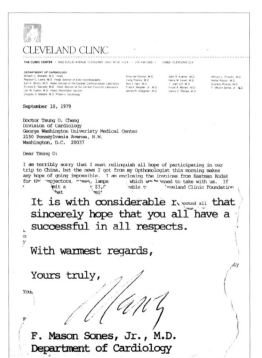

*Fig. 82. Letter of regret from F. Mason Sones announcing his last minute withdrawal from the First Teaching Delegation of the American College of Physicians to China due to a newly discovered eye problem.*

he contributed much of his time and effort in getting all the lecturing equipment ready for the delegation. The visit lasted nearly 4 weeks and covered five cities—Beijing, Chengdu, Chungking, Wuhan and Shanghai—including a 3-day cruise along the Yangtze River and the Three Gorges (Fig. 83), three decades before all these will be changed forever by the Three Gorges Dam Project, scheduled to be completed in 2009 [211].

There was a great deal of exchanges of valuable information between the American visitors and their Chinese counterparts during the visit. We utilized the 3-day cruise not only to review what we have accomplished but also to plan what more we should do. We gave lectures on the latest advances in medicine and cardiology. Among the various topics we covered were: two-dimensional real-time echocardiography, and Starling's law of the heart—its basis and relevancy to cardiology (both by E. Wood); nuclear cardiology (by Henry Wagner); the New England Regional Infant Cardiac Program, and cardiac catheterization in infants (both by A. Nadas); hypertension, and stroke (both by J. Hunt); Prinzmetal's angina and coronary artery spasm, and pitfalls in interpretation of coronary arteriograms (both by me); sudden cardiac death, and vasodilator therapy for heart failure (both by E. Amsterdam); infective endocarditis (by E. Hook); intraaortic balloon pumping, and mechanical support of the failing heart (both by D. Bregman); pericardiectomy, and management of arterial aneurysms (both by H. Shumacker); thyroid diseases (by S. Asper), rheumatic diseases, and immunosuppressive and immunomodulating therapy (both by A. Myers), and respiratory failure, and sleep apnea (both by R. Rogers)

The visit was an enormous success, so much so that at the Annual Scientific Meeting of the American College of Physicians in 1980 in New Orleans, a special China Exhibit was held to depict the various highlights of the visit (Fig. 84). It was well attended. The segment on cardiology drew the most attention. Furthermore, as a consequence of this visit, many young cardiologists from China were able to come to the United States to receive postgraduate training at various institutions where the different delegation members worked. As the

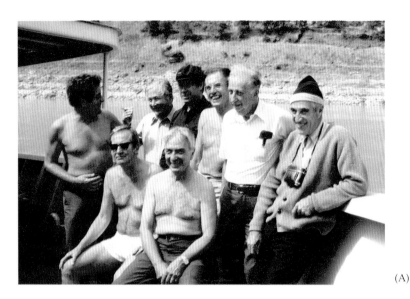

(A)

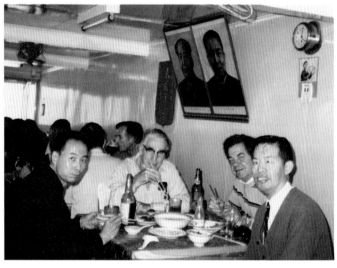

(B)

*Fig. 83. A, Some members of the American College of Physicians Teaching Delegation aboard the cruise ship along the Yangtze River past the Three Gorges. From left to right: Henry Wagner, Samuel Asper, John Salvaggio, Edward Hook, Alexander Nadas, Earl Wood (standing in back), James Hunt and Harry Shumacker (sitting in front). B, Two American cardiologists (Earl Wood and Henry Wagner) and two Chinese cardiologists (Rui-Long Sun and myself) having lunch in the ship's dining room under the watchful eyes of Chairman Tse-Tung Mao and Chairman Guo-Feng Hua.*

Chinese proverb says, "when planning for a year, sow rice; when planning for a decade, plant a tree; when planning for a life-time, train and educate people."

## National Institutes of Health–China Collaboration, 1980–2000

Soon after the formal establishment of diplomatic relation between the United States of America (USA) and the People's Republic of China (PRC), both governments signed an agreement in 1979 to cooperate in science and health. In 1980, a precious seed was planted in the area of cardiovascular research through cooperation between the USA's National Heart, Lung, and Blood Institute of National Institutes of Health and PRC's Cardiovascular Institute and Fuwai Hospital of Chinese Academy of Medical Sciences and Guangdong Provincial People's Hospital Guangdong Cardiovascular Institute of which I am an Honorary Director. The aim was to assess the prevalence and risks of cardiopulmonary diseases in more than 10,000 men and women living in urban areas in Beijing and Guangzhou and surrounding rural areas [212].

As Claude Lenfant, the USA Coordinator for USA-PRC Collaboration in Cardiopulmonary Research, said, "Our mutual interest in cardiopulmonary diseases stems from a joint concern about the growing threat that these diseases pose to the health of populations in both countries as well as many other nations. These diseases have extensive personal and social implications for large segments of the population not only in terms of unexpected deaths but also because they lead to chronic illness and loss of work capability, resulting in annual economic losses of hundreds of billions of dollars. The solutions to these health problems represent difficult challenges, and the goal of our joint studies has been to create the knowledge base and infrastructure that will allow public health leaders and policy makers to develop evidence-based risk reduction strategies and prevention programs for the future. Through exchanges of information and technology, exchange of scientists, highly standardized approaches to collection and analyses of data, and frequent joint working meetings in the USA and PRC, our scientists have produced valuable data bases and reports" [212]. Some of these have already been published in major peer-reviewed journals, in both English [213–222] and Chinese [223–232], and also presented to the world scientific community at major international meetings [233–240]. The results of these collaborative efforts are significant, because a framework of international linkage and a solid foundation for continued collaboration in research in cardiopulmonary diseases had been established. As Lenfant said, "our two decades of collaboration is no more than a small beginning in meeting the urgent cardiopulmonary health needs of our countries"[212] (Fig. 85).

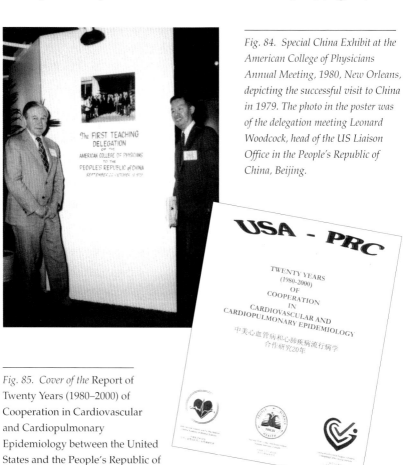

*Fig. 84. Special China Exhibit at the American College of Physicians Annual Meeting, 1980, New Orleans, depicting the successful visit to China in 1979. The photo in the poster was of the delegation meeting Leonard Woodcock, head of the US Liaison Office in the People's Republic of China, Beijing.*

*Fig. 85. Cover of the* Report of Twenty Years (1980–2000) of Cooperation in Cardiovascular and Cardiopulmonary Epidemiology between the United States and the People's Republic of China. (*Courtesy of Ruth J. Hegyeli*).

## Conclusion

In the preceding pages I briefly covered the development of cardiology in China from ancient times to modern era. Although the progress has been mostly evolutionary, the development in some fields is actually more revolutionary than evolutionary. Echocardiography is one such an example; the progress made in this subspecialty of cardiology under the able leadership of Xin-Fang Wang is truly phenomenal.

China has been called the "sleeping lion," because so little was known of many of its great accomplishments due to long periods of isolation from the rest of the world. As Napolean once said, "If China wakes, the sleeping lion will shake the world." The sleeping lion has indeed awakened, so the world better pay close attention, including cardiology in China.

## Acknowledgment

It is extremely difficult for a single individual to provide an authoritative account covering the full breadth of a rapidly evolving specialty such as cardiology in China. For this chapter I have repeatedly sought and frequently received advices and involvement of many of my colleagues, both inside and outside of China, whose invaluable assistance I wish to acknowledge. There are just too many to mention all by their names. Xie Xie!

## *References*

1. Cheng TO (2004) The current state of cardiology in China. Int J Cardiol 96:425–439.
2. Cheng TO (2001) Hippocrates and cardiology. Am Heart J 141:173–183.
3. Cheng TO (2001) Hippocrates, cardiology, Confucius and the Yellow Emperor. Int J Cardiol 81:219–233.
4. Cheng TO (1984) Glimpses of the past from the recently unearthed ancient corpses in China. Ann Intern Med 101:714–715.
5. Cheng TO (2002) Evidence of Type A personality in a Chinese lady who died of acute myocardial infarction 2,100 years ago. Texas Heart Inst J 29:154–155.
6. Bedford DE (1951) The ancient art of feeling the pulse. Br Heart J 13:423–437.
7. Cheng TO (1987) The international textbook of cardiology. New York: Pergamon Press.

8.  Cheng TO (1996) Medicine in China. Lancet 347:774.
9.  Hallstrom AP, Stein PK, Schneider R, et al. (2005) Characteristics of heart beat intervals and prediction of death. Int J Cardiol 100:37–45.
10. Cheng TO (2000) Decreased heart rate variability as a predictor for sudden death was known in China in the third century A.D. Eur Heart J 21:2081–2082.
11. Cheng TO (2000) Systolic and diastolic blood pressures and urinary sodium excretion in mainland China. Quart J Med 93:557–558.
12. Cheng TO (1989) Salt and blood pressure. Lancet 2:214–215.
13. Paul O (1986) Take heart: the life and prescription for living of Paul Dudley White, the world's premier cardiologist. Boston: Harvard University Press.
14. Hurst JW, Schlant RC (1990) The heart. New York: McGraw-Hill, p xxviii.
15. Fye WB (1996) American cardiology. Baltimore: Johns Hopkins University Press.
16. Tung CL (1931) The status of the heart in myxedema. Am Heart J 6:734–742.
17. Tung CL, Hsieh CK, Bien CW, Dieuaide FR (1934) The heart in ricksha pullers. A study of the effect of chronic exertion on the cardiovascular system. Am Heart J 10:79–100.
18. Abergel E, Chatellier G, Hagege AA, et al. (2004) Serial left ventricular adaptation in world-class professional cyclists: implications for disease screening and follow-up. J Am Coll Cardiol 44:144–149.
19. Whalley GA, Doughty RN, Gamble GD, et al. (2004) Association of fat-free mass and training status with left ventricular size and mass in endurance-trained athletes. J Am Coll Cardiol 44:892–896.
20. Abergel E, Hagege AA (2005) Detection of pathologic or physiologic left ventricular remodeling in athletes. J Am Coll Cardiol 45:1731.
21. Whalley GA, Doughty RN, Baldi JC (2005) Detection of pathologic or physiologic left ventricular remodeling in athletes—reply. J Am Coll Cardiol 45:1731.
22. Tung CL (1936) Transient auricular fibrillation as a toxic manifestation of digitalis. Am Heart J 12:272–284.
23. Tung CL (1941) The duration of electrical systole (Q-T interval) in cases of massive pericardial effusion. Am Heart J 22:35–46.
24. Tung CL (1937) The heart in severe anemia. Chin Med J 52:479–500.
25. Tung CL, Wu KH, Wang CY (1958) The relative incidence of atherosclerotic heart disease in east China and its relationship to cholesterol. Chin Med J 77:596–602.
26. Kannel WB, Castelli WP, Gordon T, McNamara PM (1971) Serum cholesterol, lipoproteins, and the risk of coronary heart disease. The Framingham Study. Ann Intern Med 74:1–12.
27. Burch GE, DePasquale NP (1964) A history of electrocardiography. Chicago: Year Book Medical.
28. Guo JH (2002) History of electrocardiology in China. Beijing: Peking Medical University Press.

29. Chen HZ, Yeh GY, Tao SC (1954) Myocardial infarction. Chin J Intern Med 3: 172–182.

30. Sun RL, Cai RS (1986) The practice of cardiac pacing and electrophysiology in Fu Wai Hospital, Beijing, China. Cardiac Impulse 7(3):9–10.

31. Cheng TO, Guo JH (2006) Catheter ablation for atrial fibrillation: the Chinese experience. Int J Cardiol 111:154.

32. Cappato R, Calkins H, Chen S A, et al. (2005) Worldwide survey on the methods, efficacy, and safety of catheter ablation for human atrial fibrillation. Circulation 111:1100–1105.

33. Chinese Society of Cardiology, Chinese Medical Association, Chinese Society of Cardiac Pacing and Electrophysiology, Chinese Society of Biomedical Engineering, Editorial Board of Chinese Journal of Cardiology (2005) The guidelines for the management of supraventricular arrhythmias. Chin J Cardiol 33:2–15.

34. Tang K, Zhang S (2005) The anatomic and electrophysiologcal characters of the coronary sinus. Chin Med J 118:404–408.

35. Cheng TO (1975) Paul D. White lecture—Cardiology in People's Republic of China. New horizons in cardiovascular practice (Russek HI, Ed.) Baltimore, University Park Press, pp 1–27.

36. Shan Q, Yang B, Chen M, et al. (2005) The electrophysiological study and implantable cardioverter defibrillator therapy for the patients with Brugada syndrome. Chin J Cardiol 33:34–36.

37. Cheng TO (1999) William Dock. Am J Cardiol 84:1215–1225.

38. Dock W, Mandelbaum H, Mandelbaum RA (1953) Ballistocardiography. The application of the direct ballistocardiograph to clinical medicine. St. Louis: Mosby.

39. Guo D, Yu G (1958) An introduction of the basic principle of ballistocardiography and construction of a prototype of a ballistocardiographic machine. Chin Med J 2:143–146.

40. Edler I, Hertz CH (1954) The use of ultrasonic reflectoscope for the continuous recording of the movement of heart walls. Kungl Fysiogr Sällsk Lund Förh 24: 40–58.

41. Feigenbaum H, Armstrong W, Ryan T (2005) Feigenbaum's echocardiography, 6th edn. Baltimore: Lippincott Williams & Wilkins, p 2.

42. Wang XF, Sheng RT (1963) Clinical application of ultrasonic cardiography—recording methodology. In: Wuhan Branch of Chinese Medical Association (ed) Corpus of ultrasonic thesis, pp 21–25.

43. Gao Y, Wang XF, Gao RY, et al. (1965) Characteristics of normal ultrasonic cardiogram and its changes in patients with mitral stenosis. Chin J Intern Med 13:710–714.

44. Hsu CC (1961) Ultrasonic diagnostics. Shang Sci Tech Press, p 167.

45. Hsu CC (1964) Preliminary studies on ultrasonics in cardiological diagnosis. I. Experimental observations on cardiac echo valves. II. The use of A-scope ultrasound apparatus in the diagnosis of heart disease. Acta Acad Med Prim Shanghai 2:251.

46. Wang XF, Wang JE (1973) First Hospital of Wuhan Medical College: The use of ultrasound in diagnosis of pericardial effusion. Chin Med J 7:411–414.

47. Feigenbaum H, Waldhausen JA, Hyde LP (1965) Ultrasound diagnosis of pericardial effusion. JAMA 191:711–714.

48. Wang XF, Xiao JP (1964) Ths use of fetal echocardiography for pregnancy diagnosis. Chin J Obstet Gynecol 109:267–269.

49. Winsberg F (1972) Echocardiography of the fetal and newborn heart. Invest Radiol 7:152–158.

50. Wang XF, Wang J, Huang Y, Cai C (1979) Contrast echocardiography with hydrogen peroxide. I. Experimental study. Chin Med J 92:595–599.

51. Wang XF, Wang JE, Lu CF, Chen HR, Huang YZ (1979) Contrast echocardiography with hydrogen peroxide. II. Clinical application. Chin Med J 92:693–702.

52. Wang XF, Wang JE, Lu CF, Chen HR, Huang YZ (1978) Contrast echocardiography with hydrogen peroxide in identifying cardiac anatomic structures. Acta Academiae Medicinae Wuhan 6:36–39.

53. Gaffney FA, Lin JC, Peshock RM, Bush L, Buja LM (1983) Hydrogen peroxide contrast echocardiography. Am J Cardiol 52:607–609.

54. Xu ZZ, Shen XD, Jiang L, Su BJ, Xu ZX (1981) Study of contrast echocardiography with $CO_2$ produced by vitamin C and sodium bicarbonate. Chin J Physical Med 3:193–199.

55. Hua ZQ, Du YZ, Qian YG, et al. (1982) Experimental study and clinical use of contrast echocardiography with acetic acid and sodium bicarbonate. Chin J Physical Med 4:1–4.

56. Meltzer RS, Serruys PW, Hugenholtz PG, Roelandt J (1981) Intravenous carbon dioxide as an echocardiographic contrast agent. J Clin Ultrasound 9:127–131.

57. Xu ZZ, Ding SZ, Zhang ZJ (November 1964) Preliminary report of limb intravascular examination by ultrasonic Doppler. Abstract corpus of national symposium on application of ultrasound, Beijing, pp 204–205.

58. Jin Y, Li X (1983) The use of ultrasonic pulse wave Doppler in diagnosis of heart diseases. Chin J Physical Med 5(3):171–176.

59. Ji R, Wang XF, Cheng TO, et al. (2002) Experimental study of assessment on ventricular activation origin and contraction sequence by Doppler tissue imaging. Journal of Huazhong University of Science and Technology [Med Sci], 22:52–57.

60. Cao QL, Jiang L (1989) The standard views and clinical use of transesophageal echocardiography. Chin J Med Imaging Technol 5(2):8–11.

61. Wang XF, Li ZA, Cheng TO, et al. (1992) Biplane transesophageal echocardiography. An anatomic-ultrasonic-clinical correlative study. Am Heart J 123:1027–1038.

62. Wang XF, Li ZA, Cheng TO, et al. (1994) Clinical application of three-dimensional transesophageal echocardiography. Am Heart J 128:380–388.

63. Cheng TO, Wang XF, Zheng LH, Li ZA, Lu P (1994) Three-dimensional transesophageal echocardiography in the diagnosis of mitral valve prolapse. Am Heart J 128:1218–1224.

64. Wang XF, Li ZA, Cheng TO, et al. (1996) Four-dimensional echocardiography: methods and clinical application. Am Heart J 132:672–684.

65. Cheng TO, Xie MX, Wang XF, Li ZA, Hu G (1997) Evaluation of mitral valve prolapse by four-dimensional echocardiography. Am Heart J 133:120–129.

66. Cheng TO, Xie MX, Wang XF, Wang Y, Lu Q (2004) Real-time 3-dimensional echocardiography in assessing atrial and ventricular septal defects: an echocardiographic-surgical correlative study. Am Heart J 148:1091–1095.

67. Xie MX, Wang XF, Cheng TO, Wang J, Lu Q (2005) Comparison of accuracy of mitral valve area in mitral stenosis by real-time three-dimensional echocardiography versus two dimensional echocardiography versus Doppler pressure half-time. Am J Cardiol 95:1496–1499.

68. Xie MX, Wang XF, Cheng TO, Lu Q, Yuan L, Liu X (2005) Real-time three-dimensional echocardiography: A review of the development of the technology and its clinical application. Progr Cardiovasc Dis 48:209–225.

69. Shen XD, Chen SB, Pan CZ, et al. (1993) To diagnose one patient with multiple aorto-arteritis and coarctation of aorta by intravascular ultrasonic imaging. Chin J Ultrasound Med 9:281.

70. Yin LX, Cai L, Li CM, et al. (2001) Cardiac conduction system excitation maps using intracardiac ultrasound catheter with tissue Doppler imaging: multiparametric imaging of electrical and mechanical activation. Chin J Ultrasonography 10:44–48.

71. Cheng LL, Shen XD, Pan CZ, et al. (1999) Echocardiographic guidance for closure of atrial septal defects with the Amplatzer occlusion device. Chin J Ultrasound Med 15:666–669.

72. Huang J, Li ZG, Wang ZG, et al. (1999) The biologic effects of myocardial ablation induced by low frequency ultrasound. Chin J Ultrasound Med 15:1–3.

73. He YL, Chen JY. Lin SG, et al. (2000). The value of percutaneous transluminal septal myocardial ablation in hypertrophic obstructive cardiomyopathy with echocardiography. Lingnan J Cardiol 6:185–187.

74. Li ZQ, Cheng TO, Zhang WW, et al. (2004) Percutaneous transluminal septal myocardial ablation for hypertrophic obstructive cardiomyopathy. The Chinese experience in 119 patients from a single center. Int J Cardiol 93:197–202.

75. Braunwald E (2005) Foreword. In: Hermann HC (ed) Interventional cardiology: percutaneous noncoronary intervention. Totowa, NJ: Humana Press, p v.

76. Huang W, Fang Q, Shao X, Sun W, Liu S (1953) Contribution of cardiac catheterization to the diagnosis of congenital heart disease. I. Principle and application of cardiac catheterization. Chin J Intern Med 3:161–174.

77. Tung CL, Tao SC, Chen HZ (1993) Practical Cardiology, 3rd edn. Shanghai Science & Technology Press, p 270.

78. Liu YQ, Xu JB, Guo DW, Wang ZY (1959) Development and achievement of contrast study of cardiovascular system during the latest 10 years in China—a review. Chin J Radiol 7:341–344.

79. Guo DW (1956) Rapid film changer for use in angiocardiography. Chin J Radiol 4:368–371.

80. Guo DW (1957) Angiocardiography. Chin J Radiol 1:10–19.

81. Liu YQ, Fang Q, Yu WN, Hu XD (1960) Angiocardiography: an analysis of 138 cases. Chin J Radiol 8:155–158.

82. Guo DW, Lin ML, Gu ZQ, Cheng TO (1984) Double-outlet right ventricle. A clinical-roentgenologic-pathologic study of 28 consecutive patients. Chest 85: 526–532.

83. Guo DW, Cheng TO, Lin ML, Gu ZQ (1986) Aneurysm of the sinus of Valsalva: a roentgenographic study of 105 cases. Circulation 74:II–403.

84. Guo DW, Cheng TO, Lin ML, Gu ZQ (1987) Aneurysm of the sinus of Valsalva: a roentgenologic study of 105 Chinese patients. Am Heart J 114:1169–1177.

85. Yu M, Gao R, Chen J, et al. (2003) Complications in selective coronary arteriography: analysis of 9196 cases. Natl Med J China 83:91–95.

86. Johnson LW, Lozner EC, Johnson S, Krone R, Pichard AD, Vetrovec GW, Noto TJ (1989) Coronary arteriography 1984–1987: a report of the Registry of the Society for Cardiac Angiography and Interventions. I. Results and complications. Cathet Cardiovasc Diagn 17:5–10.

87. Gao R (2002) Furthering the healthy development of percutaneous coronary interventions in China. Chin J Cardiol 30:705–706.

88. Section of Interventional Cardiology, Chinese Society of Cardiology, Editorial Office of Chinese Journal of Cardiology (2002) A data analysis of the Third National Coronary Intervention Registry. Chin J Cardiol 30:719–723.

89. Fleisher LA, Barash PG (2003) Treatment of coronary artery disease in the year 2003. J Cardiothorac Vasc Anesth 17:258–259.

90. Tan HQ, Liang Y, Zhu J, Liu LS (2002) Clinical characteristics of acute ischemic syndrome in China. Chin Med J 115:1123–1126.

91. Chen C, Chen J, Huang Z, Lo Z, Cheng TO (1987) Percutaneous transseptal balloon mitral valvuloplasty: the Chinese experience in 21 patients. J Am Coll Cardiol 9:83A.

92. Chen C, Lo Z, Huang Z, Inoue K, Cheng TO (1988) Percutaneous transseptal balloon mitral valvuloplasty: the Chinese experience in 30 patients. Am Heart J 115:937–947.

93. Cheng TO (1992) Percutaneous balloon valvuloplasty. New York: Igaku/Shoin.

94. Cheng TO (1994) Percutaneous balloon mitral valvuloplasty: are Chinese and Western experiences comparable? Cathet Cardiovasc Diagn 31:23–28.

95. Chen C, Cheng TO (1995) for the Multicenter Study Group: Percutaneous balloon mitral valvuloplasty using Inoue technique: a multicenter study of 4832 patients in China. Am Heart J 129:1197–1204.

96. Cheng TO (1996) Percutaneous balloon mitral valvuloplasty: the why, the when, the what and the which. Cathet Cardiovasc Diagn 37:353–354.

97. Cheng TO, Holmes DR Jr (1998) Percutaneous balloon mitral valvuloplasty by the Inoue balloon technique: the procedure of choice for treatment of mitral stenosis. Am J Cardiol 81:624–628.

98. Cheng TO, Chen CR (2000) Late results of percutaneous balloon mitral valvuloplasty: the Chinese experience. Circulation 102:e18.

99. Wang SC, Chou CE (1989) A brief overview of nuclear medicine in China. Semin Nucl Med 19:144–151.

100. Wang SC (1996) Nuclear medicine training in China. Eur J Nucl Med 23:1405–1407.

101. Wang SC, Chou C (2000) Current status of nuclear medicine in China. Chin Med J 113:387–391.

102. Liu XJ (1995) How to develop nuclear cardiology in China to a new stage? Chin J Nucl Med 15:4–5.

103. Liu XJ (1999) The advancement in nuclear cardiology. Chin J Nucl Med 19:129–130.

104. Cheng TO (1973) Medicine in modern China. J Am Geriatr Soc 21:289–313.

105. Hwang WS (1968) The rarity of pulmonary thromboembolism in Asians. Singapore Med J 9:276–279.

106. Nandi P, Wong KP, Wei WI, Ngan H, Ong GB (1980) Incidence of postoperative deep vein thrombosis in Hong Kong Chinese. Br J Surg 67:251–253.

107. Tso SC (1980) Deep vein thrombosis after strokes in Chinese. Aust N Z J Med 10:513–514.

108. Tso SC, Wong V, Chan V, Chan TK, Ma HK, Todd D (1980) Deep vein thrombosis and changes in coagulation and fibrinolysis after gynaecological operations in Chinese: the effect of oral contraceptives and malignant disease. Br J Haematol 46:603–612.

109. Woo KS, Tse LK, Tse CY, Metreweli C, Vallance-Owen J (1988) The prevalence and pattern of pulmonary thromboembolism in the Chinese in Hong Kong. Int J Cardiol 20:373–380.

110. Kueh YK, Wang TL, Teo CP, Tan YO (1992) Acute deep vein thrombosis in hospital practice. Ann Acad Med Singapore 21:345–348.

111. Liang Y, Zhao D, He S (2001) Trends of diagnosis and management of pulmonary thromboembolism in hospitalized patients in the last fifteen years. Zhonghua Jie He He Hu Xi Zazhi 24:269–272.

112. Cai B, Xu L, Guo S (2001) Trends of underline diseases of pulmonary embolism from Peking Union Medical College Hospital. Zhonghua Jie He He Hu Xi Zazhi 24:715–717.

113. Cheng TO (2007) Pulmonary embolism in the Chinese population. Int J Cardiol 116:123.

114. Ruan YM, Cheng XS, Shi WX, Zhang LZ, Liang FL (1991) A clinico-pathological analysis of 100 autopsy cases of massive or submassive pulmonary thrombo-obstruction in cardiovascular and pulmonary disease. Chin J Tuber Resp Dis 14: 5–6.

115. Cheng XS, Wang Q (1994) Experience of pulmonary embolism in China. In: Morpurgo M (ed) Pulmonary Embolism. New York: Marcel Dekker, pp 25–32.

116. Jia W, Li F, Cui T, Wang H (2002) An investigation on the misdiagnosis of pulmonary embolism in China. Chin J Cardiol 30:406–409.

117. Zhai Z, Wang C (2002) Nomenclature and defnition of pulmonary thromboembolism. Nat Med J China 82:1574–1575.

118. (2001) Guidelines to the Diagnosis and Treatment of Pulmonary Thromboembolism. Chin Tuberculosis Resp J 24:259–264.

119. Ren H, Su P, Zhang C, et al. (2005) Surgical treatment of chronic pulmonary thromboembolism. Chin J Surg 43:345–347.

120. Snapper I (1941) Chinese lessons to western medicine. New York: Interscience Publishers, p 160.

121. Cheng Y, Chen KJ, Wang CJ, Chan SH, Chang WC, Chen JH (2005) Secular trends in coronary heart disease mortality, hospitalization rates, and major cardiovascular risk factors in Taiwan, 1971–2001. Int J Cardiol 100:47–52.

122. Cheng TO (2001) Price of modernization of China. Circulation 103:e132.

123. Wang X, Fan Z, Huang J, Su S, Yu Q, Zhao J, Hui R, Yao Z, Shen Y, Qiang B, Gu D (2003) Extensive association analysis between polymorphisms of PON gene cluster with coronary heart disease in Chinese Han population. Arterioscler Thromb Vasc Biol 23:328–334.

124. Li J, Chen M, Wang S, Deng J, Zeng P, Hou L (2002) A long-term follow-up study of serum lipids and coronary heart disease in the elderly. Chin J Cardiol 30:647–650.

125. Zhao D (2003) Epidemiologic study of blood lipids in the Chinese population. Chin J Cardiol 31:74–78.

126. Chen GW, Cheng TO (2002) The textbook of modern cardiology, 2nd edn. China: Hunan Science & Technology Press, p 1546.

127. Rose G (2005) Incubation period of coronary heart disease. Int J Epidemiol 34: 242–244.

128. Luo Z (2002) Obesity: a warning to Chinese children. Beijing Review 45(26):14–16.

129. Popkin BM, Doak CM (1998) The obesity epidemic is a worldwide phenomenon. Nutrition Reviews 56:106–114.

130. Cheng TO (2003) Fast food and obesity in China. J Am Coll Cardiol 42:773.

131. Ma GS, Li YP, Hu XQ, Ma WJ, Wu J (2002) Effect of television viewing on pediatric obesity. Biomed Environ Sci 15:291–297.

132. Torpy JM, Lynm C, Glass RM (2003) JAMA patient page. Obesity. JAMA 289: 1880.

133. Yanovski JA, Yanovski SZ (2003) Treatment of pediatric and adolescent obesity. JAMA 289:1851–1853.

134. Cheng TO (2005) One-child policy and increased mechanization are additional risk factors for increased coronary artery disease in modern China. Int J Cardiol 100:333.

135. Shi H, Zhu Z (2003) Advances in research on hypertension and obesity. Program of National Congress on Prevention and Treatment of Obesity, Suzhou, China, pp 36–41.

136. Li G, Chen X, Jang Y, Wang J, Xing X, Yang W, Hu Y (2002) Obesity, coronary heart disease risk factors and diabetes in Chinese: an approach to the criteria of obesity in the Chinese population. Obes Rev 3:167–172.

137. Chinese Medical Associaton Subsection of Cardiovascular Disease, Chinese Journal of Cardiology Editorial Board (2002) Highlights of the second national conference on dyslipidemia. Chin J Cardiol 30:643–646.

138. Jia WP, Xiang KS, Chen L, Lu JX, Wu YM (2002) Epidemiological study on obesity and its comorbidities in urban Chinese older than 20 years of age in Shanghai, China. Obes Rev 3:157–165.

139. Zhou B, Wu Y, Yang J, Li Y, Zhang H, Zhao L (2002) Overweight is an independent risk factor for cardiovascular disease in Chinese populations. Obes Rev 3:147–156.

140. Cheng TO (2001) An obesity epidemic in modern China. Am J Cardiol 88:721–722.

141. Zhai F, Fu D, Du S, Ge K, Chen C, Popkin BM (2002) What is China doing in policy-making to push back the negative aspects of the nutrition transition? Public Health Nutr 5(1A):269–273.

142. Xia J, Tang D, Xia K, Tan S (1999) The achievements of medical genetic research in China during the past 50 years. Chin Med J 112:956–958.

143. Li YQ (1993) China launches genome project. Nature 365:200.

144. Cyranoski D (2001) A great leap forward. Nature 410:10–12.

145. Qiang BQ (2004) Human genome research in China. J Mol Med 82:214–222.

146. Niu T, Xu X, Cordell HJ, et al. (1999) Linkage analysis of candidate genes and gene-gene interactions in Chinese hypertensive sib pairs. Hypertension 33:1332–1337.

147. Xu X, Rogus JJ, Terwedow HA, et al. (1999) An extreme-sib-pair genome scan for genes regulating blood pressure. Am J Hum Genet 64:1694–1701.

148. Zhu DL, Wang HY, Xiong MM, et al. (2001) Linkage of hypertension to chromosome 2q14-q23 in Chinese families. J Hypertens 19:55–61.

149. Zhu D, Huang W, Wang H, et al. (2002) Linkage analysis of a region on chromosome 2 with essential hypertension in Chinese families. Chin Med J 115:654–657.

150. Chu SL, Zhu DL, Xiong MM, et al. (2002) Linkage analysis of twelve candidate gene loci regulating water and sodium metabolism and membrane ion transport in essential hypertension. Hypertens Res 25:635–639.

151. Pan WH, Chen JW, Fann C, Jou YS, Wu SY (2000) Linkage analysis with candidate genes: the Taiwan young-onset hypertension genetic study. Hum Genet 107:210–215.

152. Ge D, Yang W, Huang J, et al. (2003) Linkage analysis of 2q14-q23 and 5q32 with blood pressure quantitative traits in Chinese sib pairs. J Hypertens 21:305–310.

153. Yang W, Huang J, Ge D, et al. (2003) Variation near the region of the lipoprotein lipase gene and hypertension or blood pressure levels in Chinese. Hypertens Res 26:459–464.

154. Yang WJ, Huang JF, Yao CL, et al. (2003) Evidence for linkage and association of the markers near the LPL gene with hypertension in Chinese families. J Med Genet 40:e57.

155. Wang Q (2005) Molecular genetics of coronary artery disease. Curr Opin Cardiol 20:182–188.

156. Ridker PM (1997) Fibrinolytic and inflammatory markers for arterial occlusion: the evolving epidemiology of thrombosis and hemostasis. Thromb Haemost 78:53–59.

157. Cushman N (1999) Hemostatic risk factors for cardiovascular disease. In: Schechter GP, Hoffman R, Schrier SL, et al. (eds) Hematology 1999. Washington, DC: American Society of Hematology, pp 236–242.

158. Zhao J, Zhou X, Huang J, Chen J, Gu D (2005) Association study of the thrombomodulin −33G>A polymorphism with coronary artery disease and myocardial infarction in Chinese Han population. Int J Cardiol 100:383–388.

159. Esmon CT (1989) The roles of protein C and thrombomodulin in the regulation of blood coagulation. J Biol Chem 264:4743–4746.

160. Wen D, Dittman WA, Ye RD, Deaven LL, Majerus PW, Sadler JE (1987) Human thrombomodulin: complete cDNA sequence and chromosome localization of the gene. Biochemistry 26:4350–4357.

161. Ireland H, Kunz G, Kyriakoulis K, Stubbs PJ, Lane DA (1997) Thrombomodulin gene mutations associated with myocardial infarction. Circulation 96:15–18.

162. Li YH, Chen JH, Wu HL, et al. (2000) G-33A mutation in the promoter region of thrombomodulin gene and its association with coronary artery disease and plasma soluble thrombomodulin levels. Am J Cardiol 85:8–12.

163. Li YH, Chen JH, Tsai WC, et al. (2002) Synergistic effect of thrombomodulin promoter –33G/A polymorphism and smoking on the onset of acute myocardial infarction. Thromb Haemost 87:86–91.

164. Park HY, Nabika T, Jang Y, Kwon HM, Cho SY, Masuda J (2002) Association of G-33A polymorphism in the thrombomodulin gene with myocardial infarction in Koreans. Hypertens Res 25:389–394.

165. Yamada Y, Izawa H, Ichihara S, et al. (2002) Prediction of the risk of myocardial infarction from polymorphisms in candidate genes. N Engl J Med 347:1916–1923.

166. Normile D (2002) From standing start to sequencing superpower. Science 296:36–39.

167. Cheng TO (in press) Cardiovascular effects of Danshen. Int J Cardiol.

168. Cheng TO (1999) Warfarin danshen interaction. Ann Thorac Surg 67:894.

169. Cheng TO (1999) Herbal remedies. Am Fam Physician 60:1661.

170. Cheng TO (2000) Interaction of herbal medicine with coumadin. J Emerg Med 18:122.

171. Cheng TO (2000) Ginseng-warfarin interaction. Am Coll Cardiol Current Journal Review 9(1):84.

172. Cheng TO (2001) Comment: drug-herb interaction. Ann Pharmacotherapy 35:124.

173. Cheng TO (2004) Potential interaction between soy milk and warfarin. Am Fam Physician 70:1231.

174. Cheng TO (2005) Herbal interactions with cardiac drugs. Cardiol Rev 22:19–20.

175. Cheng TO (2006) Food-drug interactions. Int J Cardiol 106:392–393.

176. Cheng TO (2005) Herbal interaction with warfarin. South Med J 98:748. Erratum 2005;98:996.

177. Cheng TO (2005) Ginseng and other herbal medicines that interact with warfarin. Int J Cardiol 104:227.

178. Cheng TO (2000) Herbal interactions with cardiac drugs. Arch Intern Med 160:870–871.

179. Cheng TO (2000) St. John's Wort interaction with digoxin. Arch Intern Med 2000;160:2548.

180. Cheng TO (2002) Interaction of herbal drugs with digoxin. J Am Coll Cardiol 40: 838–839.

181. Cheng TO (2006) Herb digoxin interaction. Int J Cardiol 110:93.

182. Cheng TO (2000) Panax (Ginseng) is not a panacea. Arch Intern Med 160:3329.

183. Cheng TO (1973) Acupuncture anesthesia. Science 179:521.

184. Cheng TO (1973) Adequate ventilation with acupuncture anesthesia. Ann Intern Med 78:975–976.

185. Cheng TO (1974) A mini-symposium on acupuncture. JAMA 227:1123.

186. Cheng TO (1975) Acupuncture anesthesia for open heart surgery. Am J Cardiol 36:411.

187. Cheng TO (2000) Stamps in cardiology: acupuncture anaesthesia for open heart surgery. Heart 83:256.

188. Cheng TO (1998) Acupuncture treatment for angina. Cardiology 90:152.

189. Cheng TO (1998) Acupuncture for relief of angina. Circulation 98:2357–2358.

190. Cheng TO (1974) Cardiovascular Diseases. In: Quinn J (ed) China medicine as we saw it. Bethesda, Md: The Fogarty International Center, pp 261–288.

191. Yang J (1993) A doctor who laid a foundation for China's thoracic and cardiovascular surgery. Beijing Review 36(6):27–29.

192. Anonymous (1972) China's doctors on tour. Medical World News 13(47):34–48.

193. DeBakey ME (1974) A surgeon's diary of a visit to China. Phoenix, Arizona: Phoenix Newspapers, Inc.

194. Cheng TO (1997) Dr. Michael E. DeBakey is a great man. Am J Cardiol 80:394–395.

195. DeBakey ME, McCollum CH (1986) Diseases of the aorta and its branches. In: Cheng TO (ed) The international textbook of cardiology. New York: Pergamon Press, pp 829–863.

196. Zhang ZB, Cheng TO, Zhang YC (2003) Textbook of congestive heart failure. Beijing: National Science & Technology Publisher.

197. Cheng TO (1999) Doctor Y. K. Wu: father of cardiovascular surgery in China. Ann Thorac Surg 68:1439–1440.

198. Cheng TO (2005) Wu Ying-kai: Impact of one Chinese cardiothoracic surgeon and a passing star on the development of cardiology in modern China. Chin J Cardiol 32:971. Erratum 33:587.

199. Zou Y, Song L, Wang Z, et al. (2004) Prevalence of idiopathic hypertrophic cardiomyopathy in China: a population-based echocardiographic analysis of 8080 adults. Am J Med 116:14–18.

200. Ho HH, Lee KLF, Lau CP, Tse HF (2004) Clinical characteristics of and long-term outcome in Chinese patients with hypertrophic cardiomyopathy. Am J Med 116:19–23.

201. Cheng TO (2004) Prevalence of hypertrophic cardiomyopathy in China. Chin Med J 117:1600.

202. Cheng TO (2005) Hypertrophic cardiomyopathy in China: three decades of progress. Int J Cardiol 100:493–494.

203. Cheng TO (2005) Frequency of cardiac troponin I mutations in families with hypertrophic cardiomyopathy in China. J Am Coll Cardiol 46:180–181.

204. Cheng TO, Barlow JB (1989) Mitral leaflet billowing and prolapse: its prevalence around the world. Angiology 40:77–87.

205. Prevention and Treatment Region for Cardiovascular Diseases, Fanyu County, Guangdong (1983) Epidemiologic study of heart disease in 7,168 school children. Chin J Cardiol 11:33–35.

206. Du CL (1982) Prevalence of mitral valve prolapse syndrome among 1,600 healthy youngsters in Chengdu, Sichuan, China. New Med 13:10–11.

207. Zhou Y, Zu Z, Wang J, et al. (1983) Prevalence of mitral valve prolapse-click murmur syndrome among 2,001 Kazaks in Xinjiang. Chin J Cardiol 11:82.

208. Cheng TO (2004) Mitral valve prolapse. In: Conn's Current Therapy, 2004 edition. Philadelphia: Saunders 345–349.

209. Cheng TO (1988) Mitral valve prolapse. Chin J Intern Med 27:56–60 and 126–129.

210. Chen HZ, Fan WH, Jin XJ, Wang Q, Zhou J, Shi ZY (2003) Changing trends of etiologic characteristics of cardiovascular diseases among inpatients in Shanghai: a retrospective observational study from 1948 to 1999. Chin J Intern Med 42: 829–832.

211. Cheng TO (2005) Steven Nissen, Linda Butler, and Three Gorges of Yangtze in China. Am J Cardiol 95:437–438.

212. Cardiovascular Institute and Fu Wai Hospital, Chinese Academy of Medical Sciences; National Heart, Lung, and Blood Institute, National Institutes of Health; Guangdong Provincial People's Hospital, Guangdong Cardiovascular Institute (May 2001) USA-PRC Twenty Years (1980–2000) of Cooperation in Cardiovascular and Cardiopulmonary Epidemiology. Bethesda, Maryland: US Department of Health and Human Services, Public Health Service, National Institutes of Health.

213. Tao SC, Huang ZD, Wu XG, et al. (1989) CHD and its risk factors in the People's Republic of China. Int J Epidemiol 18 (Suppl. 1):S159–S163.

214. People's Republic of China–United States Cardiovascular and Cardiopulmonary Epidemiology Research Group (1992) An epidemiological study of cardiovascular and cardiopulmonary disease risk factors in four populations in the People's Republic of China. Baseline report from the P.R.C.-U.S.A. collaborative study. Circulation 85:1083–1096.

215. Tao SC, Li YH, Xiao ZK, et al. (1992) Serum lipids and their corrrelates in Chinese

urban and rural populations of Beijing and Guangzhou. Int J Epidemiol 21:893–903.

216. Folsom AR, Li YH, Rao XX, et al. (1994) Body mass, fat distribution and cardiovascular risk factors in a lean population of south China. J Clin Epidemiol 47:173–181.

217. Buist AS, Vollmer WM, Wu Y, et al. (1995) Effects of cigarette smoking on lung function in four population samples in the People's Republic of China. Am J Respir Crit Care Med 151:1393–1400.

218. Zhou B, Rao X, Dennis BH, et al. (1995) The relationship between dietary factors and serum lipids in Chinese urban and rural populations of Beijing and Guangzhou. Int J Epidemiol 24:528–534.

219. Davis CE, Williams DH, Oganov RO, et al. (1996) Sex difference in high density lipoprotein cholesterol in six countries. Am J Epidemiol 143:1100–1106.

220. Li Y, Stamler J, Xiao ZK, Folsom A, Tao SC, Zhang HY (1997) Serum uric acid and its correlates in Chinese adult populations, urban and rural, of Beijing. Int J Epidemiol 26:288–296.

221. Wu YF, Vollmer WM, Buist AS, et al. (1998) Relationship between lung function and blood pressure in Chinese men and women of Beijing and Guangzhou. Int J Epidemiol 27:49–56.

222. Rao XX, Wu XG, Folsom AR, et al. (2000) Comparison of electrocardiographic findings between Northern and Southern Chinese population samples. Int J Epidemiol 29:77–84.

223. Huang ZD, Sun JZ, He HM, et al. (1984) Epidemiologic study on hypertension, coronary heart disease, strokes and their risk factors in Guangzhou region. Guangdong Medicine 5:1–6.

224. Tao SC, Huang ZD, Lu CQ, et al. (1986) Relationship of timed overnight urinary sodium, potassium and blood pressure in middle-aged men and women in urban and rural populations of north and south China. Chin J Cardiol 14:4–7.

225. Zhou BF, Yang J, Cao TX, et al. (1986) Modified 24-hour recall dietary survey methods and its application in the study of cardiovascular epidemiology. Chin Publ Health 5:8–10.

226. Huang ZD, Zheng Y, Li YH, Cen RC, He HM, Rao XX (1987) Family inheritance of hypertension and its effect on the relationship between blood pressure and urinary sodium and potassium excretion. Guangdong Med 8:2–4.

227. Tsai RS, Chen XQ, Li YH (1987) Related problems in quality control of FVC, $FEV_1$ and $FEF_{25\%-75\%}$. Chin J Tuberculosis Resp Dis 10:10–13.

228. Deng DX, Huang ZD, Chen SG, Zhuo YL, Han WF (1987) Determination of blood lipids—standardization and quality control. Guangdong Med 8:10–14.

229. Huang ZD, Li YH, Rao XX, et al. (1988) Association of dietary intake and

hypertension, coronary heart disease, and stroke—a preliminary study in workers and farmers in Guangzhou District. Guangdong Med 9:2–6.

230. Zhou BF, Huang ZD, Li Y, et al. (1994) A comparative meta-analysis on the effects of dietary fatty acids and cholesterol on serum total cholesterol between Chinese and American population samples. Chin J Cardiol 22:20–23.

231. Wu YF, Tsai RS, Wu XG, et al. (1995) Is lung function impairment a risk factor of high blood pressure? Chin J Cardiol 23:332–335.

232. Rao XX, Tsai RS, Huang ZD, et al. (1996) Effects of smoking on lung function in populations of Beijing and Guangzhou. Chin J Tuberculosis Resp Dis 19:14–17.

233. Tao SC, Huang ZD, Taylor J, Stamler J (1986) Timed overnight urinary sodium and potassium excretion and blood pressure in two Chinese population samples. X World Congress of Cardiology, Washington, DC.

234. Tao SC, Huang ZD, Wu XG, et al. (1988) CHD and its risk factors in the People's Republic of China. Workshop on Trends and Determinants of Coronary Heart Disease Mortality, Bethesda, Maryland.

235. Huang Z, Warnick R, Zhou YL, et al. (1989) Lipid trends in south China. Second International Conference on Preventive Cardiology, Washington, DC.

236. Zhang K, Folsom A, Li Y, et al. (1992) Distribution and cardiovascular risk factors in a lean population of south China. 32nd Conference on Cardiovascular Disease Epidemiology, 1992.

237. Huang ZD, Wu XG, Rao XX, et al. (1993) North-south comparison of blood pressure in China. Third International Conference on Preventive Cardiology, Oslo.

238. Davis CE, Perova NV, Tao SC, et al. (1994) Relationship between lipids and education in women in six countries. International Symposium on Atherosclerosis.

239. Zhang HY, Li YH, Folsom A, et al. (1997) A prospective study of incidence and risk factors for stroke USA-PRC Collaborative Epidemiologic Study. 4th International Conference on Preventive Cardiology. Montreal.

240. Wu YF, Tao SC, Zhou BF, et al. (2001) Secular trends in cardiovascular disease risk factors in China: results from 15 years of the PRC-USA Collaborative Study. 5th International Conference on Preventive Cardiology, Osaka.

# Minimally Invasive Thoracic Surgery
# — A Personal Perspective

*Anthony P. C. Yim*

U nlike the other developments in cardiothoracic surgery detailed in the other chapters, minimally invasive thoracic surgery has a relatively short history. Also, unlike other innovations, minimally invasive surgery is not a procedure per se, but a new approach to the management of a wide variety of surgical diseases. This chapter is a personal reflection on the development of video-assisted thoracic surgery (VATS) in Hong Kong.

The organized adoption of the laparoscopic technique for thoracic surgery began in the late 1980s in the United States. However, this was only practiced in a few isolated centers and was not a popular approach. Therefore, during my training, I only read about this technique and had little practical experience of it.

When I returned to Hong Kong in 1992 and took up a surgical Lecturer position at The Chinese University of Hong Kong, I started to realize the potential of this technique in revolutionizing thoracic surgery in this part of the world. I was blessed to have the full support of the then Chairman of Surgery, Professor Arthur K. C. Li (who subsequently went on to become the Dean of Medicine, then Vice Chancellor of the University, and now the Secretary for Education and Manpower of the Hong Kong Special Administrative Region) to develop this technique at the Prince of Wales Hospital, the teaching hospital of The Chinese University of Hong Kong Medical School.

Together with the general surgeons (led by Professor Sydney S. C. Chung who later also became the Dean of Medicine), and the pediatric surgeons (led by Professor C. K. Yeung), we strived to develop together the minimally invasive surgery technique across different subspecialties. My first invitation to speak and operate in mainland China was in May 1993. I still have fond memories of the Second Affiliated Hospital of Hubei Medical University in Wuhan when I shared with them our results on VATS from Hong Kong. Shortly after that, I conducted a workshop with live demonstration of VATS lung resection in the People's Liberation Army General Hospital (301) in Beijing in April 1994.

The following decade saw me traveling frequently to China and other parts of the world to lecture and operate. It was a tiring but extremely gratifying time, and it became a highlight of my academic life. The first workshop on VATS in Hong Kong was organized by me at the Prince of Wales Hospital together with Professor Sydney Chung in November 1993. It was a resounding success and attracted a lot of attention not only from the surgeons, but from the chest physicians and oncologists. In 1995, we received a private donation to The Chinese University of Hong Kong from a well-known philanthropist Mr. Ka-Ping Tin to set up a visiting fellowship for thoracic surgeons in mainland China to come to Hong Kong to learn VATS. Up to 2006, twenty-five surgeons from various part of China have benefited through this program.

Apart from operating and traveling, I worked very hard in writing up this new technique. Another prolific writer in this field in Asia is Dr. Hui-Ping Liu. Hui-Ping is currently the Chief of Cardiothoracic Surgery at Chang Gung Memorial Hospital in Taipei, Taiwan. His hospital has 4,000 beds, and 80 operating rooms! I came across his papers very early on but didn't have a chance to meet him until June 1995 when we were both invited guests to the Third International Symposium of Thoracoscopic Surgery. We met inside a fast food shop lining up for order. As there were very few Chinese around, I started to chat to him and introduce myself. We soon became great friends, and have organized many symposia together since. Two symposia and workshops however worth special mention as they attracted many international delegates. The first was the First Asian Pacific Workshop on Minimally Invasive Thoracic Surgery held at the Prince of Wales Hospital on November 21–23, 1996. Drs. Rodney Landreneau, Michael Mack, Keith Naunheim, John Regan (an orthopaedic surgeon specializing in VATS spine surgery) from USA, Tsuguo Naruke and Tadasu Kohno from Japan were among the faculty (Fig. 1). Over forty talks as well as live demonstrations of VATS procedures were presented. The second meeting was the Second Minimally Invasive Thoracic Surgery Interest Group (MITSIG) International Symposium "Controversies in Cardiothoracic Surgery" held two years later, November 20–21, 1998 held at The Chinese University of Hong Kong Campus [1]. Over thirty international renowned experts serve on the faculty and they include very senior surgeons like Drs. Griffith Peason, John Benfield, Peter Pairolero and Thomas Ferguson from North America. One unique feature of this meeting was to allow pioneers in VATS and minimally invasive cardiac surgery to freely interact with the influential senior surgeons who have practiced conventional surgery throughout their

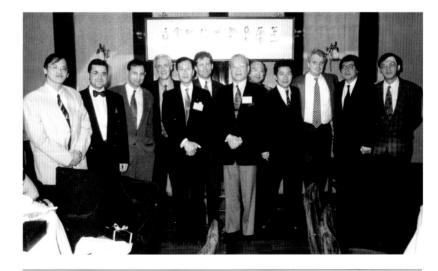

*Fig. 1.  From left: Drs. Hui-Ping Liu, Bashar Izzat, John Regan, Michael Mack, Anthony Yim, Keith Naunheim, Tsuguo Naruke, WY Lau, Tadasu Kohno, Rodney Landreneau, KM Ko, CC Ma.*

long careers. The scientific program was highly stimulating and Hong Kong was an attractive venue for the meeting. In fact, many participants still fondly remember this meeting up to this day. However, like other advances in surgery, the development of VATS was not without difficulties. The thoracic community in Asia, especially the senior surgeons tends to be highly conservative. This is understandable as operation in the mediastinum has little margin for error. These senior surgeons have spent most of their professional life learning, practicing and refining in their own way, conventional surgery through a thoracotomy. They are reluctant to change unless there is a compelling reason to do so. However, with the proven benefits of VATS, increasing demand from patients, and with the stepping down of the senior surgeons, I believe there will be a gradual adoption of VATS into mainstream thoracic surgery in China as time goes by.

One concern of adopting VATS in Asia is the high consumable costs. We have been a strong advocate of using conventional thoracic instruments. As opposed to laparoscopy, VATS on the whole, does not require carbon dioxide insufflation, and so few dedicated endoscopic instruments are absolutely necessary for VATS. Use of conventional instruments helps significantly in cutting down both consumable costs as well as time taken for the learning curve.

In recent years, we have advocated resecting a short segment of rib underneath the minithoracotomy to facilitate hilar dissection and retrival of the specimens. We have found this approach much less traumatic than rib-spreading, and we advocate to use this approach for difficult VATS cases (like re-operation) as well as to teach residents learning VATS major lung resections.

We as well as others have shown that patients who have undergone the minimal access approach for lung resection tend to survive longer than those who have undergone open surgery for cancer of the same early stage. We have researched into this intensively over the last few years. Our conclusion suggests that patients who have undergone keyhole lung resection can better preserve their body's immune function compared to open surgery. The Chinese commonly refer this to "元氣" or "internal energy" for which I believe we have now a scientific interpretation. The body's immune function is important for killing circulating tumor cells and this may be the reason why patients who have undergone minimal access surgery for cancer tend to survive longer. More work is urgently needed in this very exciting area. We are indeed witnessing a critical time of change in the practice of general thoracic surgery [2].

## *References*

1.  Yim APC, Lerut T, Wan S (eds) (1999) Proceedings of the second minimally invasive thoracic surgery interest group international symposium. Eur J Cardiothoracic Surg 16: (Supplement) S1–S130.
2.  Yim APC, Hazelrigg SR, Izzat MB, Landreneau RJ, Mack MJ, Naunheim KS (eds) (1999) Minimal access cardiothoracic surgery. USA, Philadelphia: W B Saunders.

# Heart Transplantation in China

*Wang-Fu Zang*

T he first case of orthotopic allogeneic heart transplantation in China, which was also the first one in Asia, was performed by Professor Shi-Ze Zhang and his colleagues at Ruijin Hospital of Shanghai Second Medical University on April 21, 1978. The patient lived for 109 days after the operation. Professor Zhang performed two other cases of heart transplantation thereafter, but both failed to achieve a longer survival.

In 1992 three heart transplantation operations were conducted independently at the Second Hospital of Harbin Medical University, Beijing Anzhen Hospital, and Mudanjiang Cardiovascular Hospital respectively. Only one of the three recipients survived long-term after the procedure (14 years until 2006, the longest survival in China to date). This particular operation was performed by Professor Qiu-Ming Xia of Harbin Medical University. Following this initial success,

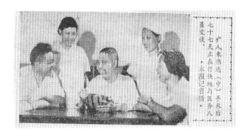

*Fig. 1. Professor Shi-Ze Zhang (left) with the patient (middle) who underwent the first heart transplantation procedure in China (1978).*

Professor Xia and his team continued their research in the field and completed the first case of bicaval orthotopic heart transplantation in China. They used both anterograde and retrograde normothermic oxygenated blood cardioplegia for donor myocardial protection. In 2001 Professor Xia won the Silver Award of Chinese National Scientific Achievement for his clinical and experimental research in heart transplantation. Their research on late coronary disease after heart transplantation is still on-going [1, 2].

By November 2006 the total number of heart transplantations in China had increased to above 450, with a 30-day success rate of around 95%, 1 year survival close to 90%, 3 year survival about 75%, and 5 year survival rate above 50% [3]. Heart transplantation has become a routine procedure at some hospitals such as Zhongshan Hospital in Shanghai, Fuwai Hospital in Beijing and the Union Hospital in Xiamen, Fujian.

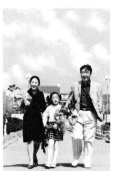

*Fig. 2. Recent picture of the patient (right) who underwent heart transplantation at the Second Hospital of Harbin Medical University on April 26, 1992.*

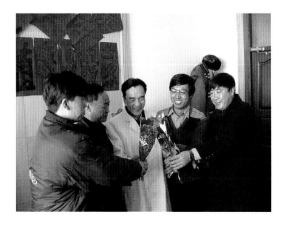

*Fig. 3. Professor Qiu-Ming Xia (middle) with four of his patients, three of them have survived more than 10 years (till early 2006).*

# *References*

1. Zang WF, Xia QM (2004) The treatment level of heart transplantation in China should be further raised. Nat Med J Chin 84 35–1586 (in Chinese).
2. Zang WF, Xia QM, Yao ZF, et al. (2000) Bicaval orthotopic heart transplantation. Chin J Org Transplant 20:55–56 (in Chinese).
3. Wang CS, Chen H, Hong T, et al. (2006) Orthotopic heart transplantations for end-stage heart diseases. Chin J Organ Transplant 27:152–155 (in Chinese).

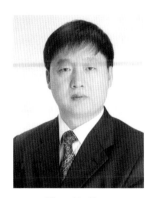

Wang-Fu Zang

# Lung Transplantation in China

*Song-Lei Ou, Song Wan*

**W**hile Norman Bethune was trying "to take peasants (boys) and young workers and make doctors out of them" in 1938 (see Editorial Comments in p. 72 of this book), probably nobody including Bethune himself seriously expected that some of these boys would become famous physicians in the years to come. The fact is, however, that one of Bethune's assistants grew up to be a leading thoracic surgeon in China and eventually performed the country's very first lung transplantation operation four decades later!

Yu-Ling Xin joined the Eighth Route Army at the age of 16 years (Fig. 1), where he had the chance to personally assist and observe Dr. Bethune saving many wounded soldiers. The impact of such a unique experience on Xin's surgical career was evident, as Bethune became his life-long role-model. He subsequently studied medicine at China Medical University (starting in Yan'an in 1942 and graduating in 1947 in Xingshan, Heilongjiang Province). In 1951 he was among the first

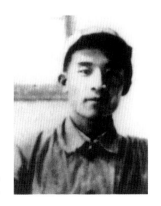

*Fig. 1. Yu-Ling Xin in 1938.*

group of students sent to Moscow, former Soviet Union, for advanced specialty training. His subject elect was thoracic surgery (Figs. 2A, B). With a doctorate degree, Xin returned to China in June 1956 and was soon appointed the chief of thoracic surgery at the Beijing Institute for Treatment of Tuberculosis and Thoracic Tumors.

During the last year of his stay in Moscow, Xin completed more than 30 lung resection operations (for pulmonary tuberculosis) under supervision, which was quite a remarkable record among the young surgeons there. However to Xin himself a more impressive experience was the repeated visits to the Laboratory for Organ Transplantation at the Sklifosovsky Emergency Institute, of which Dr. Vladimir P. Demikhov was the director. The outstanding accomplishments in the field of experimental transplantation research by Demikhov and his devoted team made exceedingly stimulating viewing for Xin. He once witnessed the whole procedure of dog head transplantation and was amazed by the immediate outcome. He was dreadfully excited to find out the "surviving signs" of the transplanted head as reflected

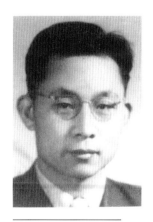

Fig. 2A. Dr. Xin in 1956.

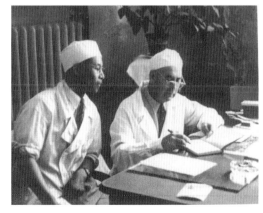

Fig. 2B. Xin with his supervisor in Moscow.

by the batting of its eyelid. Demikhov's surgical virtuosity and innovation became a driving force for Xin to embark on his dream work, namely lung transplantation.

Soon after his returning to Beijing, Xin started to plan and prepare for the experimental research. The building-up of an animal laboratory was completed in 1958. The initial project was lobar lung transplantation in dogs. However only a few dogs survived more than 10 days after surgery. Most of the other dogs died of pulmonary vein thrombosis, dehiscence of the bronchial sutures, or pneumonia. Moreover, problems were not limited to the surgical field. An unexpected "political movement" occurred in China in 1959 and every scientific activity came to a complete halt.

Xin was unable to continue his research until late 1962. This time he and his colleagues decided to try single lung transplantation in a monkey model. The first group of 50 monkeys were bought from Yunnan Province and transferred to Beijing by train. Unfortunately more than half of the monkeys died before arrival, due to inadequate care during the long-distance transportation which lasted for several days. Learning from this experience, the second group of monkeys was sent to Beijing by air and they all arrived safely. The surgical results in the monkeys appeared much better than that in the dogs. One of the surviving recipients even got pregnant after single lung transplantation and delivered a baby monkey uneventfully.

Other interesting clinical works were conducted simultaneously over this period of time. One of them that Dr. Xin was deeply involved in was the project entitled "Thoracic Surgery under Acupuncture Anesthesia." As it is under the flag of traditional Chinese medicine, this innovative technique was then widely advocated and strongly supported by the government. Xin was assigned to lead the project in Beijing and soon became a national figure in this area (Fig. 3). He and his colleagues performed 1,250 thoracic operations under acupuncture anesthesia from 1965 through 1982 [1]. Among these cases, the most famous one was a right upper lobectomy for a male patient with bronchiectasis at the Third Hospital of Beijing Medical University on February 24, 1972. The entire procedure was witnessed by an American delegation of some 30 visitors (Fig. 4), including

General Hegel and many international journalists who were accompanying President Richard Nixon on an ice-breaking visit to China. Some of the visitors even interviewed that particular patient before he was sent to the operating room to ensure that no pre-induction of anesthesia was provided on the ward. Apparently all the visitors were genuinely impressed by the effects of acupuncture anesthesia.

In the late 1970s Xin and his team continued the experimental investigation of single lung or lobar lung transplantation in dogs. In total they performed transplant operations in 90 dogs. Lung preservation techniques and postoperative monitoring and

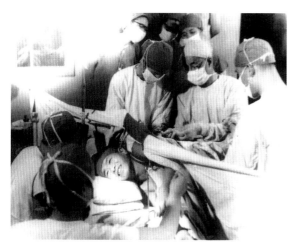

*Fig. 3. Dr. Xin (2nd from right) performing lung resection operation under acupuncture anesthesia.*

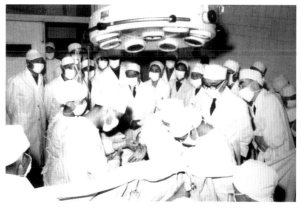

*Fig. 4. American visitors observing a lobectomy operation under acupuncture anesthesia at Beijing Medical University on February 24, 1972.*

immunosuppression were also studied [2]. Over the same period of time Jia-An Ding and colleagues [3] in Shanghai also reported their research experiences on left lung transplantation in 58 dogs, although there was only one long-term survivor in this series.

Xin and colleagues decided to explore the area of clinical lung transplantation in 1979. Within the same year they performed the first two cases in mainland China. The first patient was a 31-year-old lady with a completely damaged left lung secondary to severe pulmonary tuberculosis. She was repeatedly admitted to the hospital due to massive hemoptysis, and was found to have multiple cavities in the upper lobe of her right lung. A left lung transplant operation was scheduled on January 13, 1979. The procedure turned out to be extremely challenging as the entire diseased left lung was adherent to the chest wall, requesting extra-pleural dissection. The operation lasted 5 hours and 45 minutes, with a total blood loss of 3.8 litres. The graft ischemic time was 4 hours and 15 minutes. On the first postoperative day the patient needed tracheostomy. Her condition remained stable until postoperative day 5 when the transplanted lung deteriorated with chest X-ray signs of "white-out," despite multiple doses of steroids. The left lung was excised on postoperative day 7 and its pathology confirmed acute rejection. Eventually the patient was discharged home a few months later [4].

The second case, a 22-year-old woman, had very similar history as the first one. Since the size of the donor lung was much bigger than the lung of the recipient only a left lower lobar lung transplant procedure was performed, on November 17, 1979. The graft ischemic time was only 1 hour and 47 minutes. However the patient experienced acute rejection exactly as in the first one. Repeated high doses of steroids showed no therapeutic effects. The transplanted lobe was excised on postoperative day 12. Unfortunately, she died of acute embolism to the right pulmonary artery on postoperative day 32 [5]. Although both cases were performed before Cyclosporin A was available in China, analyzing retrospectively Dr. Xin wished some lessons had been learned earlier. In particular, the indication for lung transplantation in patients with severe pulmonary tuberculosis is debatable (personal communications).

Over the next 15 years there were several additional attempts at lung transplantation at different centers in mainland China, but none of them achieved a survival of longer than a month.

Strongly encouraged by Professor Ying-Kai Wu (Founding President of Anzhen Hospital), the thoracic surgeons at Anzhen Hospital in Beijing started their adventure in 1992. Led by Professor Yu-Ping Chen, the Anzhen team performed a left single lung transplant operation for a 48-year-old man with idiopathic pulmonary fibrosis on February 23, 1995 (Figs. 5A, B). Up to date (early 2006), this case holds the record for long-term survival after single lung transplantation in mainland China [6]. Five years and 11 months after the operation, the patient died of liver cirrhosis secondary to hepatitis B.

On January 20, 1998, Yu-Ping Chen and colleagues performed another double-lung transplant operation with the use of cardiopulmonary bypass for a 28-year-old man with primary pulmonary hypertension. The patient's wedding had occurred just

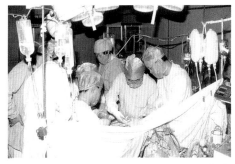

*Fig. 5A. The Anzhen Hospital team, led by Yu-Ping Chen (2nd from right), performed a single lung transplantation operation in February 1995.*

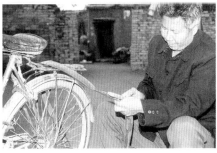

*Fig. 5B. The patient survived for almost 6 years after lung transplantation.*

months earlier. Prior to the operation, the patient's pulmonary arterial pressure measured 153/55 mmHg and his pulmonary vascular resistance was 44.4 Wood units. Despite experiencing many postoperative morbidities during his prolonged hospital stay, the patient was successfully discharged home (Fig. 6A). He survived 4 years and 3 months after the operation. During that period he enjoyed a relatively good quality of life with his wife and his son (Fig. 6B). So far this case is the first long-term survivor after double-lung transplantation in mainland China [7].

By October 2005, 93 patients had undergone single- or double-lung transplant operations in mainland China. Major centers include the 5th Hospital in Wuxi (26 cases), Anzhen Hospital in Beijing (16 cases), Shanghai Chest Hospital (15 cases), Shanghai Pulmonary Hospital (14 cases), and Guangzhou Institute for Respiratory Diseases (8 cases). Compared with the current international standard, many lung transplantation programs in China are still in the infancy stage. Nevertheless we should always bear in mind what was said by a Chinese philosopher 2,300 years ago—"without the accumulation of small steps, a 1000-mile journey cannot be finished." To catch up, keep going!

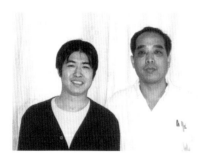

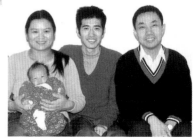

Fig. 6A. *The patient (after double-lung transplant operation) with Dr. Zhi-Tai Zhang (right) at Anzhen Hospital.*

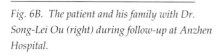

Fig. 6B. *The patient and his family with Dr. Song-Lei Ou (right) during follow-up at Anzhen Hospital.*

# References

1.  Xin YL (1985) The application of acupuncture anesthesia in lung resection operations. In: Wu YK, Peters RM (eds) International practice in cardiothoracic surgery. Beijing: Science Press, pp 75–78.
2.  Xin YL, Hu QB, Cheng XJ, Huang ZY (1981) Experimental allograft lung transplantation in dogs. Chin J Organ Transplant 2:70–72 (in Chinese).
3.  Ding JA, Gu DC, Gan XP, et al. (1985) Experimental research on lung transplantation in dogs. Chin J Organ Transplant 6:27–29 (in Chinese).
4.  Xin YL, Cai LP, Hu QB, et al. (1979) Human lung transplantation: a case report. Chin J Surg 17:328–392 (in Chinese).
5.  Xin YL, Cai LP, Zhao ZW, et al. (1981) The second case report of human lung transplantation. Chin J Organ Transplant 2:4–6 (in Chinese).
6.  Chen YP, Zhang ZT, Han L, et al. (1996) Lung transplantation for pulmonary fibrosis: a case report. Chin J Surg 34:25 (in Chinese).
7.  Chen YP, Zhou QW, Hu YS, et al. (1998) Double-lung transplantation for the treatment of primary pulmonary hypertension. Chin J Thorac Cardiovasc Surg 14: 321–323 (in Chinese).

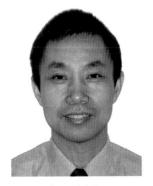

Song-Lei Ou

# Cellular Therapy for Heart Failure

*Ren-Ke Li, Chung-Dann Kan*

D espite many breakthroughs in cardiovascular medicine, congestive heart failure (CHF) secondary to ventricular remodeling post-myocardial infarction continues to be a serious medical health problem worldwide [1]. Among most developed countries, CHF affects about 0.4% to 2% of the adult general population [2, 3]. The incidence of CHF is increasing, not only because of an aging population, but also because effective palliative therapies are extending the lives of many patients [3].

After an acute myocardial infarction, the damaged myocardium usually progresses through a cascade of remodeling events including inflammation, cardiomyocyte apoptosis, non-contractile fibrous scar formation, and redistribution of the workload of the surviving myocardium (compensation). If the infarct is large, the remodeling process leads to dilatation of the ventricular lumen, and ultimately, to decompensation and deterioration of the heart [4, 5]. At the end stage, CHF is a syndrome of extremely low heart output, shortness of breath, and swelling in the extremities that cannot be effectively treated by traditional medical or surgical methods. At this stage, heart transplantation or a mechanical cardiac assisted device may be the only viable alternatives [3].

Heart transplantation has been shown to be an effective means of improving quality of life and survival in end stage heart failure patients [6], but organ shortage unfortunately limits the application of the technology [7], and the use of immunosuppressive drugs can produce major adverse effects in the recipients [8]. In patients with end-stage heart failure who were ineligible for transplantation, the Randomized Evaluation of Mechanical Assistance in the Treatment of Congestive Heart Failure (REMATCH) trial demonstrated that left-ventricular assist device (LVAD) implantation was superior to available medical therapies [9]. "Destination Therapy", which uses LVADs or artificial hearts as an alternative to transplantation has benefited patients with end-stage heart disease [6]. Although LVADs have been proposed as "a bridge to recovery", they are also associated with significant complications, such as: bleeding, infection, multi-organ failure, device dysfunction and infectious complications [9]. In addition, recurrent heart failure following the removal of the LVADs has limited this approach.

Since functional restoration of the damaged heart presents a formidable challenge, developing strategies for the prevention of post-infarction heart failure remains of utmost priority. While pre-clinical studies on gene therapy either for the prevention of heart failure or the improvement of heart function were initially promising, few such gene therapies were proven safe and effective in clinical trials [10–12].

Newts can regenerate and rebuild their damaged hearts. Taking the newt as a model for regenerating irreversibly damaged myocardium, processes such as de-differentiation, proliferation, and re-differentiation of cardiac cells might be the basis of future strategies for rebuilding the failing human heart [13]. In mammals, an efficient embryonic cardiac cell proliferation and tissue reconstruction process could lead to the reconstitution of structurally and functionally normal tissue following cardiac injury. Unfortunately, this extraordinary ability for cardiomyocyte growth and differentiation is lost at birth [14]. In adulthood, the pathophysiological reaction to myocardial infarction includes cardiomyocyte necrosis, akinetic fibrotic scar formation, and eventually heart failure. Thus, in the early 1990s, transplantation of exogenous cells with inherent contractile element forming ability was proposed as a treatment to increase contractility and cardiac performance, and as a potential cure for the syndrome of heart failure [15]. The term "cellular cardiomyoplasty" evolved based on the hypothesis that cells of myogenic ancestry or with the capacity to differentiate into myocytes can be transplanted into infarcted regions of the heart to prevent heart failure [16]. Cellular cardiomyoplasty, or cell therapy, has undergone extensive investigation and clinical trials within the last decade.

Both pre-clinical and clinical studies have demonstrated improved heart function with cell therapy after myocardial injury. However, several important practical considerations have not yet been addressed: Which cell type will be the most effective? When is the most appropriate time after injury to implant cells? What are the optimal techniques to most effectively deliver the cells to the damaged area? In this chapter, we will review the development of various types of cells for cell therapy, the current techniques for cell delivery, and the future of cell therapy for the treatment of heart failure.

## Historical Development of Cell Therapy for Myocardial Regeneration

The term "cellular cardiomyoplasty" was initiated in the early 1990s based on a hypothesis that cells of myogenic ancestry or with the capacity to differentiate into myocytes can be transplanted into infarcted regions of the heart to prevent heart failure [16]. Here, we review the characteristics and potential of a number of cell types for cell therapy currently under investigation.

### 1) Skeletal Myoblasts

Adult skeletal muscle retains an efficient regenerating mechanism. Each mature skeletal myofiber bears a few quiescent skeletal myoblasts (satellite cells), which exist in an undifferentiated state under the basal lamina (Figure 1A). Following skeletal muscle injury, the skeletal myoblasts enter the mitotic cycle, and fuse with each other and/or with damaged myofibers. The newly formed myofibers repair damaged muscle tissue and restore contractile function [17].

Skeletal myoblasts exhibit several characteristics that qualify them as potential precursor cells to repair the damaged myocardium: a capacity to proliferate and differentiate to muscle cells *in vitro* and form muscle tissue in vivo, an autologous origin, a resistance to ischemia, and a minimal risk of developing tumors. In addition, large-scale commercial clinical applicability and the lack of associated ethical issues have favored the use of skeletal myoblasts in cellular cardiomyoplasty studies.

Chiu's research team in Montreal, Canada, was the first to examine the effects of skeletal myoblast transplantation into the damaged myocardium [16], demonstrateding that the implanted cells could survive in myocardial scar tissue created by cryoinjury [16, 18]. To date, many experimental studies have been devoted to skeletal myoblast transplantation. Morphologically, the grafted myoblasts tend to differentiate into typical multinucleated myotubes and repopulate the areas of fibrotic tissue [19]. Koh et al. and Murry et al. demonstrated that skeletal myoblasts might integrate into cardiac muscle with the formation of intercalated discs [20–23]. Reinecke et al. reported that N-cadherein and connexin-43 were down-regulated in cultured skeletal myoblasts following intramyocardial implantation, and showed that the skeletal myoblasts fused with cardiac muscle cells *in vivo* in a murine model [23–24].

Several pre-clinical studies demonstrated that myoblast transplantation contributes significantly to the improvement of cardiac function—principally systolic function, but in some cases diastolic function as well [25]. In addition, the functional benefits of myoblast grafting seem to be sustained over time [26]. The mechanisms by which implanted myoblasts improve cardiac function have not yet been elucidated, but may involve the implanted cells acting as a scaffold strengthening the ventricular wall and limiting post-infarct scar expansion [19, 27]. Also, the fusion of myoblasts with cardiomyocytes and their interaction with host cardiomyocytes through the extracellular matrix serve as platforms to release growth and/or angiogenic factors [19, 27]. Although the mechanism is not completely understood, the potential usefulness of myoblasts for cellular therapy in the infarcted heart has been clearly demonstrated by studies in diverse animal models.

A phase I feasibility and safety human trial of autologous myoblast transplantation into infarcted myocardium was reported by Menasche et al. [28], who demonstrated that implanted human myoblasts formed muscle in the implanted area [29]. However, several episodes of sustained ventricular fibrillation were observed in multiple patients [28, 30, 31]. Although a direct correlation between the arrhythmia and the cell transplantation was not identified, several phase I and phase II clinical studies now include the implantation of an automatic cardio-defibrillator [25, 30].

## 2) Cardiomyocytes

Transplanting fetal or neonatal cardiomyocytes (Figure 1B) can be regarded as the primary model of cellular cardiomyoplasty [13]. These cells retain the ability to proliferate and, being of myocardial origin, might have the capacity to form contractile tissue in damaged myocardium. In the initial study, Li et al. transplanted fetal rat cardiomyocytes into the subcutaneous tissue of the rat hind limb. They found that the transplanted cells survived and beat spontaneously at the implanted area [32]. The spontaneously contracting cells formed a tissue with sarcomeres, which increased in size [33].

To evaluate the survival and integration of the implanted cells with host myocardium, Soonpaa et al. and Lero et al. grafted cardiomyocytes into normal mouse hearts and into an infarcted region of rat hearts [34, 35]. They demonstrated that the implanted cells survived and formed junctions with the host cardiomyocytes. In 1996, Li et al. reported that cardiomyocyte transplantation can improve heart function [36]. In this study, the implanted cells survived in the myocardial scar tissue and formed viable myocardial tissue, which limited scar expansion and induced blood vessel formation. Several investigators have since demonstrated that cell transplantation can improve left ventricular performance in the infarcted heart [36–39], and increase vascularization (arterioles, venules and capillaries) in the graft. Based on these findings, myogenesis and angiogenesis after cardiomyocyte transplantation have been proposed as possible mechanisms of heart failure prevention [33, 40–42].

There are still questions surrounding the transplantation of cardiomyocytes. Adult cardiomyocytes are fully differentiated cells. Can enough of these cells be grown to repair the damaged myocardium? Ethical issues and immunorejection are major barriers for fetal and neonatal cardiomyocyte cell therapy [41]. Recently, several reports have demonstrated a potential source of cardiac cells for regeneration: cardiac stem cells in the adult myocardium. The suitability of these cells will need to be determined by future studies.

### 3) Embryonic Stem Cells

Stem cells are immature, undifferentiated precursor cells with the capacity to proliferate in culture and differentiate into one or more types of specialized cells.

Embryonic stem cells were first successfully isolated from the mouse [43]. These cells and their progeny have been widely examined both *in vitro* and *in vivo* in the fields of developmental biology and regenerative medicine [44]. Many groups have reported that embryonic stem cells can differentiate into functional beating cardiomyocytes in vitro [44, 45]. Human embryonic stem cells have been established from the inner mass of the human blastocyst [46], and Kehat et al. were the first to report that functional contracting cardiomyocytes could be derived from a human embryonic stem and embryonic stem cell-derived embryoid body cell system [47].

Because of their high capacity for differentiation and their unlimited availability, embryonic stem cells are potentially very useful for cellular cardiomyoplasty. However, ethical issues, the potential for immune rejection or teratoma formation, and a restricted ability to isolate and purify desired cell types limit their application. The use of human embryonic stem cells in medical research has sparked ethical questions, and drawn much attention from the public [48]. The immunologic status of human embryonic stem cells has not been studied in great detail. Although embryonic cells have been proposed to be non-immunogenic, future studies will need to confirm whether these cells will trigger immune rejection in the recipients. It is also important to understand the mechanisms by which embryonic stem cells can proliferate and yet remain undifferentiated in culture. Will the cells become tumors after myocardial transplantation? Malignant teratomas have been reported following the transplantation of human embryonic stem cells in mice; these cells can also form "benign" teratomas in SCID mice [49, 50]. Careful evaluation of the safety issues will be required if human embryonic stem cells are to be used clinically.

## 4) Bone Marrow Stem Cells

Adult bone marrow contains mesenchymal stem cells and hematopoietic stem cells. Both types are multipotent, with the ability to replicate in the undifferentiated stage and differentiate into a mesenchymal tissue lineage [13]. Bone marrow stem cells (Figure 1C) have received attention as a cell source for cardiac regeneration because of their potential to differentiate into spontaneously beating cardiomyocytes, and to express functional adrenergic ($\beta_1$ and $\beta_2$) and muscarinic ($M_1$ and $M_2$) receptors after 5-azacytidine treatment [51, 52]. Several groups have implanted bone marrow mesenchymal stem cells into the heart after myocardial infarction and demonstrated that the implanted cells survive at the implanted area, exhibit a cardiomyogenic phenotype, and benefit cardiac function [53]. Enriched hematopoietic stem cells derived from bone marrow also improved heart function after they were implanted into the infarcted or peri-infarcted myocardium of murine hearts [54–56]. These studies suggest the possible transformation of implanted bone marrow stem cells into myocytes.

Advantages of bone marrow stem cells for clinical application in cardiac regeneration include: the possibility of autologous transplantation without the need for immunosuppression, ease of harvest from the bone marrow by aspiration, and the significant growth potential of these cells in culture. Accumulated evidence has also shown that implanted bone marrow cells stimulate angiogenesis and increase regional perfusion.

The differentiation of bone marrow stem cells is reportedly influenced significantly by their surrounding environment. For example, when implanted into a fibrotic scar, bone marrow cells become fibroblasts, or, a "scar within a scar." Several studies have also reported that bone marrow stem cells cannot differentiate into myogenic cells [57–58]. Of note, older patients possess fewer bone marrow stem cells than do younger patients, so future research into techniques to increase myogenic cell numbers in the bone marrow for transplantation should focus on enhancing beneficial effects on the recipient hearts of older patients.

## 5) Smooth Muscle Cells

To date, there is no evidence that transplanted cardiomyocytes or skeletal myoblasts can contract synchronously with the host myocardium. In bone marrow stem cell transplantation, few cells, if any, differentiated into myogenic cells. The data suggest that the benefits on cardiac function after cell transplantation are not related to the alteration of regional contractility. Rather, the improvement could be due to increased myocardial wall strength and elasticity and improved regional perfusion [36]. Experimental studies by Li et al. showed that cultured smooth muscle cells (Figure 1D) implanted into the infarcted myocardium proliferated and hypertrophied in response to the stress of cardiac contractions and ventricular pressure [59]. Engrafted smooth muscle cells have been shown to improve heart function, increase myocardial elasticity, and decrease scar expansion and thinning in the infarcted heart [59, 60]. Dr. Sakai et al. compared the results after the transplantation of fetal cardiomyocytes, smooth muscle cells, and skin fibroblasts into the infarcted myocardium of adult rats, demonstrating that smooth muscle cells and cardiomyocytes prevented ventricular dilatation and improved cardiac function similarly [59, 61]. The data strongly suggested that alteration of the infarct tissue composition is important to augment cardiac function.

A significant advantage of using smooth muscle cells to prevent the development of congestive heart failure following myocardial infarction is the growth capacity of these cells *in vitro*, which is not affected by donor age. Smooth muscle cells can be obtained from a segment of artery or vein, and the ability to culture large quantities of uniform smooth muscle cells for culture is useful for auto transplantation. In addition, smooth muscle cells secrete angiogenic factors, such as nitric oxide, fibroblast growth factors, and vascular endothelial cell growth factor; the resultant angiogenesis can alleviate angina [59, 62]. Although smooth muscle cells do not contract spontaneously after implantation into the infarcted myocardium, they do aid in its repair.

## 6) Endothelial Cells

In patients with ischemic cardiomyopathy, myocardial angiogenesis is necessary to restore hibernating cardiomyocyte function. Over the last decade, angiogenic gene and protein therapies have been studied extensively in animal models and clinical trials. Such therapies work by over-expressing angiogenic factors in the implanted area, attracting endothelial cells to form new blood vessels. The resulting neovascular structure improves blood flow in the ischemic region, contributing to the restoration of regional and global cardiac function.

Vascular endothelial cells (Figure 1E) are important components of vascular structure that can participate in vessel formation when implanted into the damaged heart [63]. Li's group has implanted endothelial cells into the infarcted myocardium of adult rats, where the cells stimulated angiogenesis, became incorporated into the new vessels, and increased regional perfusion in myocardial scar tissue. Although endothelial cells can induce the formation of an extensive capillary network, sufficient arterial conduit vessels to restore normal blood flow may not be produced. A disadvantage of endothelial cell transplantation is that the transplanted cells do not improve global function when the implanted area is fibrotic. A combination of angiogenic and myogenic cell therapies would therefore be beneficial, if prevascularization of the myocardial infarct can improve local conditions and enhance myogenic cell survival [27].

## 7) Endothelial Progenitor Cells

In 1997, Asahara et al. isolated a group of cells from human peripheral blood and demonstrated that these cells differentiated into endothelial cells [64]. Implanted into ischemic tissue, the cells induced angiogenesis and were incorporated into neo-vessels [64]. Recent studies have defined these cells, endothelial progenitor cells (EPCs; Figure 1F) as positive for both hematopoietic stem cell markers, such as CD34 or CD133, and vascular endothelial growth factor receptor 2 [65]. EPCs are mobilized from the bone marrow, play an important role in maintenance of the endothelium, and are implicated in both re-endothelialization and neo-vascularization [66].

Since they were identified as an important factor in neo-vascular formation, EPCs have been actively studied to evaluate their angiogenic capacity under pathological conditions. Kocher et al. showed that the cells can be used to directly induce new blood vessel formation (vasculogenesis) in the infarct bed, and proliferation of the preexisting vasculature (angiogenesis) in the infarcted myocardium [66]. EPCs were identified as promising cells for

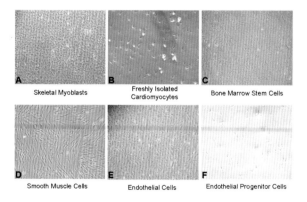

Fig. 1.  Appearance of cultured skeletal myoblasts (A), freshly isolated cardiomyocytes (B), cultured bone marrow stem cells (C), cultured smooth muscle cells (D), cultured vascular endothelial cells (E), and cultured endothelial progenitor cells.

neovascularization in patients with peripheral vascular disease or acute myocardial infarction [67, 68]. Two strategies have been used to achieve this goal [11]. The most common approach involves injection of whole or culture-expanded cells isolated from the mononuclear cell fraction of bone marrow or peripheral blood. This strategy has been applied to several animal models of myocardial ischemia, and has been used in several clinical studies [34, 56, 66, 69–72]. Another approach involves the mobilization of EPCs to ischemic regions using cytokines or conventional pharmacological agents [55, 73].

Despite the promising findings, the scarcity of EPCs in peripheral blood and their limited capacity to multiply *in vitro* are limitations on the therapeutic use of autologous EPCs in treatment of ischemic cardiomyopathy. Furthermore, the correlation between numbers of circulating EPCs and risk factors for coronary artery disease required careful evaluation.

## 8) Cardiac Stem Cells

Adult cardiomyocytes are terminally differentiated cells with a limited capacity to proliferate. The adult myocardium was originally thought to have few or no stem cells, but recent evidence demonstrates that these concepts may not be correct. Studying human myocardial biopsies, Anversa's group demonstrated cardiac stem cells in the adult myocardium that express stem cell markers and telomerase [74]. They showed that similar cells with the characteristics of myogenic stem/progenitor cells were also present in the adult rat myocardium [75]. These cardiac stem cells could be regulated by IGF-1 [76], whose receptor system induces adult rat cardiac stem cell division, enhances telomerase activity, delays senescence, preserves the reservoir of functionally competent cardiac stem cells, and delays organ aging and heart dysfunction [76]. The Schneider group identified cardiac stem cells in the injured myocardial tissue of adult mice [77]. Using a stem cell marker of isl1$^+$ to study rat, mouse and human myocardium, Chien's research team showed cardiac progenitor cells in the adult myocardium with the ability to differentiate into a mature cardiac phenotype with stable expression of myocytic markers in the absence of cell fusion. These cells also exhibited intact $Ca^{2+}$-cycling, and the ability to form action potentials [78]. These data suggest that the adult myocardium has an inherent capacity to repair; a myocardial scar forms when the endogenous repair capacity is overwhelmed by the tissue damage. Another possibility is that regenerative capacity is significantly decreased in the adult heart.

Although cardiac stem cells require further evaluation, their discovery provides a new option to repair the damaged heart. Li et al. isolated cells from endocardial biopsies of adult pig hearts [79]. The cells were cultured *in vitro* and autologously implanted into myocardial scar tissue derived by coil occlusion of the left anterior descending artery. The implanted cells survived at the implanted area, prevented scar expansion, and delayed cardiac failure. Future research is required to verify the optimal conditions under which to isolate, grow and utilize cardiac stem cells to repair the damaged heart.

## Current Cell Therapy Research

### 1) Optimal Cell Type for Myocardial Regeneration

Bone marrow stem cells and skeletal myoblasts have been identified as two major types of cells for myocardial regeneration because of their plasticity and myogenic capacity, respectively, and because of the simplicity by which samples are collected for cell isolation. Pre-clinical data have convinced clinical scientists and Regulatory Agencies to support several clinical trials using bone marrow stem cells and myoblasts to treat patients after myocardial infarction. However, the optimal cell type for cell therapy has not yet been identified because of non-satisfactory clinical results. However, several important factors in the selection of the ideal cell type for cell therapy have been identified:

(1) Nature of heart diseases: Patients with ischemic cardiomyopathy will require angiogenesis, so cells contributing to

vessel formation should be selected first. In contrast, myogenesis in the infarcted region is important for patients with scarred myocardium, for whom muscle cells or myogenic stem cells should be used. For patients in end-stage heart failure or with dilated cardiomyopathy, a combination of muscle cells and angiogenic cells may have an additive effect.

(2) Patients' health conditions: The numbers and possibly the plasticity of stem or myogenic cells are significantly decreased in older patients. Both factors could result in cell numbers insufficient to successfully repair heart damage. Patients' medications or pre-existing clinical conditions, such as diabetes, atherosclerosis, and bone marrow disease might also affect cell properties such as adhesion, proliferation, and self renewal, limiting the potential for autologous cell therapy.

(3) Cell characteristics: Autologous cell transplantation is ideal for cell therapy. Preclinical and some clinical studies have shown the potential beneficial effects of this treatment, but the limitations described above could negate its suitability for every patient.

Allogenic cell transplantation has been evaluated for its potential to regenerate the damaged myocardium. The advantages of this approach are: cell selection, flexibility in time of implantation, and quality and quantity of cells. Several stem cells have been isolated from human umbilical cord blood, and beneficial effects were observed when these cells were cultured and implanted into damaged cardiac tissue. Fetal cardiomyocytes and adult bone marrow cells could also be candidates for allogenic cell therapy, though ethical issues are a major obstruction limiting the use of embryonic stem cells and fetal cells. Immune rejection is another main barrier to the application of allogenic cell transplantation in general. Future research will be required to confirm the immune privilege reported for embryonic and fetal cells in pre-clinical and clinical studies.

Xenogenic cell transplantation could provide another source of cells for cardiac repair. However, this approach has not been well studied because of the rapid development of research into autologous cell transplantation.

## 2) Mechanisms of Action of Implanted Cells

Several mechanisms of action of cell transplantation have been proposed. Examples of these are illustrated in Figure 2:

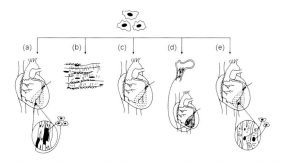

*Fig. 2. Possible mechanisms for the functional benefit of cell transplantation: (a) cell survival in host tissues; (b) extracellular matrix stabilization; (c) angiogenesis; (d) induced mobilization and homing of stem cells; (e) fusion of implanted cells with host myocardium.*

(1) Survival of implanted cells in host tissue: The original hypothesis to explain the improvement of cardiac function by cell transplantation suggested that the implantation of contractile cells, such as cardiomyocytes, improved regional contractility in the recipient tissue [14]. However, actual evidence of transplanted cell differentiation with electrical coupling and contractility is still lacking, despite preclinical and clinical reports of improved heart function [13, 35, 36, 59, 80]. This theory has met with consistently greater challenge, especially since it is also known that most transplanted cells will die within the first days after delivery [81].

(2) Extracellular matrix stabilization: Disruption of the matrix network might impair support for heart cells, resulting in ventricular dilatation and ongoing cell loss. Compounded by an imbalance of matrix-regulating enzymes, these morphological changes could lead to the gradual loss of tissue architecture [82]. Restoration of the extracellular matrix could therefore improve structural support for host heart cells, limiting infarct expansion, improving regional function, and preventing ventricular dilation [83, 84]. This theory has recently been under close investigation.

(3) Angiogenesis: The engrafted cells may stimulate angiogenesis and provide a substrate for new vessel formation, resulting in the functional restoration of hibernating cardiomyocytes, and leading to improved regional myocardial perfusion and contractility [85]. The signaling pathways that enable new blood vessel formation after cell implantation have not been rigorously assessed, but likely involve paracrine mechanisms. Vascular endothelial growth factors and their receptors (flt-1 and flk-1) may be directly involved in these mechanisms, and the magnitude of angiogenesis could be consistent with the degree of functional improvement [86].

(4) Mobilization and homing of stem cells: Stem cells and progenitor cells may home to the damaged tissue to replace lost cells. Beltrami et al. and Urbanek et al. first reported the possibility that bone marrow cells could transdifferente into cardiomyocytes; they also isolated a subset of cells from adult myocardial tissue with stem cell characteristics [74, 75]. Oh et al. provided similar evidence that such cardiac resident progenitor cells could differentiate into cardiomyocytes when cultured in the presence of 5-azacytidine, and that the cultured cells could home to the infarcted myocardium when injected intravenously [77].

(5) Fusion of implanted cells: Implanted cells might fuse with native parenchymal cells, producing hybrids that co-localize stem cell surface antigens with myocyte-specific markers. Such a combination may trigger anti-apoptotic events, leading to improved survival of the native, ischemically-damaged cardiomyocytes [87]. However, this process may be slow and limited in efficiency, and there is still no convincing evidence that cell fusion accounts for the ability of stem cells to regenerate the myocardium [14].

## 3) Optimal Time after Myocardial Infarction for Cell Transplantation

Correct timing of cell transplantation after a myocardial infarction is important to achieve the maximal beneficial effect. The optimal time frame depends on cell type, implantation technique and pathological condition of the patient. Using an animal model, our research group suggested that cell treatment might be most beneficial to cardiac function after the acute inflammatory process has subsided, but prior to the active phase of ventricular remodeling and chamber dilatation [88]. Similarly, Sakakibara et al. found that cellular cardiomyoplasty did not repair the already dilated left ventricle or augment cardiac function when injected cardiomyocytes were delivered into the myocardial scar tissue four weeks after permanent coronary artery ligation [89]. These data suggest that prevention of scar expansion and ventricular dilatation is the most likely mechanism by which the implanted cells improve cardiac function. Several clinical studies have demonstrated that cell injection into the circulation shortly after myocardial infarction does benefit cardiac function [67, 90].

### 4) Optimal Cell Dose for Cellular Cardiomyoplasty

Pouzet et al. demonstrated a linear relationship between improvement in ejection fraction and the number of autologous skeletal myoblasts injected into the infarcted area [91]. Although the most appropriate dose of cells for cellular cardiomyoplasty depends on infarct size and cell availability, accumulated pre-clinical and clinical data have demonstrated that cell number has an important role in the restoration of cardiac function, possibly because of cell loss after transplantation. Muller-Ehmsen et al. and other research groups recently showed that most transplanted cells die within the first days after implantation into damaged myocardium [81, 92]; improving the survival rate of the grafted cells is therefore an important issue. Several strategies, such as cell preconditioning, heat shock, and anti-apoptotic treatments have been evaluated, and results suggest that an efficient technique to improve survival rate could enhance cardiac functional improvement [13, 42, 73, 93–97].

### 5) Optimal Techniques for Cell Transplantation

Since cell therapy for myocardial regeneration was first proposed, various techniques for delivering implanted cells to the target myocardium have been under evaluation and modification, with the consideration of "do no harm to patients". Examples of the main techniques are illustrated in Figure 3:

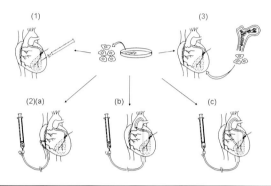

*Fig. 3. Techniques for cell delivery: (1) direct intramyocardial injection; (2) catheter-based cell delivery (a) trans-coronary sinus retrograde injection (b) trans-coronary artery antegrade injection (c) trans-catheter direct myocardial injection; (3) Intravenous systemic delivery (cell homing).*

(1) Direct intramyocardial injection: This technique was the first procedure proposed to engraft cells into damaged myocardium through multiple epicardial punctures. It ensures the cells are inserted into the targeted area, and prevents cell leakage. However it requires that patients must undergo open chest surgery. Currently, direct myocardial injection is being used in clinical trials in combination with coronary artery bypass grafts. The feasibility and efficacy have been well accepted. However, open chest surgery is limited to those patients requiring coronary bypass operation. The development of a minimal invasive surgical operation could make the procedure more widely acceptable.

(2) Catheter-based cell delivery: To reduce invasive tissue damage and to extend the application of cell therapy, percutaneous approaches are currently undergoing rapid technological development for clinical application. Using a percutaneous transcoronary artery catheter, cells can be injected directly into the target vessels and tissue. Clinical studies show that bone marrow-derived mononuclear cells can be safely delivered into the damaged area after myocardial infarction, improving cardiac function [90]. Cells can also be delivered via the transendocardial or coronary sinus routes

[30, 98, m99]. Experimentally, the endoventricular approach has been shown to cause minor cell damage after passage through the catheter, but it allows accurate injection of cells into the target areas [100]. Clinically, this approach has been used in patients receiving skeletal myoblasts and bone marrow cells [30, 72, 101].

(3) Intravenous systemic delivery—cell homing: The rationale for this technique is that circulating stem cells will home to the damaged tissue in response to stimulants such as stem cell factor or other cytokines released by the injured tissue [102], and become involved in the tissue repair. Technically, this is the most convenient and easiest route for cell delivery. However, the approach uses a nonselective distribution pattern for cell transplantation, and its effectiveness of the technique in augmenting cardiac function after myocardial infarction requires future evaluation.

## 6) Current Status of Cell Therapy Research in China

In the early 21st century, cell transplantation for the regeneration of damaged myocardium has received great attention in China, including Taiwan and Hong Kong. Using a rabbit model, several research groups have evaluated the beneficial effect of bone marrow cell or stem cell transplantation on cardiac function [103, 106], showing that implanted cells improved ischemic cardiac function. Using a rat model, Niu et al. transplanted mesenchymal stem cells into normal and infarcted adult rat myocardium. They demonstrated that the implanted cells migrated in the implanted area and differentiated into cardiac muscle cells [107, 108].

In addition to evaluating cellular therapy, several investigators have also studied a combination of cell and gene therapies to evaluate their synergistic effects. Li et al. transfected bone marrow stromal cells with an angiogenic gene [109], and then implanted the genetically modified cells into the damaged myocardium of adult rat hearts. They showed that the gene was expressed at the cell implanted area, and enhanced regional angiogenesis. Recently, Zhang et al. implanted rat bone marrow cells into the ischemic myocardium, and showed that the implanted cells up-regulated myocardial vascular endothelial growth factor and its receptor levels, as well as the levels of heat shock protein-32 and heat shock protein 70. They observed enhanced cytoprotection and angiogenesis that contributed to improvement of ischemic myocardial function [110–112]. In other studies, hepatocyte growth factor was introduced into the infarcted rat myocardium using cell transplantation technology. In those studies, the up-regulation of growth factors in combination with cell therapy restored local blood flow and regenerated the damaged myocardium, which in turn benefited cardiac function [113, 114].

The accumulated evidence for the beneficial effect of cell transplantation on cardiac repair has led to several clinical trials in China. Recently, Zhang and colleagues from Nanjing Medical University, China, reported the initial results of a phase I study of 3 patients, in which they implanted autologous satellite cells into the damaged myocardial tissue during coronary artery bypass grafting [115]. All patients survived the procedure, and recovered. Although occasional arrhythmias were observed initially, no further treatment was performed, and no further arrhythmias were observed during long-term follow-up, when improved perfusion and increased metabolic activity were found at the sites of satellite cell implantation. Significant increases in wall thickness and movement at the areas of cell injection were also observed. Tse et al from University of Hong Kong, China reported an initial phase I clinical trial in which 8 patients were implanted with autologous bone marrow cells by percutaneous catheter infusion [116]. At 3 months following cell transplantation, all patients experienced reductions in angina attack episodes and nitroglycerin tablet requirements, and improvements in their symptoms. Magnetic resonance imaging in these patients showed an increase in myocardial perfusion and regional function at the ischemic region. Chen and colleagues in Nanjiang Medial University reported a randomized phase I clinical trial [117, 118] in which autologous bone marrow mesenchymal stem cells were implanted via percutaneous coronary intervention in 69 patients. The authors concluded that bone marrow cell transplantation to improve cardiac function was safe and feasible, causing no death or malignant arrhythmia.

## *Future Research and Clinical Application of Myocardial Cell Therapy*

The first clinical case of cell transplantation into damaged myocardium was reported by Menasche et al. in 2001 [28]. In that study, skeletal myoblasts obtained from a patient's skeletal muscle biopsies were cultured *in vitro*. The cells were then autologously implanted into that patient's ischemic myocardium during a coronary artery bypass graft. The results showed that the procedure was safe and feasible. A phase I study in which cultured autologous skeletal myoblasts were directly injected into the nonviable regions of the left ventricle during coronary artery bypass grafting surgery was subsequently performed [119] in 10 patients. Regional and global perfusion and cardiac function improved in all 10 patients improved. Further, the transplanted myoblasts survived in the host ischemic myocardium and differentiated into myogenic cells in one of the patients who died 17 months after implantation [29]. Although the beneficial effects on cardiac function could not be attributed solely to the cell implantation because all patients had also received coronary artery bypass grafts, the encouraging preliminary data resulted in a phase II multicentre randomized clinical trial, designed to further examine the clinical benefits of cell implantation (the Myoblast Autologous Grafting in Ischemic Cardiomyopathy [MAGIC] trial).

Because of its potential to minimize tissue damage during cell transplantation into the ischemic myocardium, catheter delivery of autologous bone marrow stem cells and blood progenitor cells has been under clinical evaluation [30]. The first such report of bone marrow cell transplantation after myocardial infarction was published in 2002 [90]. In that study, Strauer et al. infused bone marrow mononuclear cells shortly after myocardial infarction in 10 patients, using balloon inflations to stop flow within the infarct related artery. After 3 months, cardiac function and geometry were significantly improved in the treatment group without any significant adverse events. This study showed that cell delivery may be feasible, safe, and efficacious.

A group of scientists led by Dr. Zeiher in Frankfurt, Germany, reported on their TOPCARE-AMI (Transplantation of Progenitor Cells and Regeneration Enhancement in Acute Myocardial Infarction) trial, which examined bone marrow and circulating progenitor cell therapy [67, 120–122]. Dr. Assmus et al. [67] studied 20 patients, and showed that progenitor cell transplantation resulted in a significant increase in global left ventricular ejection fraction, improved regional wall motion and myocardial viability in the infarct zone, and reduced end-systolic left ventricular volumes compared with a nonrandomized matched reference group. No differences were detected between blood-derived and bone marrow-derived progenitor cell treatments, and no malignant arrhythmias or inflammatory reactions were observed. Dr. Schachinger et al. [122] also reported that cell infusion after myocardial infarction improved cardiac function and prevented scar expansion in patients. Dr. Wollert and colleagues performed a 60-patient randomized trial (Bone Marrow Transfer to Enhance ST-Elevation Infarct Regeneration (BOOST) [123]. In that trial, patients with acute ST-elevation myocardial infarction were randomly assigned to treatment or control groups. In the treatment group, autologous bone marrow cells were intracoronarally injected, and the patients' progress was followed. There was a significant improvement of ejection fraction in the treatment group compared to the control group, with the majority of the improvement seen in the myocardial segments adjacent to the infarcted region. In contrast, other studies have reported only limited beneficial effects on cardiac function after cell implantation [71, 124].

Since safety is the main concern in clinical application, any adverse effects of cell therapy have been paid great attention. For example, arrhythmia was reported after myoblast transplantation [125]. Although the exact pathophysiology of the electrophysiological properties of transplanted cells remains unknown, this finding suggests that the development of symptomatic cardiac arrthymias within weeks of cell transfer could be a serious problem with myoblast transplantation. Restenosis has been identified as a potential side effect of delivering bone marrow cells to the heart [126]. Considering that the stented culprit lesion is the site of fresh injury, amplification of the normal inflammatory response by the bone marrow mobilizing cytokine granulocyte colony-stimulating factor could lead to an amplified restenosis response. The same cells that mediate beneficial myocardial remodeling might also mediate adverse vascular remodeling [86]. Future studies should examine the correlations between cell therapy and its adverse side effects, and identify possible techniques to overcome these problems.

## Conclusions

Cell transplantation to regenerate damaged myocardium and restore cardiac function is a relatively novel concept that has received great attention. Since it was first proposed in the early 1990s, research in this area has progressed rapidly. Over the past decade, new research focuses have been developed, including cardiac stem cells, stem cell differentiation, cell-induced angiogenesis, and embryonic stem cell technologies. Although the mechanisms by which cell transplantation restores cardiac function and myogenic differentiation are still poorly understood, the accumulated pre-clinical and clinical evidence correlates cell implantation with the augmentation of cardiac function after myocardial infarction. Cell transplantation is coming of age.

## Acknowledgements

We would like to acknowledge Ms. Heather Kinkaid for her assistance with chapter preparation and editing. Most of our own research described in this chapter was supported by grants from the Heart and Stroke Foundation of Ontario and the Canadian Institutes for Health Research to Dr. Li. RKL is a Career Investigator of the Heart and Stroke Foundation of Canada, and holds a Canada Research Chair in cardiac regeneration.

## References

1.  Caplice NM, Gersh BJ (2003) Stem cells to repair the heart: a clinical perspective. Circ Res 92:6–8.
2.  Sutton GC (1990) Epidemiologic aspects of heart failure. Am Heart J 120:1538–1540.

3.  Vitali E, Colombo T, Fratto P, Russo C, Bruschi G, Frigerio M (2003) Surgical therapy in advanced heart failure. Am J Cardiol 91:88F–94F.

4.  Pfeffer JM (1991) Progressive ventricular dilation in experimental myocardial infarction and its attenuation by angiotensin-converting enzyme inhibition. Am J Cardiol 68:17D–25D.

5.  Pfeffer JM, Pfeffer MA, Fletcher PJ, Braunwald E (1991) Progressive ventricular remodeling in rat with myocardial infarction. Am J Physiol 260:H1406–H1414.

6.  Lietz K, Miller LW (2005) Will left-ventricular assist device therapy replace heart transplantation in the foreseeable future? Curr Opin Cardiol 20:132–137.

7.  (2003) 2003 OPTN/SRTR Annual Report 1993–2002. HHS/HRSA/OSP/DOT; UNOS; URREA.

8.  Terrovitis IV, Nanas SN, Rombos AK, Tolis G, Nanas JN (1998) Reversible symmetric polyneuropathy with paraplegia after heart transplantation. Transplantation 65:1394–1395.

9.  Rose EA, Gelijns AC, Moskowitz AJ, Heitjan DF, Stevenson LW, Dembitsky W et al. (2001) Long-term mechanical left ventricular assistance for end-stage heart failure. N Engl J Med 345:1435–1443.

10. Rockman HA, Koch WJ, Lefkowitz RJ (2002) Seven-transmembrane-spanning receptors and heart function. Nature 415:206–212.

11. Melo LG, Pachori AS, Kong D, Gnecchi M, Wang K, Pratt RE et al. (2004) Molecular and cell-based therapies for protection, rescue, and repair of ischemic myocardium: reasons for cautious optimism. Circulation 109:2386–2393.

12. Okada H, Takemura G, Kosai K, Li Y, Takahashi T, Esaki M et al. (2005) Postinfarction gene therapy against transforming growth factor-beta signal modulates infarct tissue dynamics and attenuates left ventricular remodeling and heart failure. Circulation 111:2430–2437.

13. Reffelmann T, Kloner RA (2003) Cellular cardiomyoplasty—cardiomyocytes, skeletal myoblasts, or stem cells for regenerating myocardium and treatment of heart failure? Cardiovasc Res 58:358–368.

14. Leri A, Kajstura J, Anversa P (2005) Regenerating the myocardium: a reality today. Can J Cardiol 21:361–362.

15. Reffelmann T, Leor J, Muller-Ehmsen J, Kedes L, Kloner RA (2003) Cardiomyocyte transplantation into the failing heart-new therapeutic approach for heart failure? Heart Fail Rev 8:201–211.

16. Chiu RC, Zibaitis A, Kao RL (1995) Cellular cardiomyoplasty: myocardial regeneration with satellite cell implantation. Ann Thorac Surg 60:12–18.

17. Campion DR (1984) The muscle satellite cell: a review. Int Rev Cytol 87:225–251.

18. Wang JS, Shum-Tim D, Chedrawy E, Chiu RC (2001) The coronary delivery of marrow stromal cells for myocardial regeneration: pathophysiologic and therapeutic implications. J Thorac Cardiovasc Surg 122:699–705.

19. Menasche P (2003) Skeletal muscle satellite cell transplantation. Cardiovasc Res 58(2):351–357.

20. Koh GY, Soonpaa MH, Klug MG, Field LJ (1993) Long-term survival of AT-1 cardiomyocyte grafts in syngeneic myocardium. Am J Physiol 264:H1727–H1733.

21. Murry CE, Wiseman RW, Schwartz SM, Hauschka SD (1996) Skeletal myoblast transplantation for repair of myocardial necrosis. J Clin Invest 98:2512–2523.

22. Murry CE, Kay MA, Bartosek T, Hauschka SD, Schwartz SM (1996) Muscle differentiation during repair of myocardial necrosis in rats via gene transfer with MyoD. J Clin Invest 98:2209–2217.

23. Reinecke H, MacDonald GH, Hauschka SD, Murry CE (2000) Electromechanical coupling between skeletal and cardiac muscle. Implications for infarct repair. J Cell Biol 149:731–740.

24. Reinecke H, Minami E, Poppa V, Murry CE (2004) Evidence for fusion between cardiac and skeletal muscle cells. Circ Res 94:e56–e60.

25. Prosper F, Herreros J, Barba J (2004) Future perspectives in the treatment of heart failure: from cell transplantation to cardiac regeneration. Rev Esp Cardiol 57:981–988.

26. Ghostine S, Carrion C, Souza LC, Richard P, Bruneval P, Vilquin JT et al. (2002) Long-term efficacy of myoblast transplantation on regional structure and function after myocardial infarction. Circulation 106:I131–I136.

27. Chachques JC, Acar C, Herreros J, Trainini JC, Prosper F, D'Attellis N et al. (2004) Cellular cardiomyoplasty: clinical application. Ann Thorac Surg 77:1121–1130.

28. Menasche P, Hagege AA, Scorsin M, Pouzet B, Desnos M, Duboc D et al. (2001) Myoblast transplantation for heart failure. Lancet 357:279–280.

29. Hagege AA, Carrion C, Menasche P, Vilquin JT, Duboc D, Marolleau JP et al. (2003) Viability and differentiation of autologous skeletal myoblast grafts in ischaemic cardiomyopathy. Lancet 361:491–492.

30. Smits PC, van Geuns RJ, Poldermans D, Bountioukos M, Onderwater EE, Lee CH et al. (2003) Catheter-based intramyocardial injection of autologous skeletal myoblasts as a primary treatment of ischemic heart failure: clinical experience with six-month follow-up. J Am Coll Cardiol 42:2063–2069.

31. Siminiak T, Fiszer D, Jerzykowska O, Grygielska B, Rozwadowska N, Kalmucki P et al. (2005) Percutaneous trans-coronary-venous transplantation of autologous skeletal myoblasts in the treatment of post-infarction myocardial contractility impairment: the POZNAN trial. Eur Heart J 26:1188–1195.

32. Tucker DC, Snider C, Woods WT, Jr. (1988) Pacemaker development in embryonic rat heart cultured in oculo. Pediatr Res 23:637–642.

33. Li RK, Mickle DA, Weisel RD, Zhang J (1996) Mohabeer MK. In vivo survival and function of transplanted rat cardiomyocytes. Circ Res 78:283–288.

34. Soonpaa MH, Koh GY, Klug MG, Field LJ (1994) Formation of nascent

intercalated disks between grafted fetal cardiomyocytes and host myocardium. Science 264:98–101.

35. Leor J, Patterson M, Quinones MJ, Kedes LH, Kloner RA (1996) Transplantation of fetal myocardial tissue into the infarcted myocardium of rat. A potential method for repair of infarcted myocardium? Circulation 94:II332–II336.

36. Li RK, Jia ZQ, Weisel RD, Mickle DA, Zhang J, Mohabeer MK et al. (1996) Cardiomyocyte transplantation improves heart function. Ann Thorac Surg 62: 654–660.

37. Scorsin M, Hagege AA, Marotte F, Mirochnik N, Copin H, Barnoux M et al. (1997) Does transplantation of cardiomyocytes improve function of infarcted myocardium? Circulation 96:II–93.

38. Skobel E, Schuh A, Schwarz ER, Liehn EA, Franke A, Breuer S et al. (2004) Transplantation of fetal cardiomyocytes into infarcted rat hearts results in long-term functional improvement. Tissue Eng 10:849–864.

39. Muller-Ehmsen J, Peterson KL, Kedes L, Whittaker P, Dow JS, Long TI et al. (2002) Rebuilding a damaged heart: long-term survival of transplanted neonatal rat cardiomyocytes after myocardial infarction and effect on cardiac function. Circulation 105:1720–1726.

40. Etzion S, Battler A, Barbash IM, Cagnano E, Zarin P, Granot Y et al. (2001) Influence of embryonic cardiomyocyte transplantation on the progression of heart failure in a rat model of extensive myocardial infarction. J Mol Cell Cardiol 33:1321–1330.

41. Li RK, Mickle DA, Weisel RD, Mohabeer MK, Zhang J, Rao V et al. (1997) Natural history of fetal rat cardiomyocytes transplanted into adult rat myocardial scar tissue. Circulation 96:II–86.

42. Yau TM, Fung K, Weisel RD, Fujii T, Mickle DA, Li RK (2001) Enhanced myocardial angiogenesis by gene transfer with transplanted cells. Circulation 104:I218–I222.

43. Martin GR (1981) Isolation of a pluripotent cell line from early mouse embryos cultured in medium conditioned by teratocarcinoma stem cells. Proc Natl Acad Sci U S A 78:7634–7638.

44. Boheler KR, Czyz J, Tweedie D, Yang HT, Anisimov SV, Wobus AM (2002) Differentiation of pluripotent embryonic stem cells into cardiomyocytes. Circ Res 91:189–201.

45. Hescheler J, Fleischmann BK, Lentini S, Maltsev VA, Rohwedel J, Wobus AM et al. (1997) Embryonic stem cells: a model to study structural and functional properties in cardiomyogenesis. Cardiovasc Res 36:149–162.

46. Thomson JA, Itskovitz-Eldor J, Shapiro SS, Waknitz MA, Swiergiel JJ, Marshall VS et al. (1998) Embryonic stem cell lines derived from human blastocysts. Science 282:1145–1147.

47. Kehat I, Kenyagin-Karsenti D, Snir M, Segev H, Amit M, Gepstein A et al. (2001) Human embryonic stem cells can differentiate into myocytes with structural and functional properties of cardiomyocytes. J Clin Invest 108:407–414.

48. Young FE (2000) A time for restraint. Science 287:1424.

49. Papaioannou VE (1993) Ontogeny, pathology, oncology. Int J Dev Biol 37:33–37.

50. Martin GR (1980) Teratocarcinomas and mammalian embryogenesis. Science 209:768–776.

51. Makino S, Fukuda K, Miyoshi S, Konishi F, Kodama H, Pan J et al. (1999) Cardiomyocytes can be generated from marrow stromal cells in vitro. J Clin Invest 103:697–705.

52. Hakuno D, Fukuda K, Makino S, Konishi F, Tomita Y, Manabe T et al. (2002) Bone marrow-derived regenerated cardiomyocytes (CMG Cells) express functional adrenergic and muscarinic receptors. Circulation 105:380–386.

53. Wang JS, Shum-Tim D, Galipeau J, Chedrawy E, Eliopoulos N, Chiu RC (2000) Marrow stromal cells for cellular cardiomyoplasty: feasibility and potential clinical advantages. J Thorac Cardiovasc Surg 120:999–1005.

54. Jackson KA, Majka SM, Wang H, Pocius J, Hartley CJ, Majesky MW et al. (2001) Regeneration of ischemic cardiac muscle and vascular endothelium by adult stem cells. J Clin Invest 107:1395–1402.

55. Orlic D, Kajstura J, Chimenti S, Limana F, Jakoniuk I, Quaini F et al. (2001) Mobilized bone marrow cells repair the infarcted heart, improving function and survival. Proc Natl Acad Sci USA 98:10344–10349.

56. Orlic D, Kajstura J, Chimenti S, Jakoniuk I, Anderson SM, Li B et al. (2001) Bone marrow cells regenerate infarcted myocardium. Nature 410:701–705.

57. Murry CE, Soonpaa MH, Reinecke H, Nakajima H, Nakajima HO, Rubart M et al. (2004) Haematopoietic stem cells do not transdifferentiate into cardiac myocytes in myocardial infarcts. Nature 428:664–668.

58. Balsam LB, Wagers AJ, Christensen JL, Kofidis T, Weissman IL, Robbins RC (2004) Haematopoietic stem cells adopt mature haematopoietic fates in ischaemic myocardium. Nature 428:668–673.

59. Li RK, Jia ZQ, Weisel RD, Merante F, Mickle DA (1999) Smooth muscle cell transplantation into myocardial scar tissue improves heart function. J Mol Cell Cardiol 31:513–522.

60. Yoo KJ, Li RK, Weisel RD, Mickle DA, Li G, Yau TM (2000) Autologous smooth muscle cell transplantation improved heart function in dilated cardiomyopathy. Ann Thorac Surg 70:859–865.

61. Sakai T, Li RK, Weisel RD, Mickle DA, Jia ZQ, Tomita S et al. (1999) Fetal cell transplantation: a comparison of three cell types. J Thorac Cardiovasc Surg 118:715–724.

62. Yoo KJ, Li RK, Weisel RD, Mickle DA, Tomita S, Ohno N et al. (2002) Smooth muscle cells transplantation is better than heart cells transplantation for improvement of heart function in dilated cardiomyopathy. Yonsei Med J 43:296–303.

63. Kim EJ, Li RK, Weisel RD, Mickle DA, Jia ZQ, Tomita S et al. (2001) Angiogenesis by endothelial cell transplantation. J Thorac Cardiovasc Surg 122:963?971.

64. Asahara T, Murohara T, Sullivan A, Silver M, van der ZR, Li T et al. (1997) Isolation of putative progenitor endothelial cells for angiogenesis. Science 275: 964–967.

65. Urbich C, Dimmeler S (2004) Endothelial progenitor cells functional characterization. Trends Cardiovasc Med 14:318–322.

66. Kocher AA, Schuster MD, Szabolcs MJ, Takuma S, Burkhoff D, Wang J et al. (2001) Neovascularization of ischemic myocardium by human bone-marrow-derived angioblasts prevents cardiomyocyte apoptosis, reduces remodeling and improves cardiac function. Nat Med 7:430–436.

67. Assmus B, Schachinger V, Teupe C, Britten M, Lehmann R, Dobert N et al. (2002) Transplantation of Progenitor Cells and Regeneration Enhancement in Acute Myocardial Infarction (TOPCARE-AMI). Circulation 106:3009–3017.

68. Tateishi-Yuyama E, Matsubara H, Murohara T, Ikeda U, Shintani S, Masaki H et al. (2002) Therapeutic angiogenesis for patients with limb ischaemia by autologous transplantation of bone-marrow cells: a pilot study and a randomised controlled trial. Lancet 360:427–435.

69. Kawamoto A, Gwon HC, Iwaguro H, Yamaguchi JI, Uchida S, Masuda H et al. (2001) Therapeutic potential of ex vivo expanded endothelial progenitor cells for myocardial ischemia. Circulation 103:634–637.

70. Kawamoto A, Tkebuchava T, Yamaguchi J, Nishimura H, Yoon YS, Milliken C et al. (2003) Intramyocardial transplantation of autologous endothelial progenitor cells for therapeutic neovascularization of myocardial ischemia. Circulation 107: 461–468.

71. Stamm C, Westphal B, Kleine HD, Petzsch M, Kittner C, Klinge H et al. (2003) Autologous bone-marrow stem-cell transplantation for myocardial regeneration. Lancet 361:45–46.

72. Perin EC, Dohmann HF, Borojevic R, Silva SA, Sousa AL, Mesquita CT et al. (2003) Transendocardial, autologous bone marrow cell transplantation for severe, chronic ischemic heart failure. Circulation 107:2294–2302.

73. Vasa M, Fichtlscherer S, Adler K, Aicher A, Martin H, Zeiher AM et al. (2001) Increase in circulating endothelial progenitor cells by statin therapy in patients with stable coronary artery disease. Circulation 103:2885–2890.

74. Urbanek K, Quaini F, Tasca G, Torella D, Castaldo C, Nadal-Ginard B et al. (2003) Intense myocyte formation from cardiac stem cells in human cardiac hypertrophy. Proc Natl Acad Sci USA 100:10440–10445.

75. Beltrami AP, Barlucchi L, Torella D, Baker M, Limana F, Chimenti S et al. (2003) Adult cardiac stem cells are multipotent and support myocardial regeneration. Cell 114:763–776.

76. Torella D, Rota M, Nurzynska D, Musso E, Monsen A, Shiraishi I et al. (2004) Cardiac stem cell and myocyte aging, heart failure, and insulin-like growth factor-1 overexpression. Circ Res 94:514–524.

77. Oh H, Bradfute SB, Gallardo TD, Nakamura T, Gaussin V, Mishina Y et al. (2003) Cardiac progenitor cells from adult myocardium: homing, differentiation, and fusion after infarction. Proc Natl Acad Sci USA 100:12313–12318.

78. Laugwitz KL, Moretti A, Lam J, Gruber P, Chen Y, Woodard S et al. (2005) Postnatal isl1+ cardioblasts enter fully differentiated cardiomyocyte lineages. Nature 433:647–653.

79. Li RK, Weisel RD, Mickle DA, Jia ZQ, Kim EJ, Sakai T et al. (2000) Autologous porcine heart cell transplantation improved heart function after a myocardial infarction. J Thorac Cardiovasc Surg 119:62–68.

80. Scorsin M, Marotte F, Sabri A, Le Dref O, Demirag M, Samuel JL et al. (1996) Can grafted cardiomyocytes colonize peri-infarct myocardial areas? Circulation 94:II337–II340.

81. Muller-Ehmsen J, Whittaker P, Kloner RA, Dow JS, Sakoda T, Long TI, et al. (2002) Survival and development of neonatal rat cardiomyocytes transplanted into adult myocardium. J Mol Cell Cardiol 34:107–116.

82. Fedak PW, Altamentova SM, Weisel RD, Nili N, Ohno N, Verma S, et al. (2003) Matrix remodeling in experimental and human heart failure: a possible regulatory role for TIMP-3. Am J Physiol Heart Circ Physiol 284:H626–H634.

83. Fedak PW, Weisel RD, Verma S, Mickle DA, Li RK (2003) Restoration and regeneration of failing myocardium with cell transplantation and tissue engineering. Semin Thorac Cardiovasc Surg 15:277–286.

84. Thomas CV, Coker ML, Zellner JL, Handy JR, Crumbley AJ, III, Spinale FG (1998) Increased matrix metalloproteinase activity and selective upregulation in LV myocardium from patients with end-stage dilated cardiomyopathy. Circulation 97:1708–1715.

85. Angoulvant D, Fazel S, Li RK (2004) Neovascularization derived from cell transplantation in ischemic myocardium. Mol Cell Biochem 264:133–142.

86. Fazel S, Angoulvant D, Desai N, Yang S, Weisel RD, Li RK (2005) Cardiac restoration: Frontier or fantasy? Can J Cardiol 21:355–359.

87. Sam J, Angoulvant D, Fazel S, Weisel RD, Li RK (2005) Heart cell implantation after myocardial infarction. Coron Artery Dis 16:85–91.

88. Li RK, Mickle DA, Weisel RD, Rao V, Jia ZQ (2001) Optimal time for cardiomyocyte transplantation to maximize myocardial function after left ventricular injury. Ann Thorac Surg 72:1957–1963.

89. Sakakibara Y, Tambara K, Lu F, Nishina T, Nagaya N, Nishimura K et al. (2002) Cardiomyocyte transplantation does not reverse cardiac remodeling in rats with chronic myocardial infarction. Ann Thorac Surg 74:25–30.

90. Strauer BE, Brehm M, Zeus T, Kostering M, Hernandez A, Sorg RV et al. (2002) Repair of infarcted myocardium by autologous intracoronary mononuclear bone marrow cell transplantation in humans. Circulation 106:1913–1918.

91. Pouzet B, Vilquin JT, Hagege AA, Scorsin M, Messas E, Fiszman M et al. (2001) Factors affecting functional outcome after autologous skeletal myoblast transplantation. Ann Thorac Surg 71:844–850.

92. Yasuda T, Weisel RD, Kiani C, Mickle DA, Maganti M, Li RK (2005) Quantitative analysis of survival of transplanted smooth muscle cells with real-time polymerase chain reaction. J Thorac Cardiovasc Surg 129:904–911.

93. Jayakumar J, Suzuki K, Khan M, Smolenski RT, Farrell A, Latif N et al. (2000) Gene therapy for myocardial protection: transfection of donor hearts with heat shock protein 70 gene protects cardiac function against ischemia-reperfusion injury. Circulation 102:III302–III306.

94. Suzuki K, Smolenski RT, Jayakumar J, Murtuza B, Brand NJ, Yacoub MH. (2000) Heat shock treatment enhances graft cell survival in skeletal myoblast transplantation to the heart. Circulation 102:III216–III221.

95. Landmesser U, Engberding N, Bahlmann FH, Schaefer A, Wiencke A, Heineke A et al. (2004) Statin-induced improvement of endothelial progenitor cell mobilization, myocardial neovascularization, left ventricular function, and survival after experimental myocardial infarction requires endothelial nitric oxide synthase. Circulation 110:1933–1939.

96. Suzuki K, Murtuza B, Smolenski RT, Sammut IA, Suzuki N, Kaneda Y et al. (2001) Cell transplantation for the treatment of acute myocardial infarction using vascular endothelial growth factor-expressing skeletal myoblasts. Circulation 104:1207–1212.

97. Vincent KA, Feron O, Kelly RA (2002) Harnessing the response to tissue hypoxia: HIF-1 alpha and therapeutic angiogenesis. Trends Cardiovasc Med 12:362–367.

98. Brasselet C, Morichetti MC, Messas E, Carrion C, Bissery A, Bruneval P et al. (2005) Skeletal myoblast transplantation through a catheter-based coronary sinus approach: an effective means of improving function of infarcted myocardium. Eur Heart J 26:1551–1556.

99. Thompson CA, Nasseri BA, Makower J, Houser S, McGarry M, Lamson T et al. (2003) Percutaneous transvenous cellular cardiomyoplasty. A novel nonsurgical approach for myocardial cell transplantation. J Am Coll Cardiol 41:1964–1971.

100. Chazaud B, Hittinger L, Sonnet C, Champagne S, Le Corvoisier P, Benhaiem-Sigaux N et al. (2003) Endoventricular porcine autologous myoblast

transplantation can be successfully achieved with minor mechanical cell damage. Cardiovasc Res 58:444–450.

101. Fuchs S, Satler LF, Kornowski R, Okubagzi P, Weisz G, Baffour R et al. (2003) Catheter-based autologous bone marrow myocardial injection in no-option patients with advanced coronary artery disease: a feasibility study. J Am Coll Cardiol 41:1721–1724.

102. Perin EC, Geng YJ, Willerson JT (2003) Adult stem cell therapy in perspective. Circulation 107:935–938.

103. Lin GS, Lu JJ, Jiang XJ, Li XY, Li GS (2004) Autologous transplantation of bone marrow 25:876–886.

104. Sun YX, Zhao Q, Wang YQ, Yang C, Pan CZ, Han PP et al (2005) [Upregulating the expression of angiogenesis-related genes by transplanting autologous mononuclear bone marrow cells into myocardial infarction scar and the periphery]. Zhonghua Xinxueguanbing Zazhi 33:260–264.

105. Wang JA, Li CL, Fan YQ, He H, Sun Y (2004) Allograftic bone marrow-derived mesenchymal stem cells transplanted into heart infarcted model of rabbit to renovate infarcted heart. J Zhejiang Univ Sci 5:1279–1285.

106. Wang JA, Fan YQ, Li CL, He H, Sun Y, Lv BJ (2005) Human bone marrow-derived mesenchymal stem cells transplanted into damaged rabbit heart to improve heart function. J Zhejiang Univ Sci B 6:242–248.

107. Niu LL, Cao F, Zheng M, Li YH, Xie C, Zhu SJ et al. (2004) [Transplantation of exogenous mesenchymal stem cells for treatment of myocardial infarction in rat]. Zhonghua Neike Zazhi 43:186–190.

108. Niu LL, Zheng M, Cao F, Xie C, Li HM, Yue W et al. (2004) [Migration and differentiation of exogenous rat mesenchymal stem cells engrafted into normal and injured hearts of rats]. Zhonghua Yixue Zazhi 84:38–42.

109. Li Z, Mei J, Zhang B (2002) [Cell transplantation of 5-aza cytidine induced bone marrow stromal cells transfected by angiogenin gene ex vivo into infarcted myocardium, an experimental study]. Zhonghua Yixue Zazhi 82:1319–1323.

110. Zhang S, Guo J, Zhang P, Liu Y, Jia Z, Feng X et al. (2003) [Transplantation of bone marrow cells up-regulated the expressions of HSP32 and HSP70 in the acute ischemic myocardium]. Beijing Daxue Xuebao 35:476–480.

111. Zhang S, Jia Z, Guo J, Zhang P, Ma K, Wang S et al. (2003) [Transplantation of bone marrow cells upregulated vascular endothelial growth factor and its receptor and improved ischemic myocardial function]. Beijing Da Xue Xue Bao 35:429–433.

112. Zhang S, Zhang P, Guo J, Jia Z, Ma K, Liu Y et al. (2004) Enhanced cytoprotection and angiogenesis by bone marrow cell transplantation may contribute to improved ischemic myocardial function. Eur J Cardiothorac Surg 25:188–195.

113. Liu Y, Guo J, Zhang P, Zhang S, Chen P, Ma K et al. (2004) Bone marrow

mononuclear cell transplantation into heart elevates the expression of angiogenic factors. Microvasc Res 68:156–160.

114. Duan HF, Wu CT, Wu DL, Lu Y, Liu HJ, Ha XQ et al. (2003) Treatment of myocardial ischemia with bone marrow-derived mesenchymal stem cells overexpressing hepatocyte growth factor. Mol Ther 8:467–474.

115. Zhang F, Gao X, Yiang ZJ, Ma W, Li C, Kao RL (2003) Cellular cardiomyoplasty: a preliminary clinical report. Cardiovasc Radiat Med 4:39–42.

116. Tse HF, Kwong YL, Chan JK, Lo G, Ho CL, Lau CP (2003) Angiogenesis in ischaemic myocardium by intramyocardial autologous bone marrow mononuclear cell implantation. Lancet 361:47–49.

117. Chen SL, Fang WW, Qian J, Ye F, Liu YH, Shan SJ et al. (2004) Improvement of cardiac function after transplantation of autologous bone marrow mesenchymal stem cells in patients with acute myocardial infarction. Chin Med J 117:1443–1448.

118. Chen SL, Fang WW, Ye F, Liu YH, Qian J, Shan SJ et al. (2004) Effect on left ventricular function of intracoronary transplantation of autologous bone marrow mesenchymal stem cell in patients with acute myocardial infarction. Am J Cardiol 94:92–95.

119. Menasche P, Hagege AA, Vilquin JT, Desnos M, Abergel E, Pouzet B et al. (2003) Autologous skeletal myoblast transplantation for severe postinfarction left ventricular dysfunction. J Am Coll Cardiol 41:1078–1083.

120. Britten MB, Abolmaali ND, Assmus B, Lehmann R, Honold J, Schmitt J et al. (2003) Infarct remodeling after intracoronary progenitor cell treatment in patients with acute myocardial infarction (TOPCARE-AMI): mechanistic insights from serial contrast-enhanced magnetic resonance imaging. Circulation 108:2212–2218.

121. Dobert N, Britten M, Assmus B, Berner U, Menzel C, Lehmann R et al. (2004) Transplantation of progenitor cells after reperfused acute myocardial infarction: evaluation of perfusion and myocardial viability with FDG-PET and thallium SPECT. Eur J Nucl Med Mol Imaging 31:1146–1151.

122. Schachinger V, Assmus B, Britten MB, Honold J, Lehmann R, Teupe C et al. (2004) Transplantation of progenitor cells and regeneration enhancement in acute myocardial infarction: final one-year results of the TOPCARE-AMI Trial. J Am Coll Cardiol 44:1690–1699.

123. Wollert KC, Meyer GP, Lotz J, Ringes-Lichtenberg S, Lippolt P, Breidenbach C et al. (2004) Intracoronary autologous bone-marrow cell transfer after myocardial infarction: the BOOST randomised controlled clinical trial. Lancet 364:141–148.

124. Galinanes M, Loubani M, Davies J, Chin D, Pasi J, Bell PR (2004) Auto-transplantation of unmanipulated bone marrow into scarred myocardium is safe and enhances cardiac function in humans. Cell Transplant 13:7–13.

125. Bonaros N, Yang S, Ott H, Kocher A (2004) Cell therapy for ischemic heart disease. Panminerva Med 46:13–23.

126. Kang HJ, Kim HS, Zhang SY, Park KW, Cho HJ, Koo BK et al. (2004) Effects of intracoronary infusion of peripheral blood stem-cells mobilised with granulocyte-colony stimulating factor on left ventricular systolic function and restenosis after coronary stenting in myocardial infarction: the MAGIC cell randomised clinical trial. Lancet 363:751–756.

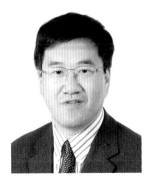

Ren-Ke Li

# The Evolution of Mitral Valve Surgery: 1902–2002

*Lawrence H. Cohn, Edward G. Soltesz*

**M**itral valve disease has been one of the most interesting human maladies to be treated in this past century from a public health, medical diagnostic and surgical technique perspective. At the beginning of the last century, mitral stenosis due to rheumatic heart disease was as virulent and prevalent as the AIDS epidemic of the 1990s and early 2000s. It was a public health problem of enormous proportions resulting from poor sanitation, lack of antibiotics, and incomplete understanding of the mode of transmission of the vectors resulting in rheumatic fever. Rheumatic fever and rheumatic heart disease affect the mitral valve by causing stenosis of both the anteromedial and posterior commissures of the valve, thus promoting obstruction to blood flow which results in pulmonary congestion, pulmonary hypertension, and eventually right heart failure. This was a common clinical picture of many young individuals affected by this disorder. The recognition and surgical treatment of this disorder is a very colorful historical legend that illustrates the many small steps taken by surgeons in the last century to treat mitral stenosis, expand the techniques learned to other disease entities involving the mitral valve, and eventually perform surgery on the mitral valve in a minimally invasive, almost atraumatic way.

This chapter will detail some of the events relating to the development of the surgical treatment of mitral valve disease from early in the last century up to the present time including robotic assisted, minimally invasive mitral valve surgery.

## Early History of Mitral Valve Surgery

The first reference to the surgical treatment of mitral stenosis in any form was written by Sir Thomas Lauder Brunton from the London Hospital in 1902 [1]. He asserted that mitral stenosis in its severest form resisted all treatment by medicine. He went on to suggest that if one could devise a mechanical or surgical method to improve the output of the heart by opening up the valve, it would be, theoretically, quite beneficial. Yet, London physicians of the time vehemently criticized him because the ongoing theory held that the myocardium was responsible for rheumatic heart disease rather than a mechanical obstruction of the mitral valve. This newfound controversy, however, was the catalyst for experimental research in mitral stenosis. From 1907 to 1914, such individuals as Cushing [2], Bernheim [3], Jeger [4], and Carrel [5] devised ingenious animal models for creating and relieving mitral stenosis.

In 1912, a talented general surgeon from Johns Hopkins, Harvey Cushing, became the first Chairman and Professor of Surgery at the new Peter Bent Brigham Hospital in Boston and a Professor of Surgery at the Harvard Medical School. Although he is known as the father of neurosurgery, he held a longstanding interest, begun at Hopkins, in experimental relief of mitral stenosis. Cushing worked with his first surgical resident, Elliot Cutler, who subsequently became the second Professor of Surgery at the Peter Bent Brigham Hospital. Cutler did some of the most important work in mitral stenosis research of that era. In the early 1920s, Cutler and his Brigham medical colleague Samuel Levine began to devise mechanical methods of treating the large number of patients with rheumatic mitral valve disease. In addition to his experiments at the Harvard Medical School relieving mitral stenosis, Cutler also performed some of the fundamental experiments in cardiac surgery, such as elevating the heart, injecting the heart and pericardium [6]. Cutler devised the cardiac valvulotome, an instrument which would resect a piece of the stenotic mitral valve in order to open the valve and improve transvalvular blood flow (Fig. 1). He did not, however, understand that he was going to create mitral regurgitation which acutely caused cardiac decompensation.

In the spring of 1923, an 11-year-old girl became the first patient ever successfully treated for mitral valve disease by a surgical operation (Fig. 2) [7]. She had been a patient at the Good Samaritan Hospital, a 7-story facility located around the corner from the Peter Bent Brigham and completely filled with young rheumatic heart disease patients. The young girl was almost comatose from low output cardiac failure and was brought over by Cutler and Levine to be operated upon at the Brigham. Fortunately, for this patient, the cardiac valvulotome had not yet been completed, so a neurosurgical tenotomy knife was inserted into the apex of the heart through a median sternotomy, and a mitral commisurotomy was performed. The patient awoke, did well postoperatively, and was discharged from the hospital 14 days later. She was later a live subject at the Surgical Grand Rounds celebrating the 10th anniversary of the

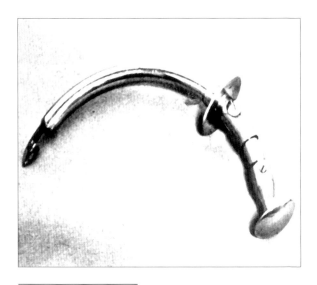

*Fig. 1. Cardiac valvulotome.*

opening of the Peter Bent Brigham Hospital. Cushing, noting this on the 1923 Annual Report of the Peter Bent Brigham Hospital, said, "Unless all signs fail, we are on the eve of a new surgical specialty of great promise—a specialty dealing with chronic diseases of the heart."

Throughout the 1920s, Cutler, Levine, and Beck, one of Cutler's students, did further work on the surgical treatment of mitral stenosis. Unfortunately, once the cardiac valvulotome was completed and in use in the operating room, the severe mitral regurgitation it caused resulted in the death of the next 7 patients Cutler operated upon. In 1929, at the American Surgical Association meeting, Cutler announced that he was declaring a moratorium on this operation due to its high mortality [8]. Interestingly, in 1925, British surgeon Henry Souttar had performed what is now considered to be the first finger-fracture valvuloplasty for mitral stenosis through the left atrial appendage via a left thoracotomy [9]. This was an operation that was soon to become relatively standard over the next 20 years. The London physicians of the era disapproved of Souttar's approach, however, and did not refer him another patient upon which to operate.

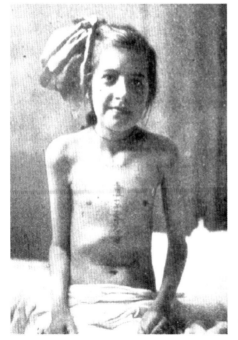

Fig. 2. *An 11-year-old girl who was the first patient ever successfully treated for mitral valve disease by a surgical operation in the spring of 1923.*

Cutler entered the Second World War as did another future Brigham surgeon, Dwight Emery Harken, who became famous for removing intrathoracic shrapnel and missiles from the chests of wounded soldiers. His ingenious techniques established the feasibility of cardiac surgery and set the stage for an illustrious career in Boston. Following the war, Cutler died and Harken assumed the role of principle cardiac surgeon at the Brigham. In a landmark paper in 1948, he was one of the first to show that the surgical treatment of mitral stenosis could be performed safely and reproducibly by closed techniques [10]. Interestingly, he originally started out using the cardiac valvulotome, but quickly realized that the resultant mitral regurgitation was too severe and switched to the finger-fracture technique of Souttar. He then commenced a large series of closed mitral valvuloplasties for mitral stenosis which were remarkably successful. His landmark studies with Lawrence Ellis, another Brigham cardiologist, were important for several reasons. They showed that closed mitral valvuloplasty could be successfully done in a large number of patients, but more importantly, they were some of the first to show in a rather preliminary way actuarial results of cardiac operations. In 1973, Harken and Ellis presented a 20 year follow-up of 710 patients showing mortality and re-operation rates, measures which became standard for cardiac surgery outcomes studies [11].

## Modern Surgical History

With the advent of the first successful cardiopulmonary bypass by Gibbon in 1953 [12], a whole new set of procedures were developed and could be performed, not only for mitral stenosis, but for mitral regurgitation, a lesion which was much more difficult to treat than mitral stenosis. Early reparative techniques failed, and most surgeons believed mitral regurgitation required valve replacement. The first artificial mitral valve was implanted by Nina Braunwald in 1960 [13]. This valve was a bileaflet, polyurethane valve with cloth chordae, not commercially available, and implanted in only a few patients (Fig. 3). The Starr-Edwards valve was the first commercially available

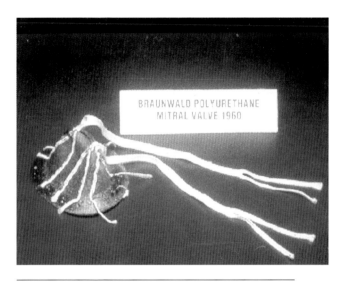

Fig. 3. Braunwald bileaflet, polyurethane mitral valve replacement.

mitral valve prosthesis implanted in humans which reproduced physiologic hemodynamics (Fig. 4). Invented by Albert Starr and Lowell Edwards in 1960, this valve quickly became the gold standard of mitral valve prosthetic devices and was utilized in tens of thousands of patients worldwide [14].

At this same time Dr. Jia-Si Huang performed the first open heart operation at Shanghai Hospital emphasizing operative valve surgery for the large rheumatic heart disease population [15]. Though mitral valve disease was primarily treated by closed mitral operations, the first mitral valve replacement operation was with a Shanghai-made mechanical valve in Shanghai in 1965 [16].

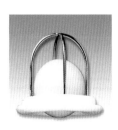

Shortly after the beginning of mitral replacement with the Starr-Edwards ball valve, a curious phenomenon was observed, particularly in patients with severe mitral

Fig. 4. Starr-Edwards mitral valve.

regurgitation: transformation of a "football"-shaped to a "basketball"-shaped heart. When mitral valve replacement was carried out in the 1960's, the tips of the papillary muscles and chordae were meticulously cut in both the anterior and posterior leaflets because of concern about prosthetic valve dysfunction if these were left intact. The mitral Starr-Edwards ball valves were carefully inserted and a good early result was demonstrated. Yet, patients, particularly those with mitral regurgitation and a somewhat borderline ejection fraction, did very poorly, and within six to twelve months, returned in congestive heart failure with a competent mitral valve, but severely cardiomyopathic. At the time, it was erroneously reasoned that shutting off the "pop-off valve" to the left atrium by the complete ablation of mitral regurgitation produced excessively high left ventricular wall tension and eventual ventricular failure. In 1964, Lillehei reported a technique of preserving the papillary muscles and chordae in patients undergoing mitral valve replacement, claiming that this would better preserve left ventricular function [17]. This created some interest in the surgical community, but because of the increased technical difficulty of performing this adjunctive step, most surgeons rejected this concept. Laboratory studies at the time were far too crude to corroborate Lillehei's theory, and it was not until Miller and his associates experimentally showed that the preservation of the papillary muscles and the entire chordal annular complex was essential to maintain normal ventricular function after valve replacement [18]. Preservation of as much of the papillary muscle chordal interaction as possible in mitral valve replacement is important, especially in patients with mitral regurgitation [19]. Subsequently, when an increasing number of patients underwent mitral valve repair for mitral regurgitation, with complete preservation of all the chordae and papillary muscles which had not ruptured, patients had very different outcomes compared to those who underwent valve replacement with resection of the papillary muscle chordal interaction. Thus, even though such a learned scholar as John Kirklin said in 1971 at the Society of Vascular Surgery that this "pop-off valve" theory was extremely important, suffice it to say that this belief has proven to be erroneous [20]. Once this had been realized, it was a rare patient that was denied mitral valve surgery, particularly mitral valve repair, because of the fear that "closing the pop-off valve" might somehow endanger the patient's life and ventricular function.

## Biologic Valves

The next major event in the evolution of mitral valve surgery was the development of the biologic porcine mitral valve by Alain Carpentier [21]. These pristine glutaraldehyde preserved mitral prostheses, however, were noted to develop calcification and become dysfunctional in 10 years (Figs. 5a–b). Several studies were done in order to gain an understanding of the pathophysiology behind this degenerative process. This phenomenon was seen more often with the mitral bioprosthetic valve in younger patients and led to an increasing hazard of re-operation [22]. Jones and his group from Emory, along with others, have shown conclusively that this dysfunction is age related [23]. Additionally, Fredrick Schoen, cardiac pathologist at the Brigham, showed that certain calcium stimulating events such as hemodialysis may prematurely influence the dysfunction of the valve [24].

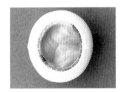

*Fig. 5a. Glutaraldehyde preserved mitral valve prosthesis prior to implantation.*

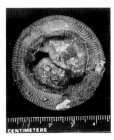

*Fig. 5b. 10-year old excised glutaraldehyde preserved mitral valve prosthesis showing extensive calcification.*

## *Development of Prosthetic Valves*

Over the ensuing years, there was a gradual progression from the high profile Starr-Edwards ball valve to the sleek, hydrodynamically efficient St. Jude valve [25]. This valve has become the largest selling prosthetic valve in the world and has been used for 20 years at the Brigham. These valves eventually gained a reputation for a relatively low risk of thromboembolism and valve thrombosis, despite the continued, although low hazard of hemorrhage [26].

## *Mitral Valve Repair for Regurgitation*

With reported series by Alain Carpentier [27] and Carlos Duran [28], it was realized in the 1970s and early 1980s that many patients undergoing mitral valve surgery for mitral regurgitation could be candidates for valve repair. Carpentier in the late 1970s had been operating upon a large number of patients immigrating from Algeria, and his classic paper on the "French Correction" is well known [29]. Thus, several factors led to an increasing use of mitral valve reconstruction for mitral regurgitation: late results showing bioprosthetic and prosthetic valves, which, though quite effective, had long-term deterioration; good long-term data supporting reconstructive techniques; improved myocardial protection; and the recognition of the importance of the papillary muscle chordal interaction.

One of our early studies from the Brigham showed that open mitral valve reconstruction for mitral stenosis is extremely effective [30]. This technique, however, has been supplanted by balloon dilatation. The vast majority of mitral valve surgery at the Brigham in 2005 was valve reconstruction in patients with regurgitant mitral valves, most of which was performed minimally invasive technique (Fig. 6). One of the key ingredients to effective mitral valve repair surgery is excellent surgical exposure. We showed that using the technique of dissection of Sondergaard's inter-atrial groove provides optimal visualization [31]. Also important in mitral valve repair is

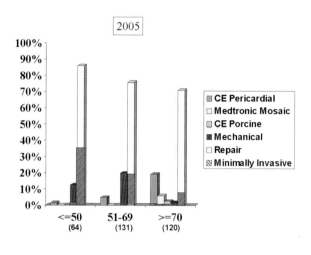

Fig. 6. *Brigham and Women's Hospital mitral valve usage, 1/1/01 through 12/31/01*

the use of a ring annuloplasty technique which Carpentier first espoused [32], but even to this day, has been somewhat controversial. In 1994, we showed that, in fact, repair of degenerative mitral valve disease was always best treated with a ring so that structural valve degeneration would be avoided in the long-term [33]. Figs. 7a and 7b show current repair techniques for the most common form of prolapse of the mitral valve: resection of the middle segment of the posterior leaflet, sliding annuloplasty apposition of P1 and P2 to each other, and the placement of an annuloplasty ring, in this case, a Cosgrove band (Fig. 8). Many other techniques may be required in mitral valve repair surgery, including chordal replacement with Gortex chordae.

## Minimally Invasive Mitral Valve Surgery

In 1996, we and others began the use of a minimally invasive approach for isolated valve surgery, both in aortic and mitral valves of patients who do not have coronary artery disease [34]. The minimally invasive

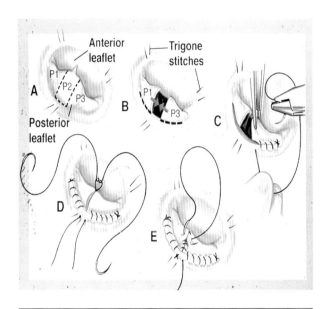

Fig. 7a. *Current techniques of mitral valve repair: resection of P2 and sliding annuloplasty of P1 and P3.*

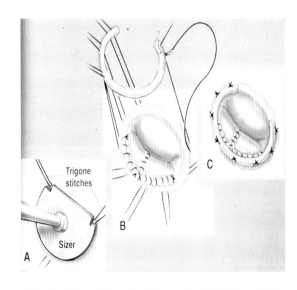

Fig. 7b. *Current techniques of mitral valve repair: placement of an annuloplasty band.*

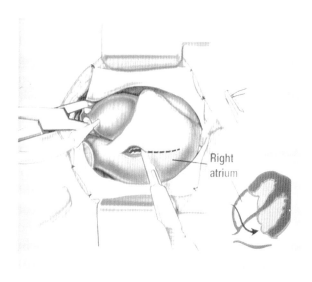

Fig. 8a. *Minimally invasive mitral valve surgery: lower mini-sternotomy incision through which the valve can approached transseptally by way of the right atrium or directly through the left atrium.*

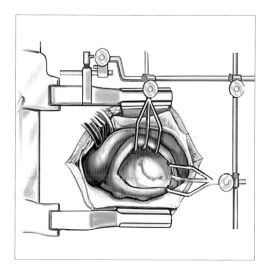

Fig. 8b. *Minimally invasive mitral valve surgery: optimal surgical exposure obtained with retractor system and approach through left-atrium.*

# Table 1 Cardiovascular Surgical Volumes in Mainland China: Annual Statistics

|  | 2003 | 2004 |
|---|---|---|
| Beijing | 10,274 (7,284) | 12,381 (9,160) |
| Shanghai | 6,457 (5,404) | 7,652 (6,292) |
| Henan Province | 5,564 (4,991) | 7,491 (6,506) |
| Shandong Province | 3,498 | 6,988 (5,907) |
| Guangdong Province | 6,024 (5,195) | 5,588 (4,963) |
| Hubei Province | 4,360 (3,995) | 5,246 (4,696) |
| Jiangsu Province | 3,380 (2,644) | 4,706 (3,820) |
| Fujian Province | 3,301 (2,496) | 3,513 (2,775) |
| Zhejiang Province | 2,736 (2,144) | 3,306 (2,526) |
| Hunan Province | 3,351 (2,685) | 3,191 (2,913) |
| ... | ... | ... |
| **Mainland China total (CPB) cases** | 76,319 (59,886) | 90,812 (74,840) |

CPB: cardiopulmonary bypass.

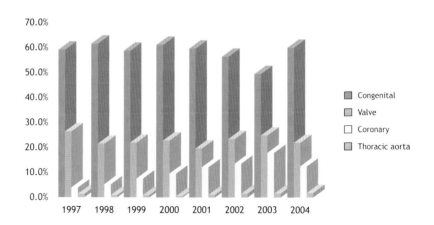

Fig. 1. The annual ratio of cardiac operations in China (1997–2004).

been the leading etiology in China. Based on some previous epidemiological investigations there are about 2.5 million patients suffering from chronic rheumatic heart disease in China. The incidence of this disease, in general, is higher in the rural areas than in the urban regions. However it also appears that such incidences were higher in Southern (i.e. 0.40/1,000 in Guangdong Province) than in the Northern China (i.e. 0.14/1,000 in Jilin Province). The recent reported incidence of rheumatic heart disease in young people aged 5 to 18 years is about 0.22/1,000 (0.03–0.40/1,000), remarkably lower than the level in 1979–1980 (0.52/1,000). Up to date, at least three out of four valvular operations in mainland China are still for chronic rheumatic lesions. This could partially explain why valve replacement, rather than repair, has been the first choice for many Chinese surgeons over the past decades.

Nevertheless, health care for an aging population has become a vital challenge worldwide, particularly in the developing world such as China. For instance, the number of elderly Chinese people (traditionally defined as aged 65 and above) is anticipated to increase from around 120 million in 2005 to more than 200 million in 2008, which will make up 14% of the total population [2]. By the year 2036, the number of elderly Chinese people may surge to over 300 million and represent up to 20% of the nation's total population [2, 3]. Chinese cardiac surgeons have a clear indicaton of such an aging trend as they are seeing much more degenerative valvular pathologies nowadays (as high as 20% of total valvular cases) than in the past (less than 5%).

In response to such a reality, at least two changes have occurred in China over the past decade. Firstly, tissue prosthesis has started to re-gain some popularity, simply because there is a wealth of knowledge supporting the use of bioprosthesis as the prosthesis of choice for the elderly. It is particularly noteworthy that a few made-in-China products have progressed amazingly well in the past few years. A bovine pericardial prosthesis (BalMedic®, Beijing, China, Fig. 2) had been implanted in over 1,200 cases at more than 70 hospitals across China with encouraging mid-term results. One of the features of this bioprosthesis is the preservation methodology, namely the

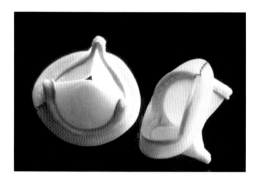

*Fig. 2.*

treatment with Hydroxyl Chromium, which may significantly enhance its durability (Jin L, PhD. Personal communication). These so-called "second generation" bioprostheses appeared promising so far and do warrant further multi-center evaluation with careful long-term monitoring.

The other notable change is the significantly enhanced nationwide experience in valve reconstruction surgery during the last 20 years. One should remember that valvular interventions in the early period of open-heart surgery were always "repair," and it was no exception in China [4, 5]. Xi-Chun Lan and his colleagues (Fig. 3, right upper inset) at the Shanghai Second Medical College performed the first closed mitral commissurotomy (using the index finger through the left atrial appendage, Fig. 3, right middle inset) on February 9, 1954. This procedure marked the beginning of intracardiac surgery in China. Within the next 10 months, this group of surgeons had performed similar operations for 34 patients (Fig. 3). The majority of the patients experienced excellent quality of life after surgery and were able to continue their active daily work (Fig. 3, left upper inset).

The largest retrospective report on closed mitral commissurotomy in China was from Fuwai Hospital in Beijing. Between 1956 and 1977, 2,037 patients had undergone different types of closed mitral commissurotomy at this institution. Up to 20-year follow-up confirmed good early- and mid-term postoperative outcome, although as expected such improvements could not be maintained during the long-term observation. It has been noted by the surgeons

# 心 臟 手 術

二尖瓣狹窄是常見的心臟病，病人每因
氣喘和咯血而喪失勞動力和生命。這種病過
去都法很怕，但在歡年前，蘇聯醫學科學院
院士巴庫列夫教授證明：施行二尖瓣分離手

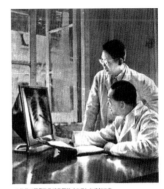

上海第二醫學院教授謝臨純（坐者）和請師過草
榮在看愛克斯光片，確定施行心臟手術的部位。　林澤洲攝影

術，使狹窄的瓣孔擴大，血液暢通，病症就
可痊癒。

上海第二醫學院的醫師們在蘇聯醫學界施
行心臟手術成功的鼓舞下，組織了研究小
組，進行多次的實驗，並得到上海市衛生局
的積極幫助。一九五四年二月九日，該院蘭
錫純教授勝利地完成了第一次心臟手術。病
人王積德在施行手術後的第五天就能起床走
動，接着就完全恢復了健康。後來該院教授梁
其琛、董方中、王一山等也先後施行過一手
術而獲得成功。在十個月內，該院已爲三十
四個病人施行了心臟手術，效果都很良好。
現在該院的醫師們，正爲醫治其他心臟病而
作進一步的研究。

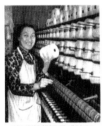

因患"二尖瓣狹窄"症而不能工作的服遠光，
施行手術後，已在去年十月到國營上海第
二棉紡織廠工作。　伊廉康攝影

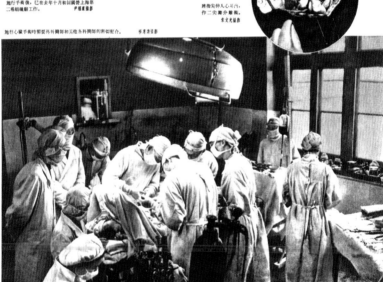

施行心臟手術時需要外科醫師和其他各科醫師的密切配合。　林澤洲攝影

將指尖伸入心耳內，
作二尖瓣分離術。　朱文光攝影

---

*Fig. 3.*

at Fuwai Hospital [6], as well as from other institutions [7], that the outcome following direct-vision mitral commissurotomy was overall much better than that after the closed approach.

In 1994 Liu and the Fuwai team [8] reported their experience in direct-vision mitral valve repair in 488 patients. Two years later, another series of valve reconstruction involving 326 cases was also reported by Zhuang and colleagues from Henan Medical University [9]. The techniques applied in these two series appeared more complex than those described previously in the Chinese literature. For instance, in addition to the commissurotomy with or without annuloplasty ring, the techniques used also included reconstruction of mitral leaflets or subvalvular structures. Combined tricuspid or aortic valve reconstructions were also reported in some cases. Nevertheless, due to the large proportion of patients with chronic rheumatic valvular lesions, the development of valve repair still progressed quite slowly in China before the mid-1990s.

The last decade witnessed a rapid growth of valvular reconstruction surgery in this country. The use of artificial materials during mitral repair for regurgitation became more common. Meng and his associates at Anzhen Hospital in Beijing described their experience in using Gore-Tex for chordae reconstruction. Xu and colleagues from Changhai Hospital in Shanghai also reported their series using an artificial (PTFE) chordae. Some other groups of surgeons also published their experiences in mitral valve repair with relatively large sample sizes [10]. The representative institutions include the Fuwai Hospital, Anzhen Hospital, PLA 301 Hospital in Beijing; Zhongshan Hospital, Changhai Hospital in Shanghai; Xijing Hospital in Xi'an; and Asian Heart Center in Wuhan. Newly advocated techniques such as the "edge-to-edge" repair have been applied by some surgeons in selected cases [10]. Different types of minimally invasive valve operations, either through smaller incisions (partial sternotomy or thoracotomy) or with thoracoscopic assistance, have been gradually adopted at many centers. The benefits of surgical treatment of atrial fibrillation during valve operations has also become widely appreciated, although still pending evaluation in larger patient population with longer-term follow-up.

Based on the initial experience in large groups of patients, indications and contraindications of valvular repair in the Chinese population were proposed and evaluated. Moreover it was acknowledged that those patients who underwent annular ring plasty may have better long-term outcome than those who received no-ring repair [8, 9]. Such observations have led to a remarkable increase in the use of annuloplasty ring during mitral valve repair. Once again, the Chinese-made annuloplasty ring showed promising potential as reflected by the latest share in the national market. Currently, among all valve cases in China, about half were mitral valve replacement or repair, followed by combined mitral and aortic operations (around 30%), and isolated aortic valve intervention (about 15%) [11].

Recently, Meng and his colleagues summarized their 12-year experience on valvular surgery at Anzhen Hospital in Beijing [12]. Between January 1, 1993 and December 31, 2004, 5,066 patients (52.8% were male) had undergone various valvular operations at this institution. Majority of the patients (94%) were younger than 65 years and with chronic rheumatic heart disease (76.7%), whereas 8.3% and 8.1% of the patients in this series had congenital or degenerative valvular lesions, respectively. Only 6.5% of the patients had previous open-heart interventions, which were predominantly valvular operations (314 out of 327 cases). Among all the valvular procedures, 51.7% were for mitral valve (n=2,621), followed by mitral plus aortic valves (30.3%, n=1,535), and isolated aortic valve (15.8%, n=800) or tricuspid valve (1.9%, n=98) operations. Approaching one third of the total cases had combined tricuspid valve intervention (32%, n=1,680). About 4.1% of the patients (n=208) received concomitant coronary artery bypass grafting. Perioperative complications occurred in 18.2% (n=921) of the cases, and the overall surgical mortality rate was 4.6% (n=235). The numbers of cases of repair versus replacement were 567/3,589 for mitral, 79/2,235 for aortic, and 1,690/88 for tricuspid positions, respectively. Among patients undergoing valve replacement operations, about 97% of them received mechanical prostheses in this series which was far different with the present status outside China (partially due to the relatively young age of these patients). Nevertheless, the ratio of the elderly patients (age of 65-year-old or above) had gradually increased to as high as 15% since the year 2000 [12]. Such an ageing trend indeed represents some new challenges as far as the perioperative care and particularly the surgical outcome are concerned (Fig. 4). On a separate note, the 10-year survival and freedom from re-operation for patients received mitral valve repair were 88% and 86%, respectively.

To summarize the current status in China of valvular surgery in general and mitral valve surgery in particular, it seems that one could not describe it better than by quoting Winston Churchill: "Now this is not the end. It is not even the beginning of the end. But it is, perhaps, the end of the beginning."

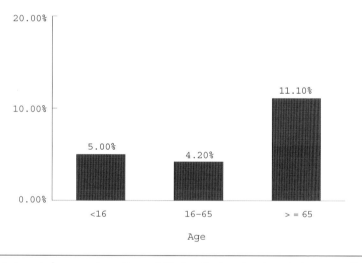

*Fig. 4. Impact of age on perioperative mortality in patients undergoing valvular surgery (from [12] with permission).*

## References

1.  Hu SS, Kong LZ (2006) Cardiovascular disease in China: report of 2005. Bulletin of the Chinese Society for Thoracic & Cardiovascular Surgery, Chinese Medical Association 10 (4):12–17 (in Chinese).
2.  Chinese Academy of Social Science. Green book of population and labor. Beijing, 2004.

3. United Nations Population Division. World population prospects: the 2002 revision. http://esa.un.org/unpp/p2k0data.asp (accessed on January 10, 2006).

4. Lan HC, Feng CJ, Huang MH, Yu KJ (1955) Surgical treatment of mitral stenosis. Chin Med J 73:278–292.

5. Wan S, Yim APC (2003) The evolution of cardiovascular surgery in China. Ann Thorac Surg 76:2147–2155.

6. Guo JQ, et al. (1963) Direct-vision surgical treatment for mitral stenosis. Chin J Surg 11:128–132 (in Chinese).

7. Sun YQ, et al. (1979) Direct-vision versus closed mitral commissurotomy: over 12-year follow-up in 65 patients. Chin J Surg 17:451–453 (in Chinese).

8. Liu YM, et al. (1994) Outcome analysis on direct-vision mitral valve repair. Chin J Surg 32:17–20 (in Chinese).

9. Zhuang SC, et al. (1996) Valvular reconstruction in 326 patients: clinical results. Chin J Thorac Cardiovasc Surg 12:100–101 (in Chinese).

10. Meng X (ed) (2005) Advanced techniques for mitral valve reconstruction in adult. Beijing Publishing House, Beijing (in Chinese).

11. Zhang BR (2005) Report on the 6th national heart valve surgical symposium. Chin J Thorac Cardiovasc Surg 21:A4.

12. Meng X, Bai T. Retrospective analysis in 5,066 patients undergoing valvular operations: impact on perioperative care. Chin J Thorac Cardiovasc Surg (in press)

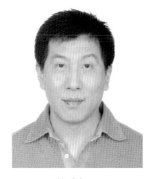

Xu Meng

# *Cardiology in China: Current Status and New Trends*

*Shu Zhang, Ming-Zhe Chen*

## Epidemiology

With the development of the economy and of medicine there have been great changes in the spectrum of diseases in China. Many diseases such as malnutrition and most infectious diseases which threatened the lives and health of the Chinese in the past have now been controlled, whereas trauma and some chronic illness (such as cardiovascular diseases and malignant tumors) are beginning to become the dominant threats to the health of the population. Data from investigations in 1985 showed that the mortality from cardiovascular diseases was 131.04/100,000 in 36 cities, and 165.80/100,000 in 72 counties, which amounted to 23.39% and 25.47% of the total deaths in urban and rural areas respectively [1]. This demonstrates that cardiovascular disease is becoming the primary cause of death in China.

There is more data illustrating the prevalence of various particular cardiovascular diseases. According to incomplete investigations in 1980s the prevalence of rheumatic heart disease and cor pulmonale were 25–110/100,000 and 470/100,000 respectively, while the prevalence of congenital heart disease was 578/100,000 in newborns and 108/100,000 in adults [1]. A study in 1991 [2] showed that the prevalence of hypertension was 13.6% in the population over 15 years old. Other data acquired in 1996 [3] showed that the prevalence of coronary atherosclerotic heart disease was 6.46% in the population over 40 years old, and its mortality (most caused by acute myocardial infarction) was 64.25/100,000 in urban and 26.62/100,000 in the rural areas respectively. It was found that the level of blood pressure in the Chinese population was higher than that in developed countries, while the level of blood lipid was lower than that in developed countries [4].

According to an investigation of 14 provinces or municipalities using cluster sampling in 2004, Zhou et al. [5] reported that the total prevalence of atrial fibrillation (AF) was 0.77% in the population over 30 years old. Subgroup analysis showed that the prevalence of AF was 0.2%–0.5% in the group between 40 and 60 years old, 1.3% in the group between 60 and 70 years old, 3.1% in the group between 70 and 80 years old, and 7.5% in the group over 80 years old. Those taking oral warfarin for anticoagulation therapy represent less than 10% of the total patients with AF.

## Academic Associations

The Chinese Society of Cardiology is the most influential academic association for cardiovascular diseases in China. There are also some academic associations for certain cardiovascular diseases or special groups in a certain field of cardiology, such as the Chinese Society of Pacing and Electrophysiology, the Chinese League of Hypertension, the Chinese Society of Biomedical Engineering, and the Section of Interventional Cardiology of the Chinese Society of Cardiology.

## Non-invasive Diagnostic Techniques

Before the 1980s, biochemical tests, electrocardiogram (ECG), chest X-ray and M-type ultrasonic cardiogram were the main techniques used the diagnosis of cardiovascular diseases. After the 1980s many types of high-tech diagnostic equipment were introduced to and used in cardiology. Stress ECG (exercise testing) and 24-hour ambulatory monitor ECG (Holter) [6] have been used to diagnose ischemic heart diseases and arrhythmias. Electronic-beam computer tomography [7] and multiple-slices computer tomography (the most advanced one in currency is 64-slices) can provide the images of each layer of transect and subsequently reconstruct the three dimensional anatomic structure of the heart. Magnetic resonance imaging [8] can also show the images of any section and reconstruct the 3-D anatomic structure of the heart. Two-dimensional B-type UCG and color-Doppler UCG are routine techniques for diagnosis of heart diseases [9–10]. Myocardial contrast echocardiogram is also used to detect the ischemic region [9]. Another valuable technique for diagnosis of CAD is radionuclide imaging, which includes single photon emitted computer tomography and positive electron computer tomography [11].

# Current Status

## *Ischemic heart disease*

Initial work on interventional diagnosis of coronary disease started in 1973 [12] when coronary angiography was performed in Zhongshan Hospital of Shanghai Medical College and Fuwai Hospital of Peking Union Medical College. In 1984 Zheng's group [13] performed the first case of percutaneous transluminal coronary angioplasty (PTCA) in Xi'an, which marked the beginning of the interventional era in China. In 1992, intracoronary stent was introduced to China [14]. The most significant progress in PTCA and stenting (the combination of the two is termed percutaneous coronary intervention, PCI) is that PCI can be used for revascularization in patients with acute myocardial infarction (AMI), which includes primary PCI and rescue PCI (when thrombolysis therapy failed). Cases of PCI have increased significantly since the mid-1990s. Data from registry [15] shows that 8,725 cases of PTCA were performed in 75 registered hospitals during the period 1997 to 1998, and the total success rate was 95.9% (8,369 cases). In 1997, 3,740 cases of PTCA were performed with a success rate of 95.0% (3,553 cases); such numbers increased in the next year to 4,985 cases and 96.6% (4,816 cases), respectively. The total amount of lesions of coronary arteries treated was 10,218, with a success rate of 94.4% (9,650 lesions). Among these 8,725 cases, 6,326 patients received 7,748 stents including 86 stents implanted in the left main coronary artery (LMCA). The success rate of intracoronary stenting was 99.1% (7,677 stents). Severe complications emerged in 510 patients (8.1%) who received intracoronary stenting, including 25 cases of death (0.40%), while severe complications in the total number of PTCA cases occurred in 959 (11.0%) cases including 32 cases of death (0.37%). Moreover, 1,054 patients with AMI underwent emergent PCI, with a success rate of 95.8% (1,001 cases). In addition, 93 cases (94 vessels) of percutaneous transluminal coronary rotational atherectomy were registered with a success rate of 93.6%.

According to the Third National Coronary Intervention Registry [16], 36,098 cases of PCI were performed in 112 registered hospitals during 1999 to 2001 with a total success rate of 97.0%. Among them, 8,000 cases were performed in 1999, 11,753 in 2000, and 16,354 in 2001. A total of 53,695 lesions of vessels were treated, and 43,304 (80.6%) lesions were implanted with stents. The success rate of stenting was 99.0%. Complications of selective PCI (a total of 30,339 cases) included: coronary arterial spasm (2.4%), severe coronary dissection (2.2%), acute coronary occlusion (0.8%), acute and sub-acute thrombosis (0.6%), AMI (0.5%), emergent coronary artery bypass graft (CABG) (0.07%), and death (0.31%). Revascularization of target vessels was 7.0% during follow-up. Emergent PCI for the treatments of AMI had increased to 5,779 cases, including 4,417 cases of primary PCI and 1,342 cases of rescue PCI, with a success rate of 96.3%. Among the total 36,098 cases of PCI there were 551 cases whose target lesions were in LMCA with a success rate of 98.4%. Death rate was 0.9% (5 patients) during the LMCA PCI procedure and 1.5% (8 cases) during follow-up. Revascularization of LMCA was 8.2%. At 46% of the registered hospitals, there were less than 75 PCI cases performed each year. At only 20% of the registered hospitals were there more than 200 cases of PCI per year, which indicated an imbalance in the development of PCI among hospitals nation-wide. Drug eluting stent has been used in clinical practice since 2001 in

China [17]. After the 1990s the value of intravascular ultrasound (IVUS) in the diagnosis of CAD has been recognized by many cardiologists. At the same time, percutaneous transluminal septal myocardial ablation for the treatment of obstructive hypertrophic cardiomyopathy has been developed in a few major centers [18].

So far no PCI registry data is available after the year 2001. However according to the data of 1999–2001 (during which period the annual increase rate of PCI procedures was over 30%), the number of PCI procedures may reach 60,000 in the year 2005. Meanwhile, an annual international symposium "China Interventional Therapy," led by Dr. Run-Lin Gao, current President of Chinese Society of Cardiology, has been launched since 2003.

## Arrhythmias

Pacing therapy was available in China since 1964, marked by the use of a transpericardial pacemaker [19]. The first transvenous pacemaker was implanted in 1973 [20]. Cases of pacing therapy have significantly increased over the past three decades. According to the pacing therapy registry in 2002 [20], 279 hospitals in China have pacemaker implantation service. In the year 2001, 10,845 pacemakers were implanted throughout the country (equal to 8 pacemakers per million population), an increase of 15.5% compared to 2000 [21]. Of these 9,858 were primary implants and 797 were replacements; 36.3% were dual-chamber pacemakers, 56.2% were single-chamber, and other types including AAI (R) and VVI(R)) represented 7.5%. Although no registry data for pacing therapy after 2002, based on the recent trends cases of pacing therapy may reach 15,000 in 2005. Current indication is not limited to sick sinus syndrome and/or atrioventricular block. Other indications include: (1) carotid sinus hypersensitive syndrome or nerve mediated syncope; (2) obstructive hypertrophic cardiomyopathy; (3) long-QT syndrome; (4) prevention of AF; and (5) heart failure caused by dilated cardiomyopathy [20]. The principle of pacing therapy for the treatment of heart failure is to restore the synchrony of systole of the two ventricles, which is termed resynchronization therapy (RCT). The first RCT pacemaker (biventricular pacemaker) was implanted in 1999. By the end of 2004, more than 150 RCT pacemakers had been implanted throughout the country [22].

In 1991 Wang et al. [23] implanted the first implantable cardioverter and defibrillator (ICD) in Suzhou. It was a transprecardial ICD implanted during open heart operation. In 1994 Yi et al. [24] implanted a transvenous third-generation ICD with single lead. The first dual-chamber ICD was implanted in 2002 [23]. The number of ICD implanted was 65 in 2000 and 77 in 2001. By the end of 2001, a total of 285 ICD had been implanted [21]. By the end of 2003 total cases were still fewer than 400 [25], which suggested that the development of ICD was limited by the economy status in China.

Early work on clinical electrophysiology began in October 1973, when Sun and Hu [23] recorded the first electrogram of the His bundle in Beijing. In 1975, Sun and Hu [23] reported for the first time the normal range of atrioventricular conduction time in the Chinese population. In 1978, Ma et al. [23] in Jiangsu performed the first case of surgery for the treatment of preexcitation syndrome by cutting off the atrioventricular accessory pathway. Ten years later, Li [23] developed the first experiment model of radiofrequency catheter ablation (RFCA) in Wuhan. Subsequently, Li reported the experimental results of RFCA of myocardium, coronary sinus and atrioventricular node in 1990 and 1991 [23]. The initial clinical work on RFCA was conducted by Li and Chen in 1991 [23]. Two years later, RFCA started to extend to other provinces and cities. Hu [23] did a great deal of work to promote the techniques of RFCA. According to data from the RFCA registry in 1995 [26], 10,035 cases of RFCA had been performed in 93 registered hospitals between January 1991 to May 1995, with a total success rate of 96.6% (9,598 cases). There were 263 cases of recurrence (2.7%), 181 cases with severe complications (1.8%), and 6 cases of RFCA-related death (0.06%) in the group. Since then the number of RFCA cases increased significantly. A recent investigation showed that 10,811 cases of RFCA were performed in 136 registered hospitals in 2000 [27], with a success rate of 96.5%. No national registry data on RFCA has been reported

12.5 mg three times per day (treating group, N= 7,468) or the matched group taking oral placebo with similar preparation (control group, N= 7,494), according to the principle of randomization. The period of treatment was 4 weeks. The total death rate in the treatment group was lower than in the control group (9.1% versus 9.7%, P=0.19). Other indexes of these 2 groups included: incidence rate of heart failure lowered by 9.5% in the treatment group compared to the control group (17.0% versus 18.7%, P=0.01); incidence rate of events of combined end-points lowered by 7.2% (21.5% versus 23.1%, P=0.02); incidence rate of shock increased by 10.7% (4.9% versus 4.4%, P= 0.11); incidence rate of hypotension increased by 38.5% (16.1% versus 10.9%, P=0.001). The death rate was lowered by 17.0% (8.6% versus 10.2%, P=0.02) in patients with AMI in the anterior wall; by 15.1% (9.2% versus 10.7%, P=0.01) in patients whose heart rates in baseline were between 60 beats per minutes (bpm) and 100 bpm; and by 36.6% (17.2% versus 24.9%, P=0.0001) in patients whose heart rates in baseline were over 100 bpm. The results suggested that clinical use of captopril at an early stage of AMI was effective and safe, especially for those patients with AMI in the anterior wall, with normal heart rate, or with too fast a heart beat.

CCS2 referrs to *Clopidogril and Metoprolol in Myocardial Infarction Trial (COMMIT)* [47], which was also a multicenter, randomized, double-blind, placebo controlled clinical trial. Its objective was to study whether clinical use of metoprolol or clopidogril could lower the mortality of AMI. This study included Clopidogril Trial and Metoprolol Trial. Between June 1999 and February 2005, 45,851 patients were enrolled in the Clopidogril Trial. They were randomly assigned to either clopidogril (N=22,960) or placebo (N=22,891) groups. Patients took oral clopidogril or placebo 75 mg per day in addition to oral aspirin 162 mg for 4 weeks. The Metoprolol Trial enrolled 45,851 patients and assigned them to metoprolol (N=22,928) and placebo (N=22,923) groups. Patients were first injected with 15 mg of the drugs (metoprolol or placebo), then took oral drugs (metoprolol or placebo) 200mg daily for 4 weeks. The results of the COMMIT trial were reported at the 54th Congress of the American College of Cardiology in 2005 [47–48], which suggested that the use of metoprolol at the acute stage of AMI does not significantly lower in-hospital mortality. However, taking clopidogril in addition to oral aspirin could decrease the in-hospital mortality rate.

# New Trends

In the new century, Chinese cardiologists are trying their best to advance both basic research and clinical practice in catching up the cutting edge development worldwide. In some research areas such as using stem cells for treating heart failure secondary to AMI, and for sick sinus syndrome or atrioventricular block ("biological pacemaker"), encouraging data have been obtained. In the clinical setting, catheter ablation of AF, prevention of sudden cardiac death, percutaneous transcatheter aortic valve replacement, and percutaneous transcatheter mitral annuloplasty are the major focuses of studies in China.

Imbalanced regional development in China is a general phenomenon in all fields of medicine, paralleling to the status of the social economy in different areas [16]. Medical resources are concentrated mainly at major hospitals in the urban areas. There is less chance for patients in rural areas to obtain high quality health care. Thus cardiologists at major centers continuously train physicians from small cities or rural areas in order to support the development of cardiology in those regions.

In addition, standardization is an important task for Chinese cardiologists. Establishing guidelines is one part of the work towards standardization. Training physicians from small cities and rural areas is another crucial part. The Ministry of Health has recently promulgated a permission system for developing PCI [49]. Standardized cardiology will be further improved in China in the new millennium.

## References

1.  Chen HZ (2001) Summary of circulatory system. In: Ye RG, Lu ZY (eds) Internal medicine, 5th edn. Beijing: People's Health Publishing House, pp 149–154.

2. Tao SC, Wu XG, Duan XF, et al. (1995) Hypertension prevalence and status of awareness, treatment and control in China. Chin Med J 108:483–489.

3. Chen HZ, Qian JY, Li Q (2005) Coronary atherosclerotic heart disease. In: Chen HZ (ed) Practice of internal medicine, 20th edn. Beijing: People's Health Publishing House, pp 1467–1493.

4. Chinese Society of Cardiology, Editorial Board of Chinese Journal of Cardiology (2005) Summary of the eighth national congress of cardiology of Chinese medical association. Chin J Cardiol 33(3):204–209.

5. Zhou ZQ, Hu DY, Chen J, et al. (2004) Epidemiology of atrial fibrillation in China. Chin J Internal Med 43(7):491–494.

6. Xu YS (2002) Dynamic electrocardiogram (Holter). In: Chen ZJ, Gao RL (eds) Coronary heart disease. Beijing: People's Health Publishing House, pp 269–285.

7. Dai RP (2002) Electronic-beam computer tomography for diagnosis of coronary atherosclerotic heart disease. In: Chen ZJ, Gao RL (eds) Coronary heart disease, pp 441–464.

8. Dai RP (2002) Magnetic resonance imaging for diagnosis of coronary atherosclerotic heart disease. In: Chen ZJ, Gao RL (eds) Coronary heart disease, pp 465–476.

9. Liu HY, Zhang JG (2002) Ultrasonic cardiogram for diagnosis of coronary atherosclerotic heart disease. In: Chen ZJ, Gao RL (eds) Coronary heart disease, pp 286–380.

10. Yang YJ (2002) Evaluation of the function of the left ventricle with ultrasonic Doppler cardiogram. In: Chen ZJ, Gao RL (eds) Coronary heart disease, pp 381–405.

11. Tian YQ, Liu XJ. Radionuclide imaging for diagnosis of coronary atherosclerotic heart disease. In: Chen ZJ, Gao RL (eds) Coronary heart disease, pp 406–426.

12. Gao RL (2002) Selective coronary angiography and left ventriculography. In: Chen ZJ, Gao RL (eds) Coronary heart disease, pp 477–521.

13. Gao RL (2002) Interventional therapy for the treatment of coronary atherosclerotic heart disease. In: Chen ZJ, Gao RL (eds) Coronary heart disease, pp 630–704.

14. Gao RL, Wu XG, Chen JL, et al. (1999) The major achievements in studying the coronary heart disease in China. Chin J Cardiol 27(5):325–332.

15. Section of Interventional Cardiology, Chinese Society of Cardiology, Editorial Board of Chinese Journal of Cardiology (2000) A data analysis of the Second National Coronary Intervention Registry. Chin J Cardiol, 28(1):10–13.

16. Section of Interventional Cardiology, Chinese Society of Cardiology, Editorial Board of Chinese Journal of Cardiology (2002) A data analysis of the Third National Coronary Intervention Registry. Chin J Cardiol 30(12):719–723.

17. The Sino-SIRUS Study Investigators. A preliminary experience with the sirolimus-eluting stent in the treatment of de novo coronary artery lesions in Chinese patients—The Sino-SIRUS study. Chin J Cardiol 31(11):814–817.

18. Li ZQ, Gao RL (2000) Summary of the first symposium on chemical ablation for the treatment of obstructive hypertrophic cardiomyopathy. Chin J Cardiol 28 (2):160.

19 Huo LK, Fang ZP, Wang ZN, et al. (1964) Experiments and initial clinical use of two kinds of self-made pacemakers. Chin Med J 50:219–224.

20. Zhang S, Wang FZ, Huang DJ, et al. (2003) Current perception and recommendation of implanted pacing therapy. Chin J Cardiac Arrhyth 7(1):8–21.

21. Wang FZ, Hua W, Zhang S, et al. (2003) Clinical survey of pacemakers 2000–2001. Chin J Cardiac Arrhyth 7(3):189–191.

22. Hua W, Wang FZ, Zhu L, et al. (2004) Analysis of complications of biventricular pacemaker implantation in patients with congestive heart failure. Chin J Cardiac Arrhyth 8(4):252–254.

23. Chen X (2003) Clinical cardiac electrophysiology thirty-three-years. Chin J Cardiac Arrhyth 7(2):70–79.

24. Yang XC, Zhang JJ, Wang AH, et al. (2005) The information from the sixth scientific congress of Chinese society of pacing and electrophysiology. Chin J Cardiac Arrhyth 9(2):159–160.

25. Hua W, Chen X (2005) Clinical application of implantable cardioverter defibrillator should be valued. Chin J Cardiac Arrhyth 9(1):5.

26. Section of Catheter Ablation, the Society of Cardiac Pacing and Electrophysiology of Chinese Society of Biomedical Engineering, the Editorial Board of Chinese Journal of Cardiac Pacing and Electrophysiology (1996) A data analysis of the national radiofequency catheter ablation registry. Chin J Cardiac Pacing Electrophysiol 10(3):120–121.

27. The Society of Cardiac Pacing and Electrophysiology of Chinese Society of Biomedical Engineering, Chinese Society of Pacing and Electrophysiology (2001) Data analysis of the national radiofequency catheter ablation registry in 2000. Chin J Cardiac Pacing Electrophysiol 15:368.

28. Fan YJ (2003) The information of the fifth scientific session of Chinese society of pacing and electrophysiology. Chin J Cardiac Arrhyth 7(1):60–62.

29. National Work Group of Atrial Fibrillation (2005) Current status and registry of catheter ablation for the treatment of atrial fibrillation. In: Papers collection of the 3rd China atrial fibrillation symposium (in Chinese). Dalian, pp 2–6.

30. Gu FS (1999) The major achievements in cardiac rheumatic fever research in China. Chinese Journal of Cardiology (in Chinese) 27(4):265–267.

31. Dai RP (2003) Current status and new trends in interventional therapy for the treatment of congenital heart diseases. Chin J Cardiol 31(11):801–805.

32. Dong ZJ, Li SH, Lu XC, et al. (1986) A report of 35 cases of percutaneous transluminal renal angioplasty for the treatment of high blood pressure caused by renal artery stenosis. Chin J Cardiol 14(1):20–22.

33. Chinese Society of Cardiology (2002) Recommendation in medication of chronic systolic heart failure. Chin J Cardiol 30(1):7–23.

34. Chinese Society of Cardiology (2001) Guideline for diagnosis and treatments of acute myocardial infarction. Chin J Cardiol 29(12):710–725.

35. Committee to Revise the 1999 Chinese Guideline for the Prevention and Treatment of Patients with Hypertension Chinese guideline for the prevention and treatment of patients with hypertension (practical edition) (2004). Chin J Cardiol 32(12):1060–1064.

36. Chinese Society of Cardiology (2000) Recommendation for diagnosis and treatments of unstable angina pectoris. Chin J Cardiol 28(6):409–412.

37. Chinese Society of Cardiology (2002) Guideline for percutaneous coronary intervention. Chin J Cardiol 30(12):707–718.

38. Chinese Society of Cardiology, Section of Medication of Heart Diseases with Anti-arrhythmias Drugs (2001) Recommendation for medication of heart diseases with anti-arrhythmias drugs. Chin J Cardiol 29(6):323–336.

39. Work Group of Percutaneous Transluminal Septal Myocardial Ablation (2001) Recommendation for Percutaneous Transluminal Septal Myocardial Ablaton (PTSMA). Chin J Cardiol 29(7):434–435.

40. Fang Q, Wang ZL, Ning TH, et al. (1997) Principles for the prevention of dyslipemia. Chin J Cardiol 25(3):169–175.

41. Liu GZ, Hu DY, Tao P, et al. (1998) Recommendation for evaluation of methodology in clinical trials of drugs for the treatment of cardiovascular diseases. Chin J Cardiol 26(1):5–11.

42. Chinese Society of Pacing and Electrophysiology (2002) Guideline of catheter ablation for the treatment of tachyarrhythmias. Chin J Cardiac Pacing Electrophysiol 16(2):81–95.

43. (2001) Recommendation for diagnosis and treatments of pulmonary embolism Chin J Med Guide (in Chinese) 3(6):401–417.

44. Chinese Cardiac Study Collaborative Group (1995) Oral captopril versus placebo among 13,634 patients with suspected acute myocardial infarction: interim report from the Chinese cardiac study (CCS-1). Lancet 345:686–687.

45. Chinese Cardiac Study (CCS-1) Collaborative Group (1997) Oral captopril versus placebo among 14,962 patients with suspected acute myocardial infarction: a multicenter, randomized, double-blind, placebo controlled clinical trial. Chin Med J 110:834–838.

46. Chinese Cardiac Study (CCS-1) Collaborative Group (2001) Long-term mortality in patients with myocardial infarction: impact of early treatment with captopril for 4 weeks. Chin Med J 114(2):15–118.

47. To see: http://www.commit-ccs2.org.

48. Zhao MZ, Huang HX (2005) Summary of CLARITY-TIMI and COMMIT/CCS-2. Chin J Med Guide 7(2):154.

49. Lü SZ, Chen YD, Song XT (2004) The information of the first salon of percutaneous coronary intervention in China. Chin J Cardiol 32(10):958.

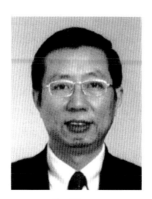

Shu Zhang

# Forging a Link*

*Thomas B. Ferguson*

**D**r. Max Cowan, a former Professor of Anatomy at Washington University School of Medicine in St. Louis, tells this vignette. A faculty member died and willed his body to the school. There was a sealed envelope, along with a covering note requesting that when his body was to be dissected, the envelope be given to the students assigned to his cadaver. Dr. Cowan opened the note and read the following: "Dear students: the greater part of my professional life has been devoted to trying to teach medical students something. This will be my last attempt."

This summarizes well what we physicians do—learn and teach, teach and learn—all for the welfare of our patients. These are life-long tasks for every one of us: forging the links not only between teachers and students, and between doctors and patients, but also among colleagues worldwide. I have had the pleasure of visiting the countries of the pacific rim on a number of occasions, but China only once, that in 1981. My wife and I look forward with eager anticipation to our mainland trip right after this meeting. It seems to me that we cannot let this opportunity to visit this great country pass without

---

* This paper was originally presented at the 2nd MITSIG International Symposium: Controversies in Cardiothoracic Surgery, Hong Kong, November 20–21, 1998.

making a few observations and predictions. Winston Churchill said it is difficult to look further ahead than you can see, but I will take that risk. After all, at my young age there should not be that many helpings of humble pie to consume if my predictions prove erroneous. Through the efforts of Dr. Ying-Kai Wu (Fig. 1), a 5-day international symposium on cardiothoracic surgery was held in Beijing in September 1981. It was said to have been the first gathering of this type in the history of Chinese medicine. There were 54 presentations by 37 lecturers, 17 of these from the People's Republic of China, and 20 from America, Canada, Europe, Scandinavia, and South America. Dr. Wu is the visual personification of the oft-quoted Chinese proverb: "To plan for a year, plant rice; to plan for a decade, plant acorns; to plan for a century, teach men." Much of what little I know about Chinese medicine I learned from Dr. Wu, and as I came to understand the "whys" the more sense the "hows" made. Let me give you a few examples.

In 1982, a year after our Beijing trip, I was privileged to be President of the American Association for Thoracic Surgery. Dr. Wu was my Honored Guest, and in his lecture he first divulged to a Western audience much of the information about the Chinese methods of diagnosis and treatment of carcinoma of the esophagus that are common knowledge to us now. They recognized that in their country this form of cancer was endemic, and in many of the mountainous areas in Northern China, epidemic. They resolved to do something about it. A reporting system was developed, where every village in the country sent updated statistics to a central office in Beijing. Recognizing that earlier diagnosis was the only hope, they instituted the now famous (or infamous) compulsory screening program, where in high-risk regions every adult over 30 was required to submit to periodic esophageal cytological examination. From this they soon learned that Stage 1 or in situ carcinomas can be diagnosed in this way, and that a remarkably high number of all cancers detected cytologically were stage 1 (78, 85 and 84% in one 3-year study). Furthermore, they found that the latent period between stage 1 and invasive carcinoma can be as long as 3–5 years. If this window of opportunity is utilized, resection rates can vary from 60 to 100%, and

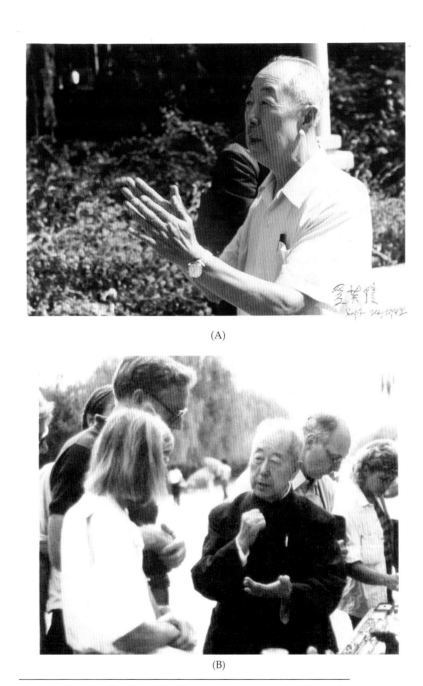

(A)

(B)

*Fig. 1. [A] Dr. Ying-Kai Wu; [B] Dr. Wu and rapt listeners at the Ming tombs.*

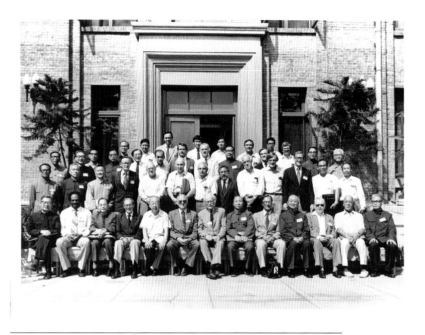

*Fig. 2. Beijing Symposium on Cardiovascular Surgery, September 20–24, 1981.*

5-year cure rates of between 30 and 80% can be achieved. But the story did not stop there. They also mounted an intensive Public Health campaign to identify and eliminate risk factors for esophageal cancer: bad oral hygiene, hot and coarse foods, and nitrosamine, a carcinogen introduced in the preparation of food. And to this list, 2 decades later, must be added tobacco abuse. In the meantime, how have we fared in the West? Since the incidence of esophageal cancer in the United States is 5/100 000 instead of the more than 20/100 000 seen in China, we have, in our wisdom, decided that the cost-benefit ratio for mass screening is too steep. Hence, we persist on focusing on such important aspects of the disease as to whether MRI scans can correctly detect metastases. As a result, overall 5-year survival rates have only increased from 5 to 10 % in the last 2 decades. Is there not a lesson to be learned from this Chinese proverb? "The superior doctor prevents sickness; the mediocre doctor attends to impending sickness; the inferior doctor treats actual sickness."

Another example is the barefoot doctor—better termed dispensary attendant—a concept poorly understood in Western thought. The need for them arose because of a few basic statistics. China occupies roughly the same latitude and has the same land mass as the Unites States, yet has a third less tillable soil, and four times the population to feed and care for. The brigade system with the so-called barefoot doctor at the entry point for medical care was a brilliant solution to what seemed an insurmountable problem. The term "barefoot doctor" is really an unfortunate misnomer that arose because their ranks were made up of peasants who were given basic medical training, and who worked barefoot in the rice paddies a half day, and then ran the dispensary a half day treating minor complaints and triaging sicker patients to hospitals and medical centers. The importance of the concept was not whether high quality care was available, but that *every* community, no matter how small or isolated, had a place where the sick person could go and receive medical attention. In the United States, where we embrace the concept that only high-end technology will suffice, we have for decades and with little success been trying to locate and man treatment centers of this type in the inner cities and the rural areas of our country.

At one time it was estimated that there more than 1,000,000 barefoot doctors in China, and it is interesting that this number has been steadily decreasing, not because the idea is not a good one, but with economic change the dispensary attendants have found that they can make more money farming. And this is occurring at a time when in the United States, again because of economic conditions, the services of the non-MD health care workers—nurse practitioners, midwives, physician assistants—are in great demand at the medical entry level, often to the purposeful exclusion of physicians. Another insight I developed from my acquaintance with Dr. Wu is the importance of keeping an open mind on all subjects, but particularly on matters of health. I lost my intolerant attitude toward acupuncture when we witnessed at the Beijing Tuberculosis Hospital a female surgeon performing a left upper lobectomy on a 35-year old woman, whose only "anesthesia"was a needle inserted in the meridian of the right forearm. Whether so-called modern medicine considers this witchcraft or a mental tour-de-force is beside the point. What is important is that this technique has been with us since 2600 BC. It was developed during the reign of the third Emperor of China, "Huang Di"(the Yellow Emperor), who authored a medical textbook that made him the Hippocrates of China. Something this enduring must have value. The same principle of "worth in longevity" can be applied to herbal medicine. Chinese physicians practicing traditional medicine have learned to work in concert with physicians using modern or "Western"methods. The roots and bark, berries and leaves that been used for centuries to treat medical ills should not be cast aside as worthless in a more sophisticated world, but rather should be plumbed even deeper for their yet undefined secrets. Confucius himself, around 500 BC, had the last word on this subject: "because newer methods of treatment are good, it does not follow that the old ones are bad: for if our honorable and worshipful ancestors had not recovered from their ailments, you and I would not be here today."

One final example from the lessons I learned from Dr. Wu relates to their mental approach to the care of the sick. It has been my observation that the people of Asia treat their fellow human beings with great respect, and, as Confucius just told us, the elderly and those that have passed on are accorded a special, almost reverential status. We obviously see elements of this attitude in Western culture, but I do not believe to the same degree. The dignity and respect accorded those that have passed on is present in great abundance in the room of the patient near death. The nuance to which I am referring is expressed well by Phillips Brooks: "Duty makes us do things well, love makes us do them beautifully" and by J. Engelbert Dunphy: "Death holds no fearful threat. Living without life is hell. Death is natural; it may be just; it is often easeful and merciful; it ought always to be dignified. Who knows, it may be paradise."

There is an invaluable little book written by Lois Wheeler Snow, entitled *A Death with Dignity*. The 148-page volume tells the story of the slow and painful death from carcinoma of the pancreas of her husband, Edgar Snow. The Snows spent many years in China, and have written books and articles about the country. She tells of their bitter, lonely experiences in clinics around the world before they

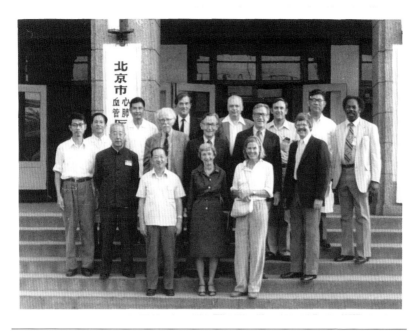

*Fig. 3. September 25, 1981—Visit to the Beijing Heart, Lung and Blood Vessel Medical Center, of which Y. K. Wu was the Director.*

decided to return to their then home in Switzerland for his last days. Then the Chinese came. They had heard of his illness, and wanted to take care of him. In paraphrase, she says: When the Chinese came, they shared all information: doctors, nurses, the patient and the family discussed problems openly. Medical personnel were freely available to the family. The patient received companionship whenever he wanted it. Emphasis was on the person, and the family, as well as the incurable illness. Then Mrs. Snow concludes with what is certainly my favorite quotation, and one that in my judgment merits a place in every physician's office: "There is yet a limit to technology, there is none to humanity, beyond our own making."

These are a few examples of the wonderful insights we learned from Dr. Wu during our visit to China almost 2 decades ago. The external face of China has surely changed, but my guess is that the important things Dr. Wu talked about have not. Eastern Culture and Eastern Medicine can certainly benefit from many things imparted by the West, but I believe the West has just as much to learn from the East. Perhaps more. For the next few minutes I would like to play Nostradamus. Benjamin Disrali in 1867 said of his times, "Change is inevitable. In a progressive country change is constant." I predict that we are on the threshold of the greatest global restructuring in history. In the business world these days the buzzwords are merger, consolidation, and bigger is better. There is no segment of the economy or social order that is not caught up in this rush to put away petty differences with rivals and join forces to survive and thrive. Examples are part of our everyday life: financial houses, media giants, clothing stores—add your own illustration. And the medical industry is caught up in whirlwind fashion, so that small supply houses, small hospitals and solo practitioners are all as endangered as the Bengal tiger. Nations, too, are involved with the process. Like all of you, I have watched with fascination as the European countries, each with its own proud heritage of customs and traditions in place for the greater part of two millennia, are coming together as a single unit, to forge a whole that will be infinitely greater than its parts. We have also seen a bellwether of this activity in medicine, where in a scant dozen years The European Association for Cardio-thoracic Surgery has become the spokesman for our specialty in that part of the world. So the thought progression here is obvious. It is not difficult to envision the day when interdependence across all the elements of modern society will be centered in the three land masses separated by the great bodies of water on this planet: They are now called Europe-Africa, North America–South America, and Asia-Australia. Some day in the distant future each may even adopt for itself a separate new name.

There will be many problems to be solved during this evolution, and many barriers that have been in place since the beginning of recorded history will need to be removed. Without question the greatest of these is the "confusion of tongues" initiated at the tower of Babel. But as the world becomes smaller and different heritages are mixed one with the other by sonic travel, and with every computer on earth linked together, this problem surely will resolve itself over the fullness of time. Except we want to hurry it along faster than that. Perhaps the world medical community will lead the way. During my lifetime I have seen the German language, once the standard for medicine, replaced by English, and have seen medical meetings all over the world discard the translator earphones and adopt English as the official language for their conferences. This trend I don't believe reflects any particular love for the English language, but is more likely rooted in the fact that most countries of the world except the English-speaking ones have long realized the importance of being conversant with a number of languages. Therefore, they have made learning these tongues a serious and sizable part of every child's education from kindergarten on.

The Chinese language represents one of the greatest challenges. It is said that Chinese culture made four great contributions to mankind: paper, movable type, compass, and gunpowder. This certainly must be a judgment that originated in an ignorant West, since, for example, a surgeon named Hua Tuo in the second century AD was using anesthesia induced by a Chinese herb called *Ma Fei San* for performing major abdominal operations and amputations. But it is unfortunate that when movable type was invented, these same individuals did not apply themselves to making the characters simpler and thus easier to carve and fire in the clay molds that were used. So the Chinese language is indeed still a barrier for the rest of us, and we need to work hard to resolve this dilemma. Mark Twain recognized the elements of this problem when he said, "Be careful about reading health books. You may die of a misprint."

But you must know that the three land masses are not the end of the story. This progression can only reach its goal when we truly have attained what, in 1940 and far ahead of his time, Wendell Willkie called, "One World." When that happy day occurs, my hope and prayer is that physicians all over the world can willingly meet the standard asked of us by Norman Cousins in 1940, when he wrote: "To practice medicine at a time when the earth has become a single geographic community calls for an enlargement of the Hippocratic oath. In today's world the physician must make his commitment not just to the individual but to the institution of life. To the extent that medical societies are concerned only with professional questions, they restrain physicians from involvement in ethical issues. Insulated in that manner from his central role, the physician can trail happily after illness while ignoring his obligation to help humanize society and to make it safe and fit for human beings."

A big order? Of course it is! But the attitude of physicians all over the world, and I'm proud to say, cardiothoracic surgeons in particular, is epitomized by this quotation: "Those who say it can't be done should never interfere with those that are doing it."

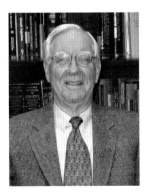

Thomas B. Ferguson

## *Appendix*

To: Professor T. B. Ferguson

June 28, 1999

Dear Tom,

　　Your letter of May 11, 1999 reached me about two weeks ago. It gave me great pleasure and made me recall our wonderful meeting in Beijing in Sept. 1981, eighteen years ago. I appreciate the copy of *Annals of Thoracic Surgery* which contained the article written by Dr. Song Wan and Dr. Yim of Hong Kong. Your lecture on "Forging a Link" reminded me of many things happened during the period 1981–1982 in Beijing and also the AATS meeting in 1982 when I was made a member of this great association under your chairmanship. Many of the friends attended both meetings have passed away. You and I are the fortunate one. Your are still carrying on the heavy jobs as editor of the *Annals of Thoracic Surgery*. I am still working on popular education on the prevention and control of CVD in Beijing, at 89! We are both the type of people you described in your lecture that we learn and teach, we teach and learn. We learned from our common teacher, Dr. Evarts Graham, when we were really young. I cannot forget what I learned from this great man and all the nice colleagues at Barnes and Robert Koch Hospital, 1941–1943.

　　As to myself, I am an Emeritus Director of the Beijing Cardiovascular Institute, at the Anzhen Hospital, since 1987. I am not involved in clinical work nor in administration. However I still come to my office in the hospital three mornings weekly to organize popular education program in the CVD prevention and to have help from the secretaries. I have written my personal story. I am also reviewing all my writings and lecture notes and all the things I want to keep for the future people, including reprints and instruments I carried back to China in 1943. I am sending you a copy of my personal memo, printed in 1997 for you to keep. You can see the few photos at the beginning and I have made some English translation for the topics of different sections.

　　I am still living in the old PUMC campus at 26, Bei-ji-ge Santiao,

Dongdan, Beijing 100005. I like the old house with wide porch and some land for gardening around the house. My wife is in good health. My health is fair for my age, chiefly atherosclerosis here and there, but no serious attach yet. Recently eye problems, cataract and glaucoma for which I had 3 operation during the past year. My eldest son and his family moved back to Beijing after working in the World Bank for nearly ten years. He now works in an International Finance Co. They live in the suburb and would come to have dinner with us once every other week.

China has changed a lot. You must come to see Beijing and China at any time convenient to you. If you will need an invitation for entry, please let me know. My last visit to the USA was in 1992 and decided not to go out of Beijing any more for health reasons.

With my best wishes to you and your family.

Cordially Yours truly,

Wu Ying-kai

# Pediatric Cardiovascular Surgery: Project Hope and the Shanghai Children's Medical Center

Richard A. Jonas

The Shanghai Children's Medical Center (SCMC), situated in the Pudong special development area of Shanghai, China, is a result of more than 20 years of close collaboration between Project Hope of Millwood, Virginia, the Shanghai Second Medical University and the Shanghai municipal government. In 2003, cardiac surgeons at the Shanghai Children's Medical Center undertook 1,579 operations with an overall mortality of approximately 2%. Of these procedures, 801 were in babies less than 2 years of age with more than 40 neonates. Thus, this center has grown to become one of the busiest pediatric cardiac programs in a freestanding tertiary level pediatric hospital in the world.This chapter will describe some personal reminiscences of the remarkable efforts of so many selfless individuals that led SCMC to where it is today.

## Personal Background

In late 1983, Dr. Aldo Castaneda, chief of cardiac surgery at Children's Hospital Boston and William E. Ladd, Professor of Surgery at Harvard Medical School, invited me to join him as his junior associate on the staff of the Children's Hospital Boston. I was at the time his chief resident working with both him and Dr. William Norwood. Dr. Norwood had recently been appointed as the new chief of cardiac surgery at the Children's Hospital of Philadelphia. 1983 had been a remarkable year to be at Children's Hospital Boston. Dr. Norwood had just published the first report of a successful outcome following surgical palliation of hypoplastic left heart syndrome, the last major challenge in the management of complex congenital heart disease. In the same year Dr. Norwood and Dr. Castaneda pioneered the neonatal surgical management of transposition of the great arteries employing the arterial switch procedure. I was familiar with the fact that Dr. Norwood had been closely involved with Project Hope and the development of pediatric cardiac surgery in Krakow, Poland. I was also aware that Dr. Norwood had been invited by Project Hope to travel to China in 1983 together with Dr. Steve Sanders and Dr. John Murphy, who were both pediatric cardiologists in Boston, to explore the possibility of establishing a similar program in the People's Republic of China. Not long after he returned from that preliminary visit Dr. Norwood sat down with me and suggested that not only should I take over his staff position in Boston but in addition suggested that I should take over the role of team leader for the new pediatric cardiac program in Shanghai. I discussed his suggestion with my chief, Dr. Castaneda, who was adamantly opposed. Despite that stern advice, I agreed to meet with John and Bill Walsh, the two sons of the founder of Project Hope, Dr. William Walsh. They had little difficulty convincing me that this was a remarkable opportunity for a young surgeon. I agreed to begin the work of putting together the equipment and personnel needs for the first working team visit to Shanghai.

It was easy to understand why I found the allure of China impossible to resist despite my chief's protestations. As a young boy growing up in Australia, my grandmother had told me stories of my grandfather's global wanderlust that had taken him as a young journalist from Adelaide South Australia to work in Chicago for several years and on his return trip to visit Shanghai. The timeframe was the 1930s, when Shanghai was known throughout the world as the Paris of the East, a fascinating mix of European and Chinese culture. My grandfather brought home with him silks and carved figures that remain in the family home in Australia even today and still evoke memories of my grandmother and her stories of China.

As I entered medical school in the late 1960s Australia was just as deeply embroiled in the Vietnam War as the United States. Indonesia had just been taken over by a communist revolution and there was no difficulty convincing the Australian people including me that the domino theory of world domination by communism posed a huge threat to Australia. After 1966 and the onset of the great Cultural Revolution of Chairman Mao, China had become a complete enigma to Australians and was greatly feared. This all had important personal implications for me as I undertook three years' mandatory ROTC military training, much of it taught by regular Army soldiers who had just returned from harrowing experiences in Vietnam. In the late 1970s following Mao's death and as I undertook my surgical training in Australia and New Zealand, tantalizing glimpses from within China began to appear with news coverage of the activities of the Gang of Four.

By the late 1970s, Australian surgeons had begun visiting China in an effort to help overcome the consequences of the Cultural Revolution. I had heard stories from Dr. Harry Windsor from St. Vincent's Hospital in Sydney, and Dr. Roger Mee from the Children's Hospital in Melbourne of the remarkable lack of surgical facilities that existed at that time. We gradually learned that not only had teachers in the universities and schools been targeted during the Cultural Revolution, but advanced technical specialties such as cardiac surgery were singled out as elitist in many hospitals and closed down. For all intents and purposes medical schools ceased to function for many years during the Cultural Revolution. And all of this was occurring in a country where the annual birth rate was estimated to be 18 million. By my calculation this meant that 144,000 children were being born each year with congenital heart disease. And yet none of these children had received adequate or even any surgical care during the years of the Cultural Revolution itself. By the late 1970s only the most courageous surgical pioneers were able to re-establish open heart surgery. So when John and Bill Walsh spoke to me in 1984 it was quite clear that there was a huge need within

China for surgical education. It seemed obvious to me from the beginning that this was an opportunity as a surgical educator to make far more of an impact than I would ever be able to achieve training surgical residents in the United States. Surely this was the mission of an academic cardiac surgeon. Coming from a family where my parents had demonstrated through their own personal examples the importance of community service it was an easy decision to begin a long-term commitment with Project Hope despite the risk it might pose to my own academic advancement in Boston.

## History of Project Hope

Project Hope is an independent, international non-profit health training organization based in a beautiful rural setting in the horse country of Millwood, Virginia. The organization was founded by Dr. William Walsh, who was personal physician to President Eisenhower. Dr. Walsh was able to convince President Eisenhower to allow funding for a military hospital ship to sail to third world countries to provide medical care and training. The SS Hope first set sail for Indonesia in 1960. From the beginning the goal was to "train the trainer" and to establish health care independence rather than dependence. Many hundreds if not thousands of dedicated physicians, nurses and healthcare technicians traveled on the SS Hope to many difference countries over the next 14 years until the SS Hope was finally retired. However this was certainly not the end of Project Hope, which remained dedicated to helping people to help themselves through education and training. Project Hope has now conducted programs in more than 80 countries worldwide and currently works in 32 nations. Over its history it is estimated that Project Hope has trained more than 2 million healthcare workers.

In the early 1980s, Dr. Walsh was invited by the Chinese government to establish a number of health training programs throughout China. At one point as many as 12 Project Hope programs were functioning throughout China including pediatric preventive density, neonatal nursery care for premature infants, and an ongoing highly successful program for the management of diabetes. But what equipment had been obtained and the infrastructure was being put into place at Xinhua Hopsital.

During 1984 and 1985, as I began to establish myself as a staff surgeon at Children's Hospital Boston including facing the daunting challenge of managing the many babies with hypoplastic left heart syndrome who were being referred to Boston in those years, I also worked on putting together a team of individuals who could join me on the first team visit to Shanghai. By March 1986 we had established a group of 15 dedicated volunteers including four intensive care cardiac nurses who would be able to man the intensive care unit around the clock, a cardiac operating room nurse, a respiratory therapist, a cath lab technician, a cath lab cardiologist, an echocardiographer, a cardiac radiologist, a cardiac anesthesiologist and myself (Fig. 1). In March 1986 we set off on Northwest Airlines bound for Shanghai, little knowing what incredible challenges lay ahead.

The view of Shanghai from the air as we arrived at night in March 1986 was quite remarkable. For a city of nearly 12 million people it was quite incredible to see no major buildings lit up at night and few street lights. The street lights appeared to be 25W bare bulbs. As we were driven from the dilapidated airport to the Peace Hotel on the Bund, we were amazed to see that there were absolutely no other cars on the street. This was at about 9:00 pm at night. We passed only an occasional cyclist. The area around the Bund was similarly deserted, a holdover as we later learned from the years of the Cultural Revolution when effectively a curfew by about 9:00 pm existed.

Although the Peace Hotel may have been a grand institution in the past, it had certainly seen better years and as we stood in the lobby with paint peeling from the walls and attempted to check in to the hotel, a process which took quite some time, I know that all the team members were wondering exactly how we were going to survive for a month in this city.

The next morning as we headed out to Xinhua Hospital it was pouring with rain, as it did for almost every day during the month that we were in Shanghai and it was frequently quite cold. The

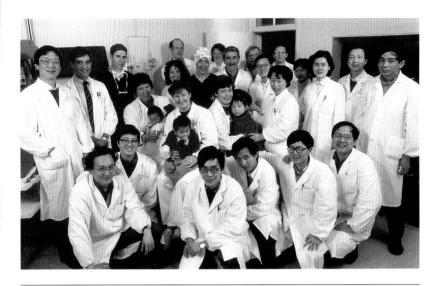

*Fig. 1. The first clinical working group of Project Hope volunteers participating in the pediatric cardiac program at Xinhua Hospital in Shanghai, China pictured in March 1986. The Hope volunteers are accompanied by their Chinese counterparts. The author is second from the left between the Dr. Ding-Fan Cao and Dr. Zhi-Wei Xu. Dr. Xu is now director of the cardiothoracic program at the new Shanghai Children's Hospital Medical Center. Second from the right and kneeling is Dr. Jin-Fen Liu who is now the president of the Shanghai Children's Medical Center and continues to practice pediatric cardiac surgery.*

entrance to the cardiac ward was through the emergency room and every morning we were shocked to see the large number of seriously ill individuals who would be lying on stretchers apparently receiving little attention. They were often there at night when we left more than 12 hours later. The cardiac ward was even more of a shock for us though we soon appreciated the efforts that Hashim and the bioengineers had made over the previous year. We also were pleased to find that the hundreds of shipping cartons containing all of the consumables and instruments that we would require had arrived safely and had survived the customs department. We spent the remainder of the first week unpacking equipment and beginning the process of instructing our peers in the use of the instruments and equipment.

In addition to setting up equipment through the first week we

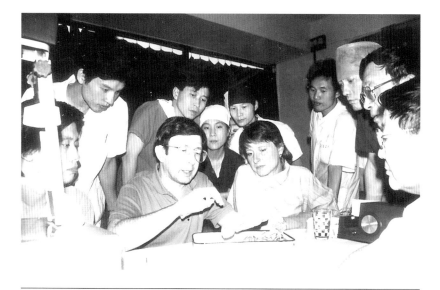

*Fig. 3. Dr. Paul Weinberg from Children's Hospital of Philadelphia conducts a teaching session with Chinese staff.*

anything other than the blue or gray Mao suits with men and women having similar haircuts and no adornments. All of this changed very rapidly over the next several years. It was quite a remarkable experience to arrive on an annual basis during this period and to see new high rise buildings popping up like mushrooms around the city. As new buildings emerged, the light level at night and the number of people and cars on the streets began to increase exponentially.

In June 1989 we were all shocked and disappointed to see the events in Tiananmen Square. There were some who even suggested that we should discontinue the visit that was planned for the following fall but I was adamantly in favor of returning. It was quite clear to me that the physicians, families and children in particular were the ones who needed us and this had to be our priority. Government politics were something we should leave to the politicians. I simply could not understand the argument that our visiting China was an endorsement of Chinese government policies. When we did return in the fall of 1989 the streets were once again deserted, it felt as if the lights had been dimmed to the gloom of 1986 and there was a hush across the city that was eerie. The 747 that flew us into Shanghai contained only 10 Americans, a handful of Japanese and a few Chinese. But over ensuing visits once again development progressed, slowly at first but then rapidly again and we watched as wealth and prosperity exploded across the city, transforming Shanghai from a sleepy backwater to regain the splendor and excitement that had characterized it in the 1930s when my grandfather had visited (Fig. 4).

Not only was progress occurring in the city of Shanghai as a whole during these years but in addition the cardiac surgery program was rapidly expanding. By 1989, 500 cardiac procedures were performed in one year. This was clearly placing a major stress on the infrastructure at Xinhua Hospital, which had simply not been

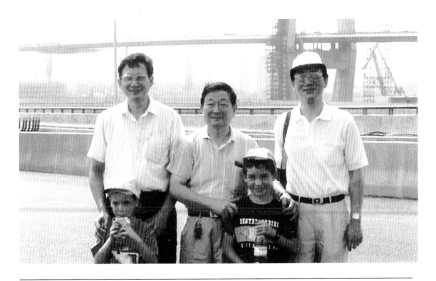

*Fig. 4. By the early 1990s construction in Shanghai was proceeding at an extraordinarily rapid pace. The author's sons Andrew and Michel are pictured in front of the new southern bridge spanning the Huangpu River between old Shanghai and the new Pudong development area. The Shanghai Children's Medical Center is situated close to the approaches of the bridge on the Pu Dong side of the river.*

designed to support a high volume complex tertiary surgical specialty like pediatric cardiovascular surgery. It was clear that if the program was to expand further to serve the needs of not only the children of Shanghai but in addition to serve as a training magnet center for the remainder of China, it would be necessary to develop a new hospital. Dr. William Walsh began discussion with the Shanghai municipal government supported by John and William Walsh.

One of the most difficult questions confronting us was where this new hospital should be situated and how the land could be obtained. Although Project Hope and I had initially suggested that a downtown location close to the campus of the Shanghai Second Medical University and the old French Concession area would be most beneficial for an academic pediatric hospital, the government insisted that they wanted the hospital to be situated in the Pudong area. In 1991 this was hard for us to accept. As we sat in the dining room at the Peace Hotel on the Bund we looked across the river each morning at breakfast to the market gardens of the Pudong area. A ferry boat ran from close to the Peace Hotel back and forth across the river bringing cyclists and pedestrians from the tenement developments in the Pudong area. Most of Pudong was still being used for growing vegetables for market across the river. It seems that this poor and inaccessible area would be quite inappropriate for a high level hospital. How wrong we were.

The Shanghai municipal government and the central government had earmarked the Pudong area as a special development area and subsequently poured billions of yuan into the development of infrastructure. A new tunnel and two new bridges were built in a remarkably short space of time to connect the old city across to Pudong. The municipal government generously donated 13 acres of land close to the freeway approaches of the southern bridge. In October 1992 Dr. Walsh and the board of Project Hope joined our team in Shanghai for a groundbreaking ceremony with the Vice Mayor of Shanghai who had been a strong supporter of the hospital from the earliest discussions. As we stood in the cabbage farm on a beautiful fall day with the fireworks going off, the Chinese children singing and the band playing it was still difficult to envision this would soon be a high tech Children's Hospital surrounded by the massive high rise developments of the Pudong area (Fig. 5).

## Development and Building of the Shanghai Children's Medial Center

Following the groundbreaking ceremony in October 1993, we faced many challenges in bringing the Shanghai Children's Medical Center to fruition. There were some in the Shanghai municipal government who preferred to focus on the concept of a large general pediatric hospital rather than a specialist hospital that would focus on a highly technical area such as pediatric cardiovascular surgery and pediatric hematology/oncology which was the other planned area of focus of the hospital. There was also the not inconsiderable problem of raising 37 million dollars, which was the commitment of Project Hope to the

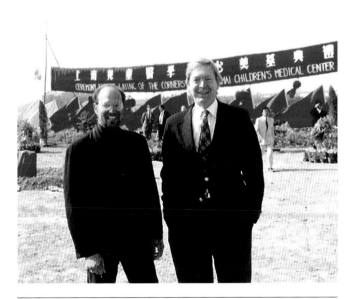

*Fig. 5. Long-time Project Hope volunteers Dr. Henry Issenberg and Dr. David Wessel at the groundbreaking for the new Shanghai Children's Medical Center. The hospital is situated in the Pudong development area in an area that was previously a cabbage farm.*

new hospital. By this time Dr. William Walsh's health had failed and his son William Walsh Jr had taken over as president of the organization. Through the tireless efforts of William Walsh Jr the $37 million was gradually raised. Bill and I made many visits to US corporations to seek their assistance and through their generous contributions the hospital gradually came to fruition.

In addition to the challenge of raising the financial backing for the hospital, there were numerous architectural and engineering challenges to be faced. Shanghai is built on the Yangtze river delta and has an extremely low level relative to sea level with a frequent risk of flooding. The ground water level is remarkably high, only a few feet below the surface, so that deep pilings had to be placed and there was no chance of building the usual basement for engineering support. By 1996, however, the plans had been finalized and on March 13, 1996, exactly 10 years since we had first arrived in Shanghai, we were able to attend the ceremonial driving of the first pile into the muddy grounds of the former cabbage farm.

Over the next two years the hospital took shape surrounded by a shroud of bamboo scaffolding (Fig. 6). By June 1998, the hospital had been completed. We were honored that First Lady Hillary Clinton (Figs. 7–10) was able to officially open the hospital together with the Vice Mayor of Shanghai, who had played a hugely important role in supporting the development of the hospital. Cardiac surgery was rapidly transitioned from Xinhua Hospital across to SCMC during late 1998 and 1999. The accompanying graph (Fig. 11) illustrates the rapid increase in procedures that occurred between 1999, when 717 procedures were undertaken, to 1,579 procedures in 2003.

## Shanghai Children's Medical Center in 2005

The rapid expansion of pediatric cardiac surgery at Shanghai Children's Medical Center has been accompanied by an equally dramatic increase in the diagnostic workload in the echocardiography laboratory as well as interventional catheterization procedures in the cardiac catheterization lab (Fig. 12). Outpatient and inpatient activity have increased in parallel. Dr. Jin-Fen Liu, himself a highly successful

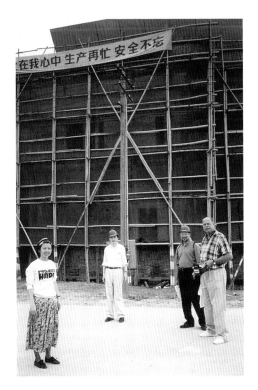

Fig. 6. *Dr. Freida Law (left) pictured in front of the bamboo scaffolding surrounding the new Shanghai Children's Medical Center during its construction. To Dr. Law's left is Dr. Shu-Bao Chen who was the first president of SCMC as well as Project Hope volunteers Henry Issenberg and Lyle Smith. Dr. Law, who is originally from Australia and was the onsite director for Project Hope for more than five years played an extremely important role in establishing the pediatric cardiac program at SCMC.*

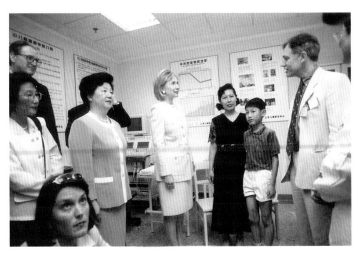

Fig. 7. *First Lady Hillary Clinton with the Vice-Mayor of Shanghai to her right and the author at the opening of SCMC in June 1998.*

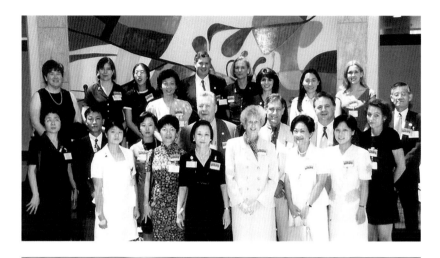

Fig. 8. *Project Hope staff and volunteers in the atrium of Shanghai Children's Medical Center at the time of the official opening by First Lady Hillary Clinton. At center back is Mr. William Walsh, president of Project Hope. Directly in front of him is Mr. Bob Burastero, who was regional director for Project Hope in Asia for many years.*

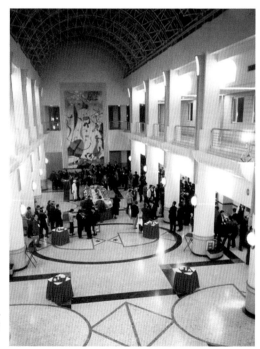

Fig. 9. *The atrium of the Shanghai Children's Medical Center.*

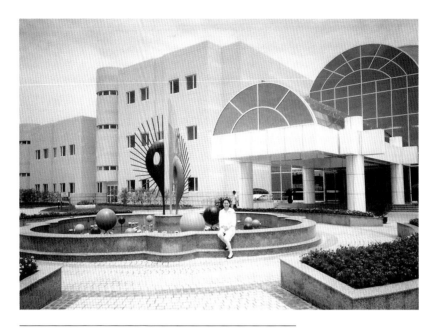

*Fig. 10. The main entrance to Shanghai Children's Medical Center.*

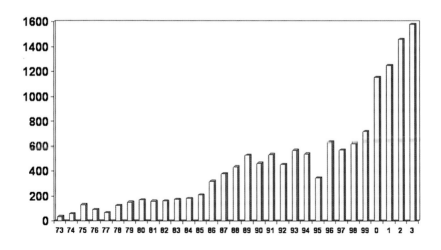

*Fig. 11. Number of cases performed annually at Xinhua Hospital and Shanghai Children's Medical Center.*

pediatric cardiac surgeon, has been president of the hospital for several years and works in close collaboration with Dr. Xiao-Ming Shen who is president of the Shanghai Second Medical University, having previously been president of SCMC prior to Dr. Liu. Dr. Shu-Bao Chen (Fig. 13) and Dr. Wen-Xiang Ding continue to provide incredibly important support to the cardiac program which is now directed by Dr. Zhi-Wei Xu. Dr. Ding-Fan Cao as well as Dr. Zhao-Kang Su and Dr. Yan have also provided incredibly important support within the surgical department. Dr. De-Ming Zhu has provided superb support with the cardiac perfusion services. Perhaps one of the most rewarding areas of the entire experience from my perspective has been to watch the development of the pediatric cardiac nursing program in the operating room, intensive care unit and ward. Over the years these educational activities have been coordinated by Ms

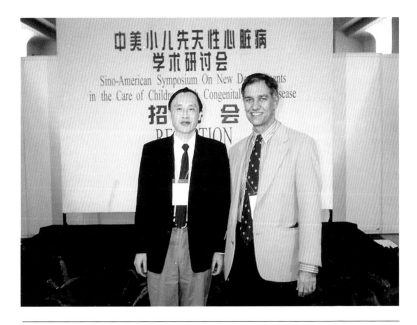

*Fig. 12. The author and Dr. Shu-Bao Chen, Chief of Cardiology, at the opening of the Sino-American Symposium on New Developments in the Care of Children with Congenital Heart Disease held at SCMC, November 1999.*

Patricia Hickey, the Vice President for Intensive Care Nursing and cardiovascular Services at Children's Hospital Boston. Working with many outstanding nurse educators, Ms Hickey has put together a superb team of nurses who manage patients with the same independence, meticulous attention to detail and yet caring and compassionate family centered care as her nursing team in Boston.

## *The Future*

Shanghai Children's Medical Center demonstrates the success of the Project Hope philosophy of "Train the Trainer." The Shanghai Children's Medical Center is now a magnet teaching center for much of China with many surgical teams from regional centers visiting the hospital as well as teams from SCMC visiting other centers where

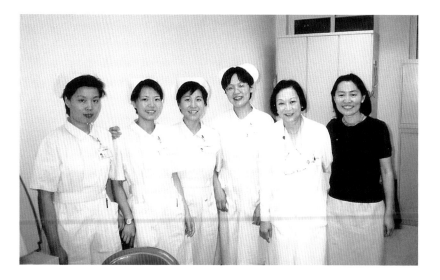

*Fig. 13. Project Hope maintained a full time nurse educator on site at Shanghai Children's Medical Center. Nursing education and empowering senior nurses in administrative decisions within the hospital were important components of the Project Hope program at Shanghai Children's Medical Center. Lin-Ti Chang (right) was the Project Hope chief nurse educator for several years.*

they assist and train others. Project Hope under the inspirational leadership of Dr. John Howe continues to provide support and education for the cardiac program at SCMC. It has been an honor and a privilege to have had the opportunity to participate in this highly successful collaboration between the United States and China.

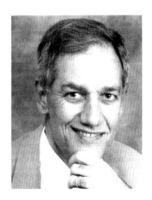

Richard A. Jonas

# My Relationship with China's Cardiac Surgery

*Albert Starr*

t is a great honour for me to be involved in writing a chapter in *Cardiothoracic Surgery in China*. I have been most interested in that great country and in getting to know their medical system. I hope my stories may shed some interesting light on what the potential readers really know about the development of China's adult cardiac surgery. Adult cardiac surgery in China has shown significant changes in the last decade or so, especially in coronary artery bypass grafting (CABG). At the time of my first visit to China in the early 1990s, there were only a few cardiac surgeons in a few of institutes who were able to perform CABG, which now becomes a norm in most prestigious cardiac centers.

My first trip to China was in the winter of 1994, when I had a chance to give lectures and to demonstrate cardiac operations in an educational meeting and visit several top cardiac centers in China. In Shanghai, I visited Shanghai Chest Hospital, Zhongshan Hospital, Changhai Hospital and demonstrated cardiac operations in Zhongshan Hospital. In Beijing, I visited Cardiovascular Institute and Fuwai Hospital, the biggest cardiac center in China (Fig. 1). I gave two lectures in Fuwai Hospital—Mechanical valve comparative data: features and benefits; Valve repair vs. replacement: risk benefit analysis. I also demonstrated two surgical procedures: mitral valve repair and aortic valve repair. I was impressed with Fuwai's excellent work. The hospital had 8 cardiac operating suites generating 10–12 cardiac cases per day, approximately 2,500 cardiac cases per year. At this visit, I met with the hospital president, Dr. Xiao-Dong Zhu, who performed the first aortic valve replacement with a self-made bovine pericardial prosthesis in 1976 in China (Fig. 2). This center established a heart valve prosthesis research lab and a company that produces pericardial valve with standard producing and testing system. His pioneer work prompted the use of tissue valve in heart valve replacement. It is well-known that pericardial valve gained its popularity for its improved durability due to decreased stress-induced structural deterioration and better tissue orientation combined with improved tissue preservation techniques. There has been increasing interest in Carpentier-Edwards pericardial valve since it gained FDA approval for aortic use in the US in 1991. In our institution, Carpentier-Edwards pericardial valve was used in 90% of aortic valve replacement recipients. The rationales for using

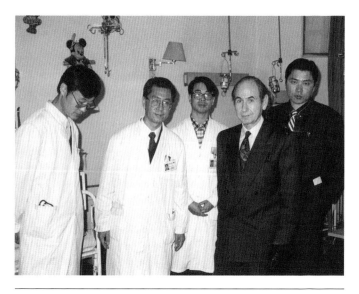

*Fig. 1. At Pediatric ICU of Fuwai Hospital, Beijing. From left to right: Dr. Ming-Di Xiao (2nd from left) and Dr. Feng Wan (first from right).*

this type of valve are its improved durability and their low thrombogenicity, which does not require anticoagulation *per se*. Our recent study demonstrated 10-year actual freedom from explant for structural valve deterioration was 98.9% for aortic valve replacement with Carpentier-Edwards pericardial valve. Chinese patients may be reluctant to receive tissue valve fearing to have a second operation for valve failure. However, appropriate patient education based upon scientific and evidence-based knowledge is very important in directing patients to select optimal valve prosthesis. I appreciated Dr. Xiao-Dong Zhu's pioneer work in promoting tissue valve use in China.

At my first visit to China, I experienced Chinese people's hospitality and friendship. Before I first went to visit China, I anticipated that China's cardiac surgery was underdeveloped due to a long-term termination for a historic reason. We initially intended to provide them with our surgical techniques by frequently

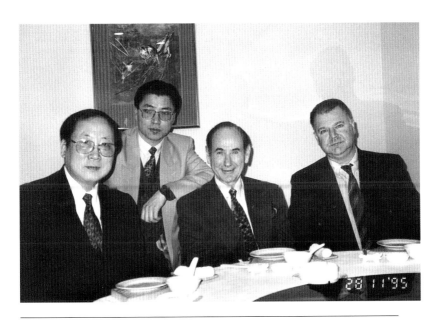

*Fig. 2. Meeting with Dr. Xiao-Dong Zhu (1st from left) and Dr. Feng Wan (2nd from left).*

demonstrating cardiac operations in China. After visiting several prestigious cardiac centers in China, I realized that their cardiac surgery was keeping up with the most updated surgical techniques of the world. Through a profound academic exchange with Chinese cardiac surgeons, I was quite impressed by their excellent surgical skills and patient care. It came up to my mind that offering unilateral education to Chinese cardiac surgeons is unnecessary. They were doing a good job. But I felt that it would be wonderful if we could establish a bilateral, reciprocal, and cooperative academic exchange program. Returning to Portland, we started to initiate a cardiac program in China. At that time, we already had affiliate professional corporations in three states, Washington, Oregon and California. We planned to develop new one in China as opportunities arise. Soon after, Starr-Wood Cardiac Group, China was established and based in Beijing. Ex-trainee, Dr. Feng Wan acted as executive officer for Starr-Wood Cardiac Group, China. We began to do some investigation and explore cooperation from Chinese Hospital. We were happy that many top cardiac centers expressed their wishes to work with us. Those were Beijing Fuwai Hospital, Shanghai Chest Hospital, and Shanghai Renji Hospital. First, Starr-Wood Cardiac Group, China signed contract with Post and Telecommunications General Hospital in Beijing. Later on, Qingdao-Starr international cardiac surgery center was established in Qingdao (Fig. 3). The responsibilities of Starr-Wood Cardiac Group, China included lending its full effort to developing and advancing the surgical service to the contracted hospital by academic interchange, performance of surgery and lectures by Starr-Wood Cardiac Group, China and the training of personnel including surgeons, perfusionists, nurses and administrators. Contracted hospital provided physical plant, support structure, and equipment necessary for cardiac surgery and ancillary services. In 1995, Changhai-Baxter-Starr international cardiovascular surgery technology exchange center was established in Changhai Hospital, Shanghai (Fig. 4). I participated in the opening ceremony and was nominated as a guest professor of Shanghai Second Military Medical University at this meeting (Figs. 5A, B). I was glad to know that it was in this university hospital that China's first successful

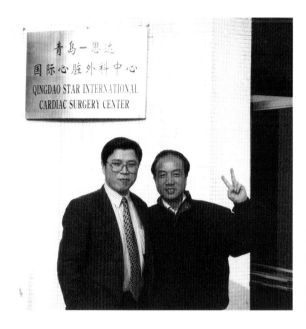

Fig. 3. *Qingdao Starr International Cardiac Surgery Center. Dr. Feng Wan, CEO of Starr-Wood China (left).*

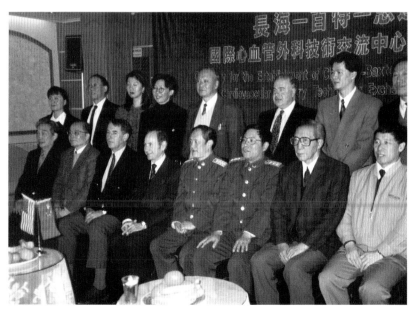

Fig. 4. *Ceremony of the establishment of Changhai-Baxter-Starr International Cardiovascular Surgery Technology Exchange Center.*

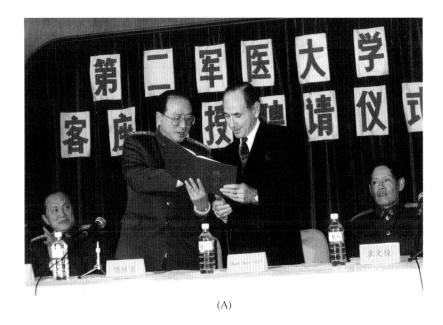

(A)

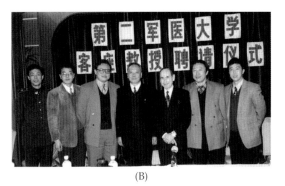

(B)

*Fig. 5. [A, B] Nomination of guest professor for Dr. Albert Starr.*

mitral valve replacement with a locally made ball and cage mechanical prosthesis took place, 5 years after we performed the world's first successful mechanical mitral valve replacement. That important event initiated heart valve replacement in China. It has been known that heart valve replacement prolongs patient's survival and improve patient's quality of life. Since the first heart valve replacement, large numbers of heart valve replacement has been performed all over China. Our research team recently analyzed the value of heart valve replacement in an economist's view. From 1960 through 2003, 7,194 adult patients underwent heart valve replacement in our institute. A statistic model was used to generate the future life-years of patients who are currently alive. The value of life-years proposed by economists was applied to determine the economic value of the additional life given to these patients by heart valve replacement. The heart valve replacement generated a net value of $13.5 billion. Should this method be applied to the analysis of the value of heart replacement in China in the past, its economic value would be huge. At 1995 visit, I also met with Chinese famous pediatric cardiac surgeon, Dr. Wen-Xiang Ding, Director of Institute of Pediatric Heart Disease, Shanghai Children's Medical Center (Fig. 6).

Through many visits, I established a friendly relationship with Chinese cardiac surgeons. Some of them were invited to visit our institute. We really enjoyed Dr. Xiao-Cheng Liu and Dr. Qing-Yu Wu's visit to our institution. I also have a good friendship with the Chinese Society for Thoracic and Cardiovascular Surgery. I was frequently invited by the Society to attend their meetings. In 2000, I was invited

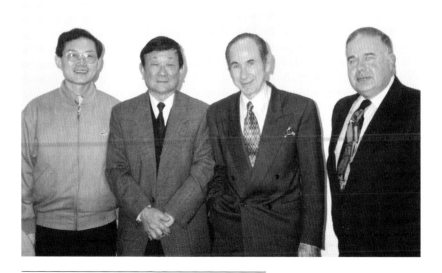

*Fig. 6. Meeting with Dr. Wen-Xiang Ding (2nd from left).*

as an honorary president of the Fifth China International Congress on Thoracic and Cardiovascular Surgery in Beijing. Unfortunately, an unexpected event prevented me from attending that meeting. I look forward to future opportunity to interact with Chinese cardiac surgeons.

At last, I would like to thank all Chinese cardiac surgeons trained at Starr-Wood Cardiac Group, Providence St. Vincent Medical Center for their contributions to our cardiac program. Since the establishment of our cardiac fellowship program, 18 Chinese cardiac surgeons have been trained in our heart center (Fig. 7). Most of them returned back to China and became a leader at their cardiac centers. A few of them are continuing their training or practicing medicine in the United States. Some of these surgeons revisited our cardiac center. Our team members were often invited to visit their hospital in China. I am proud of the many Chinese surgeons who have trained with us in Portland (Addendum).

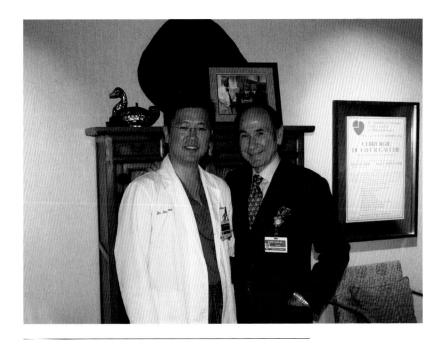

Fig. 7. Dr. Starr with current cardiac fellow, Dr. Guang-Qiang Gao.

## Addendum: List of Chinese Cardiac Surgeons Trained in Portland and Their Whereabouts

Chen, Hai-Quan, MD.: No. 6 People's Hospital, Shanghai, China

Ding, Zhi-Xiang, MD.: Shanghai, China

Gao, Guang-Qiang, MD: Oregon Health & Science University, Portland, Oregon, USA

He, Guo-Wei, MD: The Chinese University, Hong Kong, China

Kong, Ye-Kong, MD: Ruijin Hospital, Shanghai, China

Li, Ying-Ze, MD: Chest Hospital, Shanghai, China

Liu, Ming-Hui, MD: Oregon Health & Science University, Portland, Oregon, USA

Pi, Kai-Duan, MD: Yale School of Medicine, New Haven, CT, USA

Ren, Zhen, MD: Mayo Clinic, Rochester, Minnesota, USA

Sun, Han-Song, MD: Cardiovascular Institute & Fuwai Hospital, Beijing, China

Wan, Feng, MD: Beijing University People's Hospital, Beijing, China

Wang, William Gang, MD: California Pacific Medical Center, San Francisco, California, USA

Wang, Xiao-Zhou, MD: Chest Hospital, Shanghai, China

Xu, Zhi-Yun, MD: Changhai Hospital, Shanghai, China

Yang, Bi-Bo, MD: Beijing University Hospital, Beijing, China

Yeh, John, MD: Asia Pacific Heart Institute, University of California, San Francisco, CA, USA

Zhao, Qiang, MD: Zhongshan Hospital, Shanghai, China

Zhu, Zhi-Gang, MD: USA

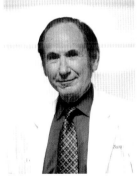

Albert Starr

# China: Personal Reminiscences

*W. Gerald Rainer*

I am honored by having been asked to write a few lines about my personal thoughts of the time that I have spent observing and savoring the relationships that I have had with some of the Chinese Medical Community. Having had the opportunity to visit China early (1978), and returning again in 1985 and 1997 I have sensed a broad overview of a dynamic and powerful score of years in the development of China and its people.

## July 1978

The first visit that my wife and I had the privilege of participating in was in July of 1978 with a group from the Educational Department of Long Beach Memorial Hospital. This was an eclectic group and all of us were curious and excited about what lay ahead of us. Following a brief scientific meeting in Kyoto, Japan, we took the only route available to American visitors in those days and that was via train from Hong Kong to Kwangchow (Canton) stopping at the border of the New Territories with mainland China and disembarking the train, carrying our luggage across the bridge, and re-boarding the train on the other side. It was hot and there were innumerable formalities (security checks) all along the way. At that time Kwangchow was nothing more than a city that had been virtually destroyed from the long period of military action and the lack of infrastructure maintenance of what we would look upon as normal facilities. Our travel guides and advisors did the best they could to see that we had passable accommodations but these were not always possible and we were frequently bumped from the nicer hotels by some visiting agricultural or farm delegation or some governmental dignitaries. Nonetheless, at every point we were treated with great hospitality and graciousness. Throughout this trip we were struck by the enormous number of bicycles and the virtual absence of automobiles. We were fortunate enough to have arranged for us visits to a farm commune with its medical facility and an industrial urban commune with its medical facilities (which were much nicer because of a more lucrative productivity). We were exposed firsthand to "traditional" medicine including acupuncture, cupping, moxibustion, and the like.

Shanghai was our next stop where we were welcomed with great courtesy (Fig. 1). We were treated to a tour of the facilities of the Shanghai Chest Hospital, thanks to the courtesy of Dr. Zhi Pan, Chairman of the Thoracic Surgery Department (Fig. 2). We had the privilege of observing an open heart surgical procedure consisting of the closure of a ventricular septal defect in a 23 year old male

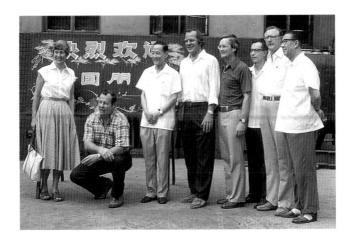

*Fig. 1. Greeting our delegation in Shanghai 1978.*

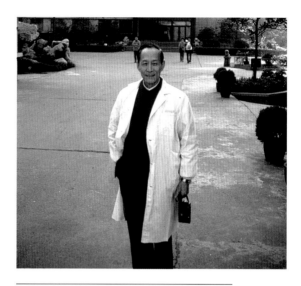

*Fig. 2. Dr. Zhi Pan at the Shanghai Chest Hospital.*

(Fig. 3). Fig. 4 shows the heart-lung machine and disposable bubble oxygenator that was used. It was interesting to note the heat exchanger that was used (a green plastic bucket with either hot or cold water poured around the tubing as the need may dictate) and the lack of any postoperative invasive monitoring. However, the techniques employed were executed with facility and I was particularly amazed at the ability of the Chinese surgeons to accomplish their work in an excellent fashion with a minimal amount of surgical equipment.

In every major city that we visited we had the opportunity to see some of the structures of interest outside the medical area and one in particular was the beautiful Shanghai Exhibition Hall. Herein were included all sorts of products of Chinese industry from operating tables to farm tractors and pianos. It was an enormous exhibit and most impressive.

The last stop on our first visit to China was Beijing where we were guests of the Fuwai Hospital and our host was Professor Ying-Kai Wu. From the very first moment that I met Professor Wu I was impressed with his vision, his ambitions, and his dedication to the

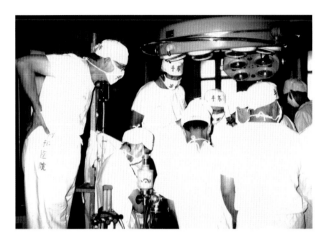

Fig. 3. *Observing open heart surgery at Shanghai Chest Hospital, 1978.*

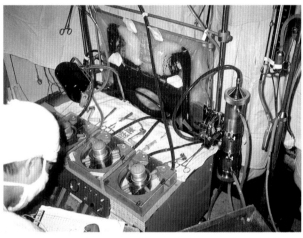

Fig. 4. *Heart-lung machine with disposable bubble oxygenator, Shanghai Chest Hospital, 1978.*

training of younger surgeons in thoracic surgery (Fig. 5). We learned that Professor Wu had spent time training with Dr. Evarts Graham in St. Louis immediately before World War II and upon his return to China in the early 1940s he performed the first ligation of a patent ductus arteriosus in China. We also met a young staff surgeon, Dr. Xiao-Dong Zhu (Fig. 6), who we would meet again on a later trip in 1997 when he was President of the Chinese Society of Thoracic and Cardiovascular Surgery. We were given a tour of scientific exhibits showing vascular prosthetic grafts made of silk and locally made porcine heart valves (Fig. 7).

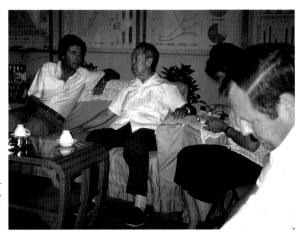

Fig. 5. *Our first meeting with Professor Ying-Kai Wu.*

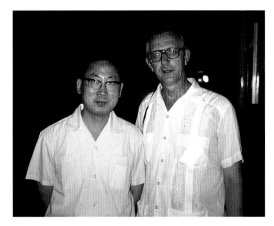

Fig. 6. *Meeting a young Staff Surgeon, Dr. Xiao-Dong Zhu, Fuwai Hospital, 1978.*

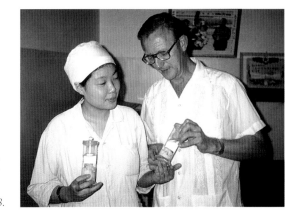

Fig. 7. *Technician showing locally made porcine heart valve, Fuwai Hospital, 1978.*

Following the usual sightseeing ventures around Beijing we returned home and were fortunate enough to have several Chinese trainees spend time with us over the next ten years. In 1981 Dr. Zhi Pan visited us in Denver a few days prior to attending the annual meeting of the Society of Thoracic Surgeons in Los Angeles. When he left Denver there was a hiatus of about five days before we saw him again at the meeting in Los Angeles and I asked Dr. Pan, "What have you done since I saw you a few days ago in Denver"? He replied, "I visited Dr. Cooley in Houston and Disneyland—they were very similar." Dr. Pan then delivered the first lecture at a major United States thoracic surgical society meeting as a representative from China. The title of his presentation was "Surgical Treatment of Ruptured Aneurysm of the Aortic Sinuses" which was well received.

Thus the foundation was laid for a long-standing, close relationship between some of the thoracic surgeons from the United States and our compatriots in China.

## October 1985

We were invited by Professor Ying-Kai Wu to come to Beijing at the time of introduction of the book entitled "International Practice of Cardiothoracic Surgery" which was a compilation of papers from surgeons around the world. The delegation at this time was composed of well-known and respected surgeons from many countries. This was also commemorating the opening of the Beijing Heart, Lung and Blood Vessel Institute (a Chinese NIH) and Anzhen Hospital of which Professor Wu was deservedly very proud.

Following a wonderful visit to Beijing, five couples from the United States embarked upon a visit to Chengdu, and thence by train back to Chongqing where we went aboard the "East is Red" ferry for a trip down the Yangtze River. It being October, the climate was somewhat chilly, rainy, and cloudy for the most part. The accommodations were somewhat less than first class but the group with whom we traveled made it one of the most memorable experiences of our entire traveling career. Fortunately upon approaching the Three Gorges the weather lifted and we were treated to a spectacular site that will be forever etched upon our memory. We debarked at Wuhan and flew a Sharps 123 plane to Shanghai where we again visited the Shanghai Chest Hospital this time under more favorable circumstances with much less security than had been present seven years previously. My wife and I had the distinct pleasure of being guests in the home of Dr. and Mrs. Zhi Pan (Fig. 8) and we have remained very close friends since that time.

## *October 1998*

In October of 1998 our delegation consisted of three couples as representatives from the Society of Thoracic Surgeons and the American Board of Thoracic Surgery to the Chinese Society for Thoracic and Cardiovascular Surgery. We were guests of Academician Zhu Xiao-Dong, who was also the President of the Chinese Society and Advisor to the Fuwai Hospital. Our delegation consisted of Dr. Marvin Pomerantz, the Chairman of the American Board of Thoracic Surgery, Dr. Richard Cleveland, the Secretary of the American Board of Thoracic Surgery, and Dr. Gerald Rainer, a representative from the Society of Thoracic Surgeons. Our spouses accompanied us on this memorable occasion and the high point of this visit was the

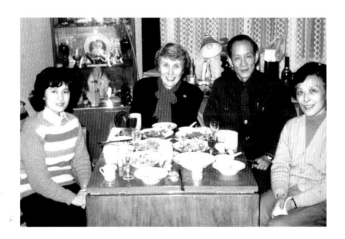

*Fig. 8. Visitors in the home of Dr. Pan-Chih 1985.*

signing of a document declaring the intent for increased collaboration and cooperation between our two societies in an educational exchange program and in the assisting of the development of an accreditation program in thoracic and cardiovascular surgery in China (Fig. 9). As always, our hosts were incredibly hospitable and gracious and we had a wonderful exchange of scientific papers during a symposium at that time. We also had the opportunity to revisit Professor Hong-Xi Su who had spent time at Northwestern University in Chicago at the same time that I interned at the Northwestern Wesley Memorial Hospital.

## *Epilogue*

Having been fortunate enough to see much of China during this period of enormous importance in its development both technically and industrially, we were impressed by the thousands upon thousands of bicycles that we saw in 1978 being replaced by thousands upon thousands of automobiles in 1997. Along with this has not been only an enormous building of technical facilities and much improved infrastructure but also a continued improvement in

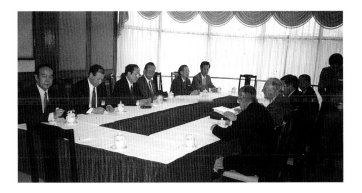

*Fig. 9. Signing ceremony of declaration of intent of cooperation between the Society of Thoracic Surgeons and the Chinese Society of Thoracic and Cardiovascular Surgery 1997.*

thoracic and cardiovascular surgery both from the standpoint of training and execution.

The relationship that we have had with the Chinese Surgical Community has been most rewarding and, as is so often the case, colleagues in medicine can overcome any obstacles presented by political and philosophical differences.

We shall always treasure memories of our visits to China and the relationships that we have had with the surgeons who were not only extremely technically competent but were deeply concerned with the care given to the Chinese people and in the humanitarian aspects of the practice of medicine.

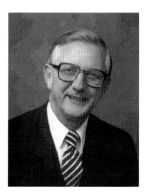

W. Gerald Rainer

# Leo Eloesser: An American Cardiothoracic Surgeon in China

*Yi-Shan Wang, Tsung O. Cheng*

We present a historical vignette of one of the pioneer cardiothoracic surgeons as well as one of the most extraordinary surgeons of the 20th century with a deep-rooted connection with China. Leo Eloesser (1881–1976) was an inveterate traveller and fluent in ten languages [1]. It was in September, 1945, soon after the end of World War II that Yi-Shan Wang (YSW) met Leo Eloesser in the National Central Hospital in Nanjing (Nanking), China where YSW was a resident in the department of surgery (Fig. 1). Dr. Eloesser appeared as a short-statured but strong and high-spirited man over 60 years of age, with a warm smiling face, piercing light grayish-blue eyes, and a short and concisely shaped mustache (Fig. 2). The director of the department of surgery at the hospital introduced YSW to Eloesser for training in thoracic and cardio-vascular surgery under his direction and tutelage. Eloesser was, of course, already a world-renowned figure in thoracic surgery at the time, as one of the leading pioneers in the field in the United States, a professor of surgery at Stanford University, and editor-in-chief of the prestigious *Journal of Thoracic Surgery* which was the predecessor of the *Journal of Thoracic and Cardiovascular Surgery*. Eloesser went to China in 1945 with the United Nations Relief and Rehabilitation Administration (UNRRA) as a specialist in thoracic surgery.

Eloesser made teaching ward rounds with the surgical staff at

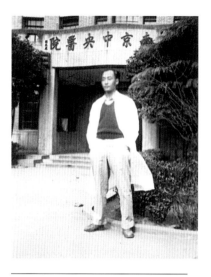

Fig. 1. *Yi-Shan Wang in National Central Hospital, Nanjing, China.*

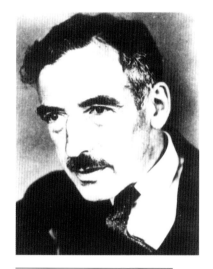

Fig. 2. *Leo Eloesser (Reproduced with permission from [4]).*

the National Central Hospital in Nanjing every Friday morning. YSW was deeply inspired and impressed by his mentor's teaching capabilities, especially in collecting facts, analyzing causes and effects of each disease, and discussing the differential diagnosis in great detail. His approach was scientific and objective. His planning for perioperative care was meticulous with great attention to every minute detail. For instance, in preoperative preparation of every thoracic surgical patient, he used to teach the patient the importance of an "effective cough." He routinely would come to each patient's bedside to demonstrate the exact technique of an "effective cough" until the patient could perform it correctly. In order to reduce the incisional chest pain, he usually instructed the patient to practice abdominal breathing before the operation.

He used to check on the effectiveness of chest drainage in the early postoperative period by squeezing the chest tubes repeatedly himself to ensure their patency. He often encouraged his patients to lie in bed in a high Fowler's position if patient's condition allowed so that it would be good for both the breathing and chest drainage. Quite often he would come back in late evenings to the postoperative intensive care unit to check on the condition of his patients. For designing a skin tube or flap for plastic surgery he usually spent much time in measuring and calculating in order to secure the proper length to reach a new site (Fig. 3). During the wartime he performed many limb amputations. He taught YSW to perform a mid-thigh amputation by using a long, sharp, pointed-tip knife, so that the procedure could usually be completed within 20 minutes. He was very imaginative and dextrous in using bamboo peel strips to plait a prosthesis for a patient's amputated lower limb. The patient could wear the prosthesis comfortably and walk with a steady gait. A photograph taken with such a patient standing next to YSW was published in *TIME* magazine with the following caption "This shows what Chinese doctors are doing."

During an operation Eloesser would demonstrate all the operative steps in great details. He would emphasize repeatedly his five doctrines:

– good exposure of operative field
– good light to exposed area
– good hemostasis
– good drainage
– good closure of incision

He often warned his assistants: "If you don't respect the tissue, then the tissue will not respect you!" His ingenious chest "flap" procedures for tuberculous empyema, which enabled pus to be drained out but prevented air from entering the chest cavity, was very widely adopted. Indeed, the Eloesser "flap" operation brought him worldwide recognition. His technique was well described in the first five editions of *Christopher's Textbook of Surgery* [2]. He was also very good in demonstrating how to do a drainage for pericardial effusion and to safely ligate a patent ductus arteriosus.

Eloesser was still single and continued to lead a very active life while in China. He often drove a Jeep smoking a pipe held tightly between his lips. On most Sundays, he would be accompanied by YSW to go sightseeing, visiting ancient tombs of the emperors of the Ming Dynasty and old temples with antiques which he loved. He paid special attention to the historical inscriptions engraved on the tombstones. He took photographs for records and asked YSW to translate or interpret word by word. He would say to YSW: "I am your student now and you are my teacher!" He liked to climb mountains and used to race with YSW. He chose one peak of Qi Ya Mountain (400 ft high and very steep). His speed was amazingly fast: he could reach the top in 30 minutes, while going down with jumps like a monkey in only 15 minutes. YSW often could not catch up with him. Sometimes he would like to ride on a bicycle along with YSW in the countryside for a very long distance as a form of exercise (Fig. 4). His riding speed was amazingly fast; YSW often could not catch up with him. On weekends, Eloesser often asked YSW to help in organizing dancing parties for social recreation for doctors and nurses in the hospital. He donated chocolates, fruits, cakes, drinks and canned food. He played both violin and viola beautifully. His performances always received thunderous applause from the audience. His dance steps were steady, elegant and rhythmic. The onlookers often clapped

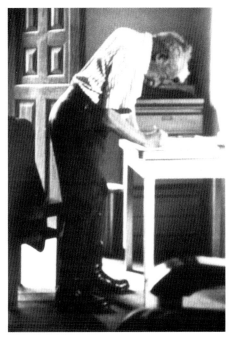

Fig. 3. *Leo Eloesser designing a skin tube or flap for plastic surgery.*

hands enthusiastically in admiration; Eloesser in return showed his appreciation by frequent nodding of his head and a slight smile on his face.

Eloesser left China in the Fall of 1949 to move to New York City to serve with the United Nations International Children's Emergency Fund (UNICEF). Three years later, he retired to Mexico, returning to the United States annually for the meetings of the American Association of Thoracic Surgery [1]. YSW left Nanjing for Shanghai in December 1948 to work in the department of thoracic and cardiovascular surgery of the Shanghai Second Medical University. Twenty five years later (1973), YSW by chance met Eloesser again in Mexico City. YSW was a member of a Chinese medical delegation visiting Latin American countries, and Eloesser represented the Mexican Medical Association in welcoming the Chinese medical delegation. Eloesser recognized YSW instantly and they embraced emotionally. Eloesser said: "Wang, I challenge you to climb a mountain!" Older and shorter, he was still physically fit. He had been happily married then. Eloesser passed away in Mexico City in 1975 at the age of 95.

Although this article deals mainly with Eloesser's time in China during his close association with YSW, Eloesser undoubtedly led one of the most peripatetic and extraordinary lives of any American surgeon [1]. Eloesser was president of the American Association for Thoracic Surgery in 1937. In the same year, when the

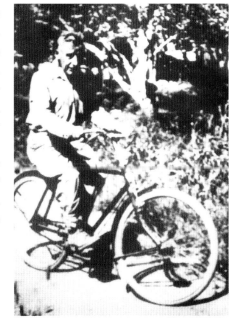

Fig. 4. *Leo Eloesser riding on his bicycle.*

American Board of Surgery was being established, he served on a committee of the American Association for Thoracic Surgery to consider founding an examining board of thoracic surgery. Although his surgical interests were varied, it was in thoracic surgery that his major contributions were found. Eloesser, Graham, Bigger and Churchill were pioneers in emphasizing at the outset of World War II the role of pericardiocentesis in the management of cardiac tamponade resulting from cardiac wounds [3]. There were other major contributions Eloesser made in thoracic surgery, too many to be enumerated in this article. In 1982, Harris Shumacker authored a full-length biography of Eloesser to which the readers are referred for more details of this remarkable man's life [4].

## Acknowledgement

This is an updated version of our article with the same title originally published in the Annals of Thoracic Surgery 2001; 71:1387–1388.

## References

1.  Rutkow IM (1998) American surgery: an illustrated history. Philadelphia: Lippincott-Raven.
2.  Eloesser L (1936–1949) Surgery of the pleura. In: Christopher's textbook of surgery. 1st, 2nd, 3rd, 4th & 5th eds. Philadelphia: Saunders, pp 991–1003.
3.  Shumacker HB Jr (1992) The evolution of cardiac surgery. Bloomington, Indianapolis: Indiana University Press, p 170.
4.  Shumacker HB Jr (1982) Leo Eloesser, M.D.: eulogy for a free spirit. New York: Philosophical Library, p 483.

# Forging Global Links: Asian Perspectives

*Chuen-Neng Lee*

C ardiothoracic surgery in China began to open to the outside world from the later half of the 1980s. China is the biggest country in Asia. It has always held a special place in the global view of countries in Asia with a Chinese heritage. With a common language (Mandarin) and shared traits of culture, close relationships developed naturally. Singapore, Hong Kong and Taiwan have been particularly closely linked to China in the development of cardiothoracic surgery.

Several groups from Singapore have been involved in this field: Dr. Huat Seong Saw and Dr. Chuen-Neng Lee went to Beijing in 1987 and 1988 to lecture and to perform surgery with Chinese surgeons in Beijing Medical University's People's Hospital and 3rd Hospital, Beijing Region Military Hospital and Beijing Heart and Lung Institute (Anzhen Hospital), as well as to visit Fuwai Hospital. The team also visited Xi'an and Guangzhou. This was the start of a series of visits by various surgeons from Singapore to China, focusing on the cities of Beijing, Shanghai and Guangzhou.

Appointments as Clinical Professors to universities like Beijing Medical University were conferred. Subsequent repeat visits over the next six years included demonstration of operations using close circuit TV to the auditorium, particularly of coronary artery surgery. This brought together groups of cardiac surgeons from around the country. Lectures and discussions were conducted in Mandarin. The usage of a common language enabled easier exchange of information compared to exchanges with non-Chinese speaking foreign surgeons. The bonds and relationships developed also tended to be closer and more lasting. It was during these visits that long-term friendships were forged. Bright young surgeons such as Dr. Song Wan from Beijing Medical University were identified. Arrangements were made for him to do his PhD in Brussels. The mentor was a good friend of Dr. Chuen-Neng Lee and a fellow Mayo alumus, Dr. Jean-Marie Desmet. Dr. Wan did very well in Brussels and was considered an asset to the university there. He subsequently moved to Hong Kong. International contacts for Beijing were made through the introduction of other close friends like Dr. Carlos Mestres of Barcelona. Dr. Mestres had since made many trips to China, contributing substantially to the development of cardiac surgery. Like many European surgeons, he has a natural affinity with the oriental cultures and the humility to make the effort to get to know the people.

It is through these visits that foreigners with a keen eye and good heart have learned to appreciate China for what it is, and what it can be, understanding the deficiencies inherent in a very big and complex developing country. One cannot know China through a short visit. It takes multiple visits, making time, making friends and learning the basic traditions, culture, people and political-economic realities to get a glimpse of China and its cardiothoracic surgery. What is definitely not welcome is the pompous, self-important foreigner who comes to China to "Teach the Natives" cardiac surgery. China has immense talents and is not to be underestimated.

A cardiologist, Prof Yeng Leng Lim from Singapore, founded the Xiamen University Medical College and Xiamen Heart Center in Xiamen City, Fujian Province. He became the Founder as well as Director of the Heart Center from 1999 to 2000. He arranged for many cardiac surgical teams to visit and operate in various cities in China in the 1990s.

Dr. Dar Ching Wu and his colleagues from Mount Elizabeth Hospital, Singapore conducted regular visits and performed surgery at the Fujian Provincial Research Institute for Cardiovascular Disease, Fuzhou City from 1986 onwards. He also arranged for training in

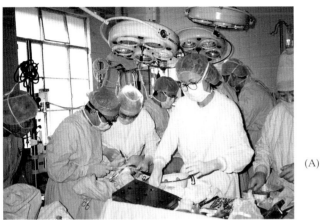

(A)

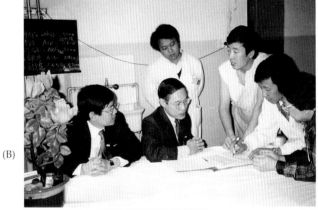

(B)

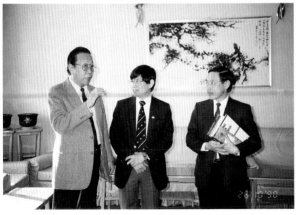

(C)

Fig. 1. [A–I] Singapore team visited Beijing Anzhen Hospital in 1990.

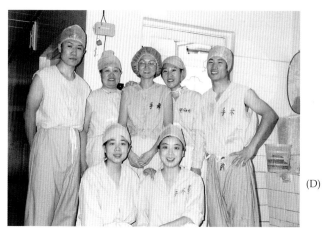

(D)

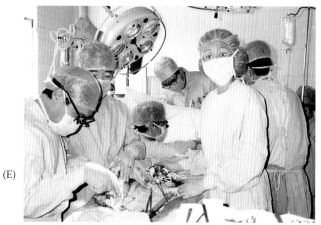

(E)

(F)

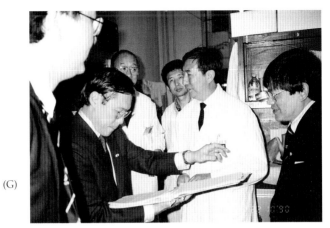

(G)

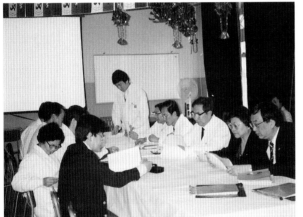

(H)

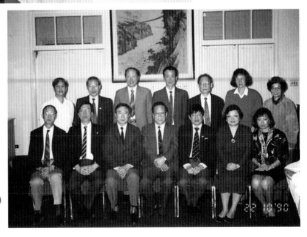

(I)

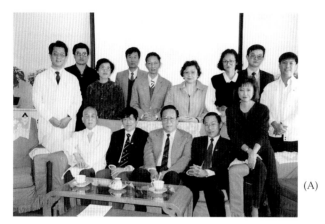

(A)

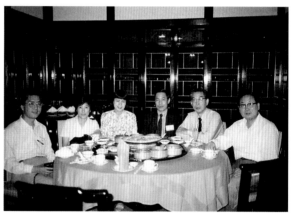

(B)

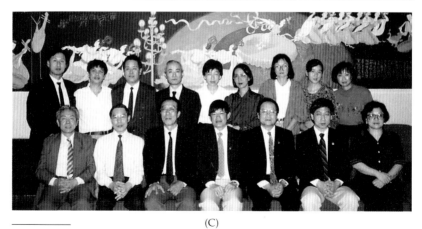

(C)

*Fig. 2. [A–D]*

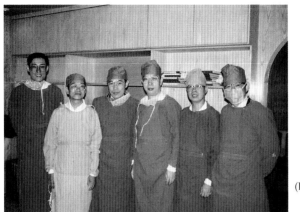

(D)

Singapore for Dr. Wen-Lin Liu and Dr. Fu-Rui Lin in 1989 and 1997. Collaboration also comprised a Joint International Symposium between Mount Elizabeth Hospital and Fuwai Hospital, Beijing in 1995, and performing surgery in Beijing Friendship Hospital. Dr. Wu helped to develop the Wuhan Asia Heart Hospital, becoming Medical Director in 1998 and later Advisor. This hospital has become a major center in central China. Dr. Liang Tao, who was trained in Singapore, became the main surgeon at this hospital.

Over the years from 1987, many young Chinese surgeons spent a period of their training in Singapore at the National University Hospital and at Singapore General Hospital. The surgeons include:

Dr. Ming Jie Zhang, who had since moved on to be Medical Director of the security hospital in Beijing.

Dr. Hong He Luo, who became full professor at Zhongshan Medical University, Guangzhou.

Dr. Li Zhang, who received a Master's degree in cardiac surgical research at the National University of Singapore before moving on to Germany to do further research.

Dr. Yue Hong Shan, who leads cardiac surgery in Suzhou Provincial Hospital.

Dr. Wei Li, who returned to Shanghai.

In the area of research, several joint projects were carried out,

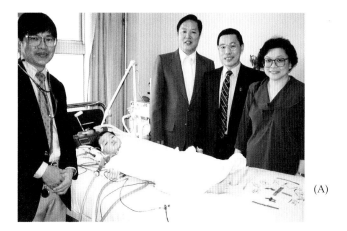

(A)

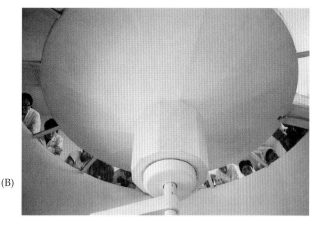

(B)

*Fig. 3. [A, B] Singapore team visited Beijing Medical University in 1991.*

including a project between Professor Tony Yeo of the Nanyang Technological University of Singapore, Zhonghsan University of Guangzhou and the Montana Heart Institute under Dr. Carlos Duran to develop pericardial moulds for aortic valve replacement. Professor Hong He Luo was the key surgeon involved in this project, having spent time as a Clinical Fellow at the National University Hospital, Singapore in 1992 and having developed contacts in Singapore.

Visiting teams of hospital administrators, cardiac surgeons, cardiologists, nurses and perfusionists have made multiple visits to hospitals in Singapore to exchange knowledge on healthcare systems, techniques, protocols, care paths, healthcare delivery and training. A few Hong Kong perfusionists have graduated from the Perfusion Course conducted by the National University Hospital of Singapore. Batches of nurses who had worked in Singapore have also returned to serve in cardiothoracic ICUs and operating rooms in Chinese cities. Over the past two decades, the development of cardiac surgery in China has been remarkable. Having the advantage of observing the changes from regular visits, it is impressive how standards have improved despite the limitations of the structure of healthcare delivery, financial constraints, and a fragmented system. The heavy emphasis on multiple percutaneous therapy hindered development of coronary surgery, often presenting the cardiac surgeon with very high risk patients. It contributed to a relatively slow growth in the number of coronary bypass surgery operations in China as a whole. Given the large population, the absolute number of surgeons and the results, coronary bypass surgery will continue to evolve and the number of centers of excellence will increase.

What is required over the next decade is the evolution of a more efficient system of delivery of cardiac surgical care, and better coordination between cardiac anaesthesia, perfusion, surgical departments and other areas. Adequate financial recognition of cardiac surgeons' work is needed. Currently the surgeons are under-compensated for their long hours and hard work. An increased number of international publication/presentation of the work being done in China is necessary to showcase the quality of this work. There are tremendous possibilities for the development of cardiothoracic surgery in China.

# Forging Global Links: European Perspectives

*Carlos-A. Mestres*

*"Brotherhood sworn under the Peach tree"*

*Episode 1*
*The Romance of the Three Kingdoms*

## The First Question

China, the Middle Kingdom, the country of the biggest human work, like the Great Wall, the Beijing-Hangzhou Grand Canal and the Karez irrigation systems. The first question about China often refers to her location, size and population. We all heard about China but we, foreigners, must confess our general lack of knowledge when first facing this huge country. This is almost a rule regardless of the professional affiliation and experience. We then need to quickly have a look at some books to have a glimpse of what China is. I believe this has been true for all of us before our first visit to China. What we know about geography, history, politics and economics? Intensive study brings us some answers, some perspective about the country. At the end, it is roughly the same information that we had when we were in the school.

Asia is a region of that claims the attention of the international community. Asia as a whole is tremendously diverse. China is an incredible part of it and also diverse. There are remarkable contrasts in terms of physical geography, rich ethnicity, economics and even language. We need to go to the basics and read old and new books that will be useful to us to understand what is going on in this part of the world.

To gain some knowledge we need simple tools that may help to explain the historical evolution and current situation of China. We need to know that China is geographically included in what it is called East Asia together with Japan and Korea. This is a consolidated area with these pieces being complementary as a physical space and with strong links in many ways throughout the history. Going a little bit more deeply into our basic knowledge we realize that there are physical criteria (mountains, valleys, gorges, etc.) administrative criteria (borders, administrative regions) and functional criteria (urban conglomerates, etc) that define such an incredibly large area [1–3].

The now excited foreigner needs to know what we are going to find upon landing in China. The usual arrival points today will probably be the renovated Beijing Capital International Airport, the recently built Shanghai Pudong International Airport or the superb Hong Kong Chek Lap Kok International Airport. Before, they were the ancient Beijing Capital Airport, the old Hongqiao International Airport in Shanghai or the incredible one-runway Kai Tak International Airport in Hong Kong surrounded by all types of skyscrapers. In a quick look to the map, from Qinghai province at an average height of 4,000 m. as in the entire plateau of the Tibet, to the harsh northwestern province of Xinjiang that includes the Taklamakan desert, the Turpan depression in the Tarim basin and the northern Tianshan mountains one will be easily lost. Moreover, the *Huang* ("Yellow") and *Chang* ("Long") rivers will define a huge plane that separates these regions from the cold areas of the north and northeast, namely Inner Mongolia and the Manchurian block with Heilongjiang, Jilin and Liaoning, accessing from the west through the Gansu corridor.

And this is before reaching the East Coast where close to 80% of the population of China lives in a booming belt that extends from Shenyang in the north to Guangdong in the south, a really crowded area [4]. In other words, from the western Pamir mountains to the southeastern island of Hainan, we easily will meet one out of four inhabitants in what we call planet Earth. So simple and realistic.

For those, surgeons or not, who like geography, history, languages, culture in general, it is therefore advisable to spend some time learning what happened in China from the precambric era to the more modern contemporary times that we live today. We have neither time nor room to deal with history, climate, ethnicity (what a rich one here in China...), language (guess how many languages and dialects...) and domestic politics, however the critical point is the astonishing fast pace of changes in China. This is well depicted in a number of publications. We should remember the most recent times that we have also been able to live. This particularly applies after June 1997, the landmark year of the historic Hong Kong handover [5]. Just to remind that Chinese economy grew by 8.8% that particular year.

Whatever happened, nowadays we are forced to recognize that this fast pace is getting even faster. This is all in newspapers, magazines, books that keep flooding us with a nonstopable storm of news and information. Another remarkable moment in recent history was November 2002 when the Sixteenth Congress of the Chinese Communist Party announced the newly elected Party General Secretary, Jin-Tao Hu. The ultimate message is that of an extraordinary number of challenges for China in current days, so well depicted by Nolan [6]. So fast changes do include tremendous market forces, the gradual development of private business activities and the coexistence of a surprising "one country, two systems" that we have seen exploding over the past decade.

As foreigners, surgeons or not, must definitely consider the impact of everything related to China in our daily lives. What will happen in the near future? Will the revaluation of the Renminbi (*Yuan*), the Chinese currency, be a critical factor soon? Will a 9.4% increase in gross domestic product on a year-to-year basis get bigger? Is a prudent monetary policy needed in China? This is what we see and read everyday and many questions and doubts come to our mind [7–11]. Are we ordinary people ready to understand if it is good or bad that China economy may show some signs of cooling [12]?

We still have to come across many more events.

## The Second Question

Now, let's go for surgery and try cardiothoracic and vascular surgery. The second question to the foreign surgeon is very simple. What do I know about cardiothoracic and vascular surgery in Asia and particularly in China? Not only this question but also some other simple ones like: what do I need to know about cardiothoracic and vascular surgery in China? Again back to the same. For the generality of professionals, we must assume and confess again and again that our level of knowledge is, or has been, by far limited, to say something polite.

Today there are lots of activities in China regarding our specialty. One example is the International Heart Forum Beijing 2005 organized by the Cardiovascular Institute and Fuwai Hospital [13] which is a sample of big projects that interlink Cardiovascular Surgery and Cardiology. This kind of meetings is nowadays frequent and reflects the advancements made in China over the past two decades. This is in opposition to the very scanty activities that some of us were able to witness years ago. The Beijing Cardiothoracic Symposium [14] is credited as the probably first major meeting organized by Chinese surgeons in cooperation with foreign colleagues, in this case, American, very early during the 1980s. Time has shown us the enormous changes seen in China and around the world.

The paper published by Wan and Yim [15], the editors of this book, had the merit of bringing the attention of cardiothoracic and vascular surgeons towards China. It has been instrumental in modifying the perception of foreign surgeons with regards the evolution of cardiothoracic surgery in this huge country. We, the Europeans, are no exception and have been caught amidst the expanding wave of emerging China. In any case we are still far from a decent knowledge of what is going on in cardiothoracic and vascular surgery in China. The increasing number of hospitals active in our field represents the final take-off of the specialty in a country with an incredible potential for all types of surgery within the chest and the vascular system. What is advisable, then, is to get personal exposure in to realize about what has been achieved and what we do expect in the future.

## Personal Exposure

By the mid-1970s in the past century, the number of hospitals capable of performing open-heart operations was in the range of 30 and the number of procedures around 5,000 in China. There was shortage of advanced equipment. Because of the political situation it was difficult to access to anything made abroad. Equipment was home-made and included valves [16], local technology that followed the early developments of heart-lung machines [15]. Information about China was limited for us and we always talked about a country that seemed to be very far away. As far away as the countries we could not get access at that time. To say something that may sound bizarre today, my first Spanish passport was valid for all countries of the world exception made of "... Albania, Outer Mongolia, People's Republic of Korea, Democratic Republic of Vietnam, People's Republic of China and the USSR" (Fig. 1). We are talking about 1975 ... and China sounded to us as far as those prohibited countries. There were the times where we, the foreigners, needed to get the Foreign Exchange Certificates (FEC) for shopping as there was no way of using the Yuan.

Promotion of foreign medical products started by 1976, mostly in Guangzhou, the former Canton for us in Europe. I came across basic information regarding the cardiovascular market years later through the incredible help of Ms. Lindy Shuk-Kam Chan, a native of Guangzhou and an entrepreneurial lady who spent her professional career traveling throughout China. Purchase of anything from abroad had to go through tedious procedures and imported by the National Import & Exports Corporations. The own Chinese clinical judgment was the key tool for the care of the patients.

I had my first contact with "the surgical China" when I first read the paper of Sloan et al. that summarized the Beijing Cardiothoracic Symposium [14]. I was then a junior trainee in cardiovascular surgery under Marcos Murtra MD, former president and current historian of the European Association for Cardio-thoracic Surgery (EACTS) and Alberto Igual MD, my senior resident at the time when I was in training, and used to read as much as I could. Then I became impressed about a meeting hold in China with Chinese surgeons and prominent American surgeons attending the meeting led by the late Lyman Brewer III. The list of attendees was impressive for this young trainee. Later I became acquainted with a number of them like Thomas B. Ferguson, former editor of *The Annals of Thoracic Surgery* and a beloved person or D. Craig Miller, a highly respected and esteemed colleague from Stanford University. The late Ying-Kai Wu emerged as a prominent Chinese surgeon for the foreigners. Although this brief report from Sloan, Tashian and Lu [14] did not provide much information about surgery, I started to understand Chinese culture and food (Fig. 2). This Beijing Cardiothoracic Symposium probably marked the beginning of the evolution of China getting opened to the outside world. Companies from Hong Kong started going to the mainland to introduce foreign medical products. The import system began to decentralize and simplify. At the end of the 1980s, the number of open-heart procedures had risen to about 10,000 a year with the same number of hospitals. Surgery for congenital heart disease represented 60% and valve disease around 35% of the caseload. Coronary artery bypass grafting (CABG) was not developed at all.

## The first visit

I had later the chance of visiting China for the first time. It was with the occasion of the International Conference on Thoracic and Cardiovascular Surgery sponsored by the Chinese Society for Thoracic and Cardiovascular Surgery. It was hold in the outskirts of Beijing on 28–30 October 1986, at the beautiful Fragrant Hills Hotel, located about 70 km from *Tian-An-Men* Square. This is another piece of art of I. M. Pei, the Sino-American architect credited with beautiful

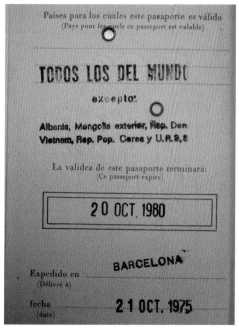

Fig. 1. *The author's Spanish 1975 passport showing all the restrictions of the time. We used to see China as far as all "forbidden" countries.*

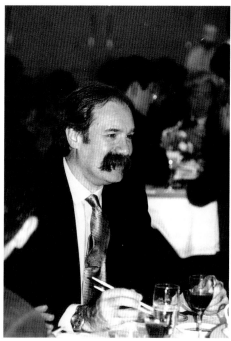

Fig. 2. *The author with a key instrument in China: The chopsticks.*

buildings like the Pyramid at the Louver Museum in Paris, the Bank of China building in Hong Kong or the Gateway building in Singapore. The President of the Conference was Hong-Xi Su with Ying-Kai Wu as the Honorary President and the Vice Presidents Yan-Ching Sun, Mei-Xin Shi and Guo-Jun Huang. Thoracic and Cardiovascular Surgery were covered in full. We had the chance to present a couple of papers. What really impressed me so much was the large Chinese experience in thoracic surgery and I specifically recall a paper from Shao et al. from Henan, reporting their experience with surgery for esophageal and cardial carcinoma in a series of 6,123 cases [17]. All the 21 papers on esophageal surgery were from China and Japan. A second paper that impressed me so much was that of Qian from Urumqi, in the Western province of Xinjiang, who reported a series of 842 cases of thoracic hydatidosis [18].

This Conference was well attended and gave me the chance to learn on the spot about China and Chinese surgery. Many of the foreign delegates came from North America. Some Europeans also attended and for the first time there was a gathering from many parts of the world in China. Overall 219 papers were presented, 98 (44.7%) from almost all provinces in China, 41 (18.7%) from the USA, 14 (6.4%) from Japan, 6 (2.7%) from India, 4 (1.8%) from Canada, 2 (0.9%) from Singapore, 2 from Qatar and the remaining 53 (24.2%) from European countries including 5 from my own country Spain. Therefore we, in Europe, started to realize about the importance of Chinese contributions although the impact of the Cultural Revolution on the scientific practice was so strong that sent the level of these contributions fifty years back as it has been shown in previous reports [15, 19]. Regardless of this Conference it was true that due to political relations, our American colleagues had already started exchanging programs with the Chinese counterparts much earlier and the renowned visit by the late Leo Eloesser endorsed by the United Nations years before [20] was a good example.

## *The Relations with the Chinese World*

A critical moment for me was to gain a broader perspective of Asia in general and the Chinese world of influence in particular. In fact, my first visits to Asia were to Mumbai, India in February 1985 to attend the World Congress in Cardiovascular Surgery organized by K. R. Shetty and later in November of the same year to Bangkok, Thailand to attend the Association of Thoracic and Cardiovascular Surgeons of Asia (ATCVSA) biennial congress and becoming the only Spanish active member since then. These were followed by a number of visits to other countries. In 1990 I was offered an attractive opportunity to work at the National University of Singapore as Foreign Teaching Staff and practicing at the Division of Cardiothoracic and Vascular Surgery at the National University Hospital under Professor Chuen-Neng Lee, a young, thorough, enthusiastic and skillful Singaporean surgeon. This was a good time for a European with just some exposure to the Asian world. This represented an unusual move in Europe as most of my senior and junior colleagues would have chosen to spend time at different Institutions in Europe, the USA or Canada. However, this stay contributed to the following:

1. To gain more experience in Asia, China and the Chinese world;
2. To dig deep inside Chinese culture;
3. To get exposed to the language;
4. To have the chance of formally practice cardiothoracic and vascular surgery and to teach at an Asian University.

Singapore is a small, multilingual and multicultural country that serves as a major hub in South East Asia. It has a strong Chinese influence as 75% of the population is ethnic Chinese. Some southern Chinese dialects, Hokkien, Hakka and Teochew, are predominantly spoken in Singapore and the neighbour countries like Malaysia and Indonesia but Mandarin, Cantonese and Hainanese can also be heard. Our practice was interesting, with a multiethnic team headed by Prof. Chuen-Neng Lee, together with a senior and experienced Nigerian surgeon, Oluwole A. Adebo from Ibadan, and junior doctors that joined on a rotation basis like Pek-Lan Khong, Jitt-Teng Chua and others. During my stay, a junior surgeon decided to join Cardiothoracic Surgery, Eugene Kwang-Wei Sim, who later became Associate Professor of Surgery and is currently the Secretary General of ACVTSA and a personal friend. These were a good team and a great time. Interestingly enough, a junior fellow from Beijing, Ming-Jie Zhang, with exposure in cardiology, joined our division for two years. He learnt how to work in cardiothoracic surgery and improved his English very much. He later went back to Beijing and his Institution, the 3rd Teaching Hospital of Beijing Medical University.

During my stay in Singapore I had the chance to give lectures in China as early as in 1991, lecturing in Shanghai and Beijing to a gathering of experienced local surgeons. The key part of it is to have a European speaking in English with simultaneous translation into Mandarin and Shanghainese. In addition I visited for the first time two of the most prestigious Institutions in China, the Fuwai Hospital and the Anzhen Hospital in Beijing, visits that were repeated over the years. This represented the consolidation my personal interest on China and everything related to this country, its people and its culture. That included the management of just a handful of words in Hokkien to able to ask the patients about pain. Not bad for a foreign European…. Worth trying, no doubt.

Some time later, the Singaporean team started a regular exchange of visits to Beijing Medical University in 1993 and 1994 with Chuen-Neng Lee, Jean-Marie DeSmet, a friend Belgian surgeon and I attending. We were proud to assist the local crew performing coronary surgery (Figs. 3–6). This cooperation was later transformed in a very humble paper that was published in the *Asian Cardiovascular & Thoracic Annals* in 1995 [21]. These were times to consolidate individual and institutional relations for a win-win situation. The most important is the friendship that started there and lasted until today. One of the editors of this book, Song Wan (Fig. 7), was an acquaintance of those days. He was instrumental in making my stays in Beijing pleasant to unexpected levels, showing me around off the usual places reserved for tourists. A remarkable visit to the Great Wall at the distant site of *Shi-Ma-Tai* continues to be an exceptional memory. Later, Song Wan went for extended training in Brussels under Jean-Marie DeSmet and Jean-Louis Vincent and produced a number of top quality papers on biological reactions of the body to

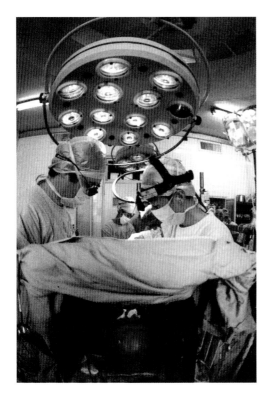

Fig. 3. *Performing a coronary bypass operation. Third Hospital, Beijing Medical University, July 1993.*

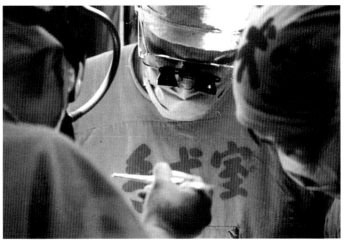

Fig. 4. *The author during a coronary bypass operation. Third Hospital, Beijing Medical University, July 1993.*

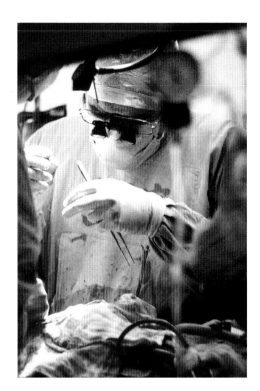

*Fig. 5. Conducting a coronary operation. Third Hospital, Beijing Medical University, August 1994.*

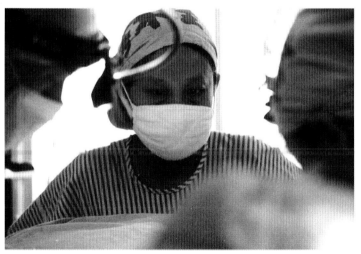

*Fig. 6. The anesthetist observing a coronary case. Third Hospital, Beijing Medical University, August 1994.*

cardiopulmonary bypass [22–24]. I was definitely proud to be in Brussels when he defended his thesis in 1997.

Those visits in 1993 and 1994 to Beijing Medical University allowed me to increase my knowledge and to observe the local skills. I was given a visiting professorship (Fig. 8) and a temporary permit to practice CABG (Fig. 9), the documents that I proudly and carefully keep in file today. At that time China was booming and its economy was already in the double digit annual growth, something that still seems extraordinary today [12]. From my first visits in 1986, one could easily see incredible changes. In 1986 there were only a handful of five-star hotels in Beijing including the Beijing Hotel, the Shangri-La Hotel and the Fragrant Hills Hotel as described earlier. Years later, high-rise buildings, all sorts of skyscrapers were mushrooming throughout a huge municipality of more than 11,000 km$^2$. In 1986 there were about two million bicycles, thousands of old Chinese buses packed with people of all ages, a scanty number of the old, black and very heavy *Zhong Guo* official cars and a handful of Toyota taxis for the foreign tourists to be driven back and forth the Great Wall at the close *Ba-Da-Ling* site. When we performed surgery at Beijing Medical University in 1993 and 1994, the streets of Beijing were packed with millions of the small yellow "*mian bao*" that were later replaced with the current taxis scattered through this huge country. I was, by the way, greeted once upon a time by the driver of one of them in the former Chinese capital of Xi'an asking me about the players of the Barcelona Football Club. In the Southeast, Shanghai underwent a profound transformation. In my first visit to this nice city in 1991, we could only see the old buildings in the Bund, an interesting mix of Russian and French architectural style from late the 19th century. Years later, on 16th July of 2002, I was having dinner with my wife on her birthday at the restaurant on top of the Oriental Pearl TV tower, 468 m above the Huangpu River at Lujiazui, Pudong New Area, opposite to the almost centennial Peace Hotel, a beautiful piece of art-déco style, in the heart of a bustling city like the modern Shanghai.Whatever happens, it is understandable the mixture of personal memories and thoughts when writing a text like this. Knowledge is associated to experience, experience associated with

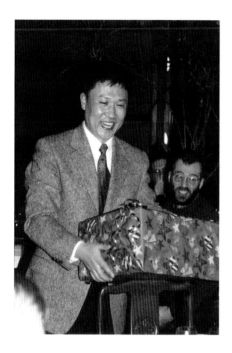

*Fig. 7. Dr. Song Wan in Brussels, Belgium, 1998.*

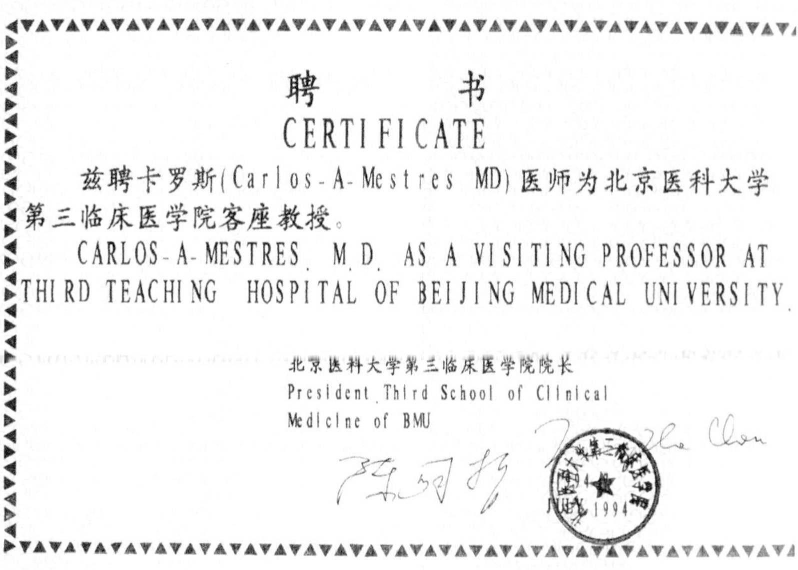

聘　　　书
CERTIFICATE

兹聘卡罗斯(Carlos-A-Mestres MD) 医师为北京医科大学
第三临床医学院客座教授。

CARLOS-A-MESTRES M.D. AS A VISITING PROFESSOR AT
THIRD TEACHING HOSPITAL OF BEIJING MEDICAL UNIVERSITY.

北京医科大学第三临床医学院院长
President Third School of Clinical
Medicine of BMU

1994

*Fig. 8. Certificate of Visiting Professor. Third Hospital, Beijing Medical University, 1994.*

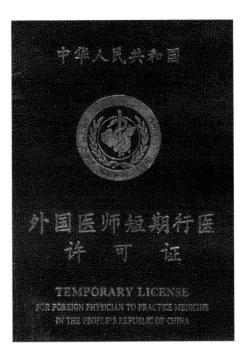

*Fig. 9. Temporary license for foreign physicians to practice medicine in the People's Republic of China, 1994.*

individual exposure. At the end, there is always a subjective component when describing any history, especially if this is your own history. And this section is no exception to the rule. I continue to visit China on a regular basis, attending meetings and exchanging thoughts and experiences with my counterparts. Also, I do take advantage of incorporating more knowledge on China, its people and its culture. And will continue to do so as long as I have the chances of doing it.

## *The Past*

These past sections have been useful to understand the individual engagement of a European with a distant China and its culture. What then about Cardiovascular and Thoracic Surgery? We just had a glimpse of previous times after the "table tennis diplomacy" when Richard Nixon first visited China in 1972, a landmark in recent history well depicted by Kissinger in an extensive text [25]. Sino-American relations were for years a notable reference to the world. We, in Europe, closely watched possible developments at all levels. Some facts mentioned earlier in this text marked the definite take-off of relations in Cardiovascular and Thoracic Surgery. A historical fact was the way in which Chinese diplomacy works, by insinuating rather than bullying. These are the words of an expert [25]. Foreign visitors were flattered by being admitted to the "Chinese club" as guests. People like me or like many others who went to China for the first time expected a kind of application for "membership" in China. And in some cases this ended up in a strong link and I consider myself lucky enough to be given a kind of wildcard to gain local knowledge in the years that came.

In these early days of the 1990s, there were tremendous changes. The Ministry of Health implemented between 1992 and 1994 a policy to classify the hospitals into three categories, with 3 being the top and 1 the lowest. Each had three grades, i.e. 3A, 3B and 3C. The main criteria for this classification were the number of medical specialties and the number of beds. The top was 3A and Cardiovascular and Thoracic surgery was the prime specialty among the specialties in order to qualify for 3A. Due to the interest of the hospitals in getting approved for 3A level, many institutions decided to increase their capabilities to perform open-heart surgery and this represented a 2–3 fold increase in the number of procedures throughout the country. The overall caseload grew to about 15,000 a year with 60% congenital hearts and an increasing evidence of more coronary surgery being performed in up to 10% of the cases. By the mid-90s, state-of-the-art technology was fully available and the number of hospitals with an open-heart program rose up to about 100 with just about 50% of them doing more than 100 cases a year. At this time, Fuwai Hospital was doing around 3,000 cases a year and Anzhen Hospital, again in Beijing, in the range of 1,000.

By early 2004, there were about 200 hospitals performing open-heart surgery. The national caseload of about 40,000 cases a year at the end of the 20th century rose up to around 50,000 in 2004. Fuwai Hospital and Anzhen Hospital in Beijing took close to 5,000 and

3,500 respectively. The old days were over and this included the way of handling equipment as we have seen in some old pictures (Figs. 10–17) that I have been lucky to collect over the years. Reminiscences from old days, those days being probably not better than today but full of good memories.

## The Present

At present time there are around 20 hospitals which perform over 1,000 cardiac cases a year besides Fuwai and Anzhen Hospitals in Beijing. Due to the growth of the population, currently around 1.3 billion, 50% continues to be surgery for congenital hearts. Valve surgery still represents 30% of the caseload and the remaining 20% includes CABG, surgery of the aorta and miscellaneous work. Coronary surgery has increased to around 7,000 cases a year and off-pump CABG seems to become more popular among young surgeons, although its actual value still needs to be confirmed.

Some limitations apply to surgery in China. There is no national medical registry except for infectious diseases. It is very hard to establish the actual number of cardiovascular and thoracic operations performed yearly throughout the country. Estimations are made from rough data presented at local or international meetings. As in other countries, most of the medical products companies use to exchange information on unit sales in previous years, especially oxygenators and stabilizers for off-pump operations. Industry estimates the number of open-heart procedures based on the numbers of these products being sold. This is also a current practice worldwide and in my country, Spain, there is a published registry from industry data [26] that matches the national Registry of the Spanish Society of Thoracic and Cardiovascular Surgery [27].

The current infrastructure in China makes very difficult to establish a National Registry. Hospitals need to reconsider joining efforts to look for consistent data from their collective and individual performances. The Chinese Society for Thoracic and Cardiovascular Surgery had never been able to coordinate in an efficient manner data collection at the national level. Important institutions like Fuwai

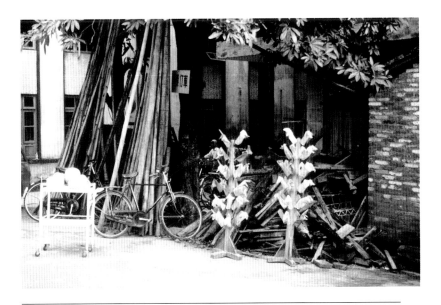

Fig. 10. *Surgical gloves drying under the sun after cleansing in the courtyard of a Hospital, 1985. (Courtesy of Dr. David C. Johnson, Westmead, NSW, Australia).*

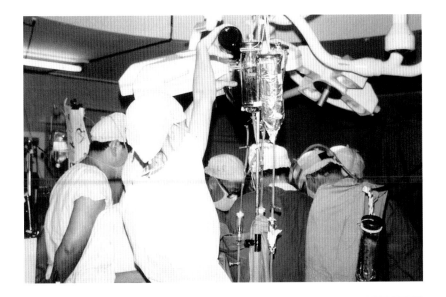

Fig. 11. *Surgical and anaesthetic teams at work. Blood tansfusion and old equipment. (Courtesy of Dr. David C. Johnson, Westmead, NSW, Australia).*

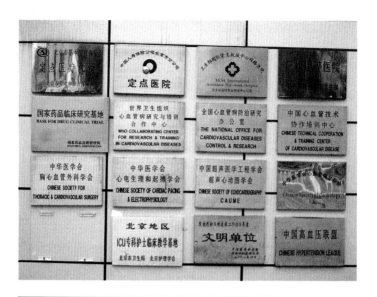

*Fig. 12. A number of organizations are based at Fuwai Hospital. These plaques hang in the wall at the main entry of Fuwai at 167 Bei Li Shi Lu.*

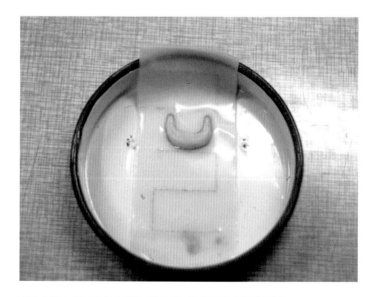

*Fig. 13. Work done at Renji Hospital, Shanghai. A pericardial monocusp patch, March 1991.*

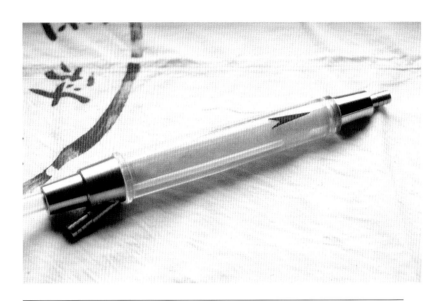

*Fig. 14. The pulsatile assist device (PAD) prototype. Renji Hospital, Shanghai, March 1991.*

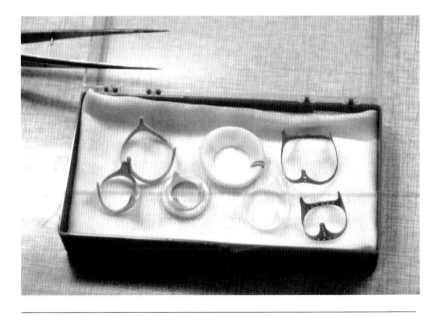

*Fig. 15. Different stents to be used in manufacturing heart valves. Renji Hospital, March 1991.*

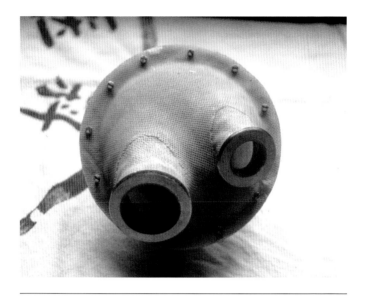

Fig. 16. *The artificial ventricle. Work done at Renji Hospital, Shanghai, March 1991.*

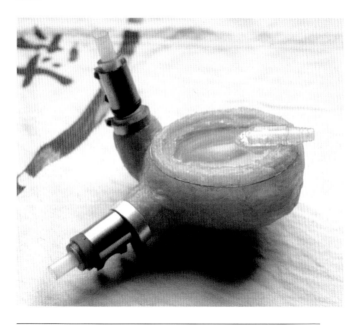

Fig. 17. *Another example of a paracorporeal assist device. Renji Hospital, Shanghai, March 1991.*

Hospital produced some amount of local information. Some important changes in the teaching structure have been taken place recently. For years, China used to be the only country in the world with medical universities. All the university Hospitals were under the Ministry of Health. By 1998, the Central Government in Beijing decided to eliminate all medical universities which were to merge with local universities to become medical schools. The government of universities and its affiliated hospitals were transferred to the provincial level. The only sector maintaining medical universities is the People's Liberation Army (PLA) and currently there are four military medical universities in China, in Guangzhou, Shanghai, Xi'an and Chongqing, the immense urban conglomerate where cardiovascular surgery started early in 1940s [15, 28]. Each of them has affiliated hospitals and the PLA also has its hospitals in four divisions, navy, air force, ground army and armed police.

What is the reality of Chinese cardiovascular and thoracic surgery today? These briefly reviewed rough data on cardiac surgery are just an example of how does it work today. My own perspective of the current status of the specialty is very clear. In about a decade China has emerged as the strongest competitor in economics and trade. The USA and the European Union have realized about this. The same applies in surgery. We have seen many Chinese "firsts" while visiting and reading and the entire scope of intrathoracic surgery is covered as anywhere in the world. The former halt of cardiovascular and thoracic surgery in China due to the Cultural Revolution is part of the history and now to deal with Chinese colleagues is to deal with our peers. Let's have a quick look to the specialty.

## *Vascular Surgery*

### 1. Endovascular surgery

Endovascular surgery has emerged in recent years as a booming subspecialty due to the following reasons: (1) Expected lower periprocedural mortality and morbidity; (2) Reduced surgical trauma; (3) Shorter hospital stay; (4) Faster patient recovery and (5) Reduced costs.

Some issues have not been solved yet as there still are morbidity and mortality and the issue of costs has not been properly addressed based on the still very high cost of the stent-graft and the annual reintervention rate due to graft malfunction, migration, endoleaks, etc. It is true, however, that the trends are towards an increasing use of these endovascular techniques both in the thoracic and abdominal aorta. China is not an exception to this. Some recent publications endorse the feelings of Chinese authors with this regard [29]. Endovascular surgery is then considered as a promising treatment, especially in critical issues like aortic dissection.

## 2. Carotid endarterectomy

Carotid endarterectomy (CEA) is a routine and popular procedure used to treat extracranial cerebrovascular disease for prevention of stroke in westernized countries. Brain atherosclerosis has been associated to ethnic differences and the Chinese population seems to be different from Caucasians as some studies have shown that intracranial disease is more extensive than extracranial involvement [30]. This fact may represent a cause of discussion when addressing the possible benefit of CEA. Current results with still limited series indicate that CEA in ethnic Chinese can be performed with acceptable morbidity and mortality and long-term results [31].

## 3. Peripheral vascular disease

When dealing with infrainguinal atherosclerotic involvement, there are no consistent data from the Far East regarding epidemiology or clinical work. It is said that the possible incidence of infrainguinal occlusive disease may involve 50–60 cases/800,000 people. Interestingly enough, Chinese people hardly suffer from deep venous thrombosis. Published data suggest that overall, that patients with infrainguinal occlusive disease are usually diabetic and female. Other than that no other major differences in early or intermediate results with western patients [32].

These are interesting data considering the evolution of Chinese population. An ageing population seems to be common in the southeast of China and Hong Kong is the best example. Bearing in mind population and economic patterns, the entire East and Southeast of China may behave in a similar way. Trustable data from the Hong Kong Census and Statistics Department by 1998 indicated that the average life expectancy for men was 77 and for women 82 years, which is exactly the same than in Spain and generally speaking, in Western Europe. These data may not significantly differ in the East Coast from Guangdong province up to the north through Fujian, Zhejiang, Jiangsu and Shandong provinces, as geography, climate and economics are closely related. Rural areas can be different. If this would be so, there is a tendency towards an increase in the prevalence of peripheral occlusive disease. However, there are still some limitations for revascularization procedures that seem to be available in large tertiary institutions thus indicating a delayed consultation [32]. Regardless of the pattern of disease, the reported results for surgical revascularization are satisfactory for the region in terms of operative mortality and mid-term survival, including gender differences that negatively affect women [33]. The fact that, according to available literature, there are no major differences in disease pattern and treatment between Chinese and western patients, represents a positive issue [32].

## Thoracic Surgery

### 1. Video-assisted thoracic surgery

One of the most striking changes seen in general thoracic surgery has been the widespread availability of video-assisted thoracoscopic surgery (VATS). Diagnosis and treatment of thoracic diseases has greatly benefited from this approach. Its major advantages are safety, effectiveness and prompt recovery. One of the first to actively promote VATS in Asia was the co-editor of this book Anthony Yim, who almost a decade ago presented with an elegant analysis of cost-containment of VATS from the Asian perspective [34]. Together with the intrinsic benefits of VATS, cost issues were, and of course are, very important in medical practice throughout the world. This particular paper was of interest to open the eyes of the reader to non-medical problems that are of extreme importance in our practice. As in Spain, where socialized medicine is the predominant system, we have seen a number of changes that make the practice of medicine more complex for the attending doctors, with increasing institutional and public pressure, an expected higher efficiency despite of the lack of adequate equipment and resources and so on. A few years ago, we were not aware of how important non-medical issues would become in medical practice.

This initial paper by Yim described interesting local strategies to reduce the cost of VATS therefore enhancing its use by thoracic surgeons with fewer restrictions [34]. I do believe that local and regional practices in Asia have evolved in an appropriate way. Today, major institutions in China provide up-to-date treatment for thoracic diseases and VATS is a routine technology. It was that the actual role of VATS was to be defined out of the treatment of spontaneous pneumothorax, wedge resection for small nodules, pleural biopsies, etc. To date, the scope of VATS has expanded and covers an important part of thoracic surgery that includes lobectomy, pneumonectomy or the treatment of pulmonary metastases to say just some procedures.

Some time later, Ren from Beijing came up with an interesting contribution that presented the community with updated information from mainland China [35]. He gave a broad presentation of VATS analyzing an institutional experience from Peking Union Medical College and reviewing the indications for such a surgery. This was of interest to me as stressed on key factors, the resistance to be used by surgeons and, obviously, cost issues. The test of time showed when and how a technique should be used and VATS has been no exception. Today is well accepted by the majority for a large number of indications and it is performed with very good results throughout China [36–39].

It is always good to periodically perform a retrospective analysis of our activities as this gives us a perspective of where we were and towards we do head. Although there is a general agreement that prospective evaluation including an eventual randomized allocation of treatment groups sounds more scientific for the evaluation of newer technologies, drugs or procedures, a review is positive as it brings back us to the origin of the problems and experiences and allows us to positively face the present and the future. The example of VATS is self-explanatory.

## 2. The esophagus

We cannot neglect the evolution of thoracic surgery in China and should remind the reader that there are some fields in which the contributions from the region and particularly from China have been very important. This especially refers to the surgery of the esophagus and the gastric cardia. For a European like me, those immense figures that I saw for the first time 20 years ago when reading abstracts or papers or attending presentations from Chinese colleagues were far beyond my expectations [17]. As epidemiology is totally different along the Asian part of the Pacific Rim, we had to learn from our colleagues from this region that the esophagus was a routine part of thoracic surgery here even though my very senior European ancestors, decades ago, were credited with the description of significant advancements in surgical technique [40, 41]. The esophagus was also mastered by American surgeons like Henry Ellis [42] and there was also extensive experience in South Africa [43] where Le Roux published significant data for the time. Perhaps the latest impact in this surgery was the work of Mark Orringer from Ann Arbor, Michigan who made popular blunt esophagectomy [44]. I still can recall one of his first presentations in Europe back in 1979 before the formerly popular Coventry Conference although that time showing very interesting data on benign strictures [45]. However, the esophagus later became a problem as many centers did not have cases enough to certify most of the thoracic surgeons in this particular field. Hence, one realizes about the amount of work silently done in China in esophageal disease and especially esophageal carcinoma. We should pay tribute to this as memories can go back as far as to the fifties in the 20th century [46].

## The Budd-Chiari Syndrome

The Budd-Chiari syndrome or coartaction of the inferior vena cava is a fascinating disease caused by blood flow obstruction of the main hepatic veins and the outlet of the inferior vena cava, characterized by retrohepatic portal hypertension or inferior vena cava hypertension. The consolidation of liver transplantation as a routine form of treatment for end-stage liver diseases has changed the approach to the Budd-Chiari syndrome in many western countries where solid organ transplant programs are active. However, in many countries, the Budd-Chairi syndrome has to be treated using a number of complex surgical techniques, from membranotomies to shunts from all types. According to Xu et al. [46] more than 3,000 cases of this disease have been reported in China in the last ten years. China and India seem to be the countries with the largest experience in the world and this has been confirmed by Victor, Jayanthi and Madanagopalan [47]. The results from Xu et al. working at Zhengzhou University are extremely good with hospital mortality of 3.1% [46]. These authors confirm correct diagnosis following an adequate staging as key for good surgical results. This is a good example of good vascular work [48, 49].

## Cardiac Surgery

### 1. Surgery for congenital heart defects

As stated, the year by year caseload is growing nationwide. Many new centers are now operational although not all of them perform large number of cases. However, the quality of the work is also getting better and has in certain cases, reached international standards. Surgery for congenital heart defects continues to be number one in percentage due to the population growth even though the strict limitations in terms of childbearing by couple set by the central government in Beijing for the Han population. A number of interesting publications are available now and many focus attention on pathologies that we seldom see in western countries, like ruptured aneurysms of the sinus of Valsalva, a congenital defect that is a rarity in Europe but well known in China. The Fuwai series is credited as one of the largest published so far [50]. The same applies to a number of complex congenital defects as Chinese surgeons produced significant information at the national and international level [51].

## 2. Valve surgery

There have been a number of contributions by Chinese surgeons mentioned earlier in this original. A number of valve designs have been tested although no one of them went on public knowledge in the western world. From mechanical valves as designed by Cai et al. early in the 1960s, to tissue valves made of bovine pericardium at Fuwai Hospital by Zhu and his team or from porcine valves as implanted by Luo et al. in Guangzhou, a large number of operations with these Chinese-made devices were performed [15]. China has always attracted foreign investors due to the immense swine production, which is one of the most developed industries in China. Furthermore, there is a large gap between swine production in China and the US, Germany or Denmark. This is the reason why large North American corporations have for years purchased pig hearts for their manufacturing plants. Pork output in China was 40.57 million tons in 1996, ranking 67.5% of total meat production [52] being 32.93 kg meat in per capita, more than twice the production in the world. The *Taihu* pigs are credited for their high quality meat. Therefore, Chinese abattoirs supplied porcine valve manufacturers abroad for decades. Some foreign investors made efforts to establish factories in China as it was the case of Pacific Biomedical Enterprises, a Singapore-based company. This was one of the most interesting projects involving China that I came across during my early visits, a company formed through the efforts of the late Shanghai-born Dr. Victor Chang of Sydney, Australia and Frank L. Tamru, an enterprising American medical device salesman who covered the entire region for a leading heart valve manufacturer. Two of his colleagues from the same device company, specialists in valve manufacturing, became equal partners in the venture and the company was officially launched in 1986.

Richard Martin headed mechanical valve operations and Brij Gupta, the production of porcine and pericardial. Although the company was established and based in Singapore, a major link to China was the key ingredient in the business plan due to the interest to produce tissue valves because such an important swine production. Pacific Biomedical formed a partnership with an ongoing valve facility based in Guangzhou under the leadership of Dr. Zheng-Xiang Luo, chief heart surgeon at Guangdong Provincial People's Hospital. The underlying credo was that of heart valves made in Asia for Asian patients at a substantially lower cost than the imported valves. A number of difficulties including the horrific murder of Dr. Chang in 1991, whose name and reputation were associated to the project made impossible to the project alive on the long-term.

What is more important today is that Chinese surgeons have made a step forward and nowadays start working on a cooperative way. It is difficult to find examples of this in China today but the already existent may eventually pave the way for subsequent studies and trials in the future. Although just a handful of trials have been conducted in the past by Chinese cardiologists, not much information is available with regards to surgical cooperative trials [53]. The Chinese cooperative prospective trial on low-dose administration of warfarin for patients with prosthetic heart valves [54], presented before the American Society of Hematology in Philadelphia late in 2002, was to me an important study for the following reasons: 1. It was probably the first time a cooperative study of these characteristics was designed and conducted in China; 2. It was able to produce data on the current INR therapeutic range in China that seems to be different from other parts of the world; 3. It concluded that Chinese patients, on the average, require 50% lower maintenance doses of warfarin than those reported for Caucasians with very low reported incidence of thromboembolic events (1/488); 4. It raised the point of a possible genetic predisposition to warfarin sensitivity [54].

This is the way to go. Some information from this study and extensive review of available data confirmed ethnic differences that were later reported by the same group [55]. Another interesting aspect of this cooperative work is that it brought together a group of eleven hospitals from all over China, also for the first time, including important institutions like Xijing Hospital from Xi'an, West China Hospital from Chengdu, Xinqiao Hospital from Chongqing, Fuwai Hospital from Beijing, Changhai Hospital and Shanghai Chest Hospital from Shanghai, the Hunan Medical University from Changsha, Union Hospital from Tongji, Zhejiang University from Hangzhou, Fujian Institute of Cardiothoracic Surgery at the Medical College from Fuzhou and Zhongshan University from Guangzhou. A selected group of institutions from such a large country. An example for the future.

## 3. Coronary artery surgery

This is the weakest part of cardiothoracic and vascular surgery in China today. Coronary surgery is still developing in China. There are many reasons for this. One seems to be the epidemiology and treatment of coronary artery disease. The largest group of ethnic Chinese studied with regards to acute coronary syndrome comes from the China branch of the OASIS (Organization to Assess Strategies for Ischemic Syndrome) study. These data were published in the *Chinese Medical Journal* [56]. The reader was informed that the usage of lipid-lowering drugs was less than in other countries, that nitrates and anti-platelet medications were most commonly used and that around 50% took beta-blockers or ACE inhibitors. Coronary angiography was performed in 35% of the patients, percutaneous transluminal coronary angioplasty (PTCA) in 16.8% and only 4.1% underwent coronary artery surgery.

This is rather interesting as coronary artery disease has become the probably most common form of heart disease in a lapse of about 50 years [53]. This is despite the fact that Chinese population has just an annual coronary mortality of one sixth of that reported in western countries [57]. A prestigious cardiologist like the Shanghai-born Tsung O. Cheng, Professor of Medicine at the George Washington University has pointed out a number of factors like changes in dietary habits, smoking and the increase in obese people like in many other countries of the world including Spain. Obesity in China, as defined by a body mass index >30, is present in 10% of the population in the North and 5% in the South whereas is 14.5% in the smaller Spanish population according to recent data from the Spanish Society for the Study of Obesity in 2002 [58].

However, coronary surgery has not developed in China in the way we are used in western countries. The first CABG operation using saphenous vein autograft was performed in China in 1974 at Fuwai Hospital in Beijing by Dr. Jia-Qiang Guo [15, 16]. The current estimation is that around 20,000 such operations have been performed in China since, with a rate of 20 per million people population. There are scanty data about CABG in China and even very large series of patients like this reported by Pan from Shanghai Chest Hospital back in 1989 [59] were able to produce just 36 patients undergoing such a operation. Incredible but true.

Although not reliable data are available today, CABG still ranks last in cardiothoracic and vascular surgery as an individual procedure in China. Compared to the rate of 2000 cases per million people population in the US or 900 cases in Europe [60] this minuscule percentage of patients undergoing CABG has to increase in the future. The prospects for the future are not bad. Cultural burdens have also to be overtaken as control of pain has been the key issue from the individual point of view as the perception of the disease by the individual [61].

### The Fuwai system

Over the past three decades, cardiovascular surgery in China has necessarily been associated with the name of Fuwai Hospital. This is why I have to contemplate a subsection that has to refer to the current level of performance of this institution. The Fuwai Hospital is the largest institution in China specialized in the prevention, diagnosis and treatment of cardiovascular diseases. Owned by the government, it is located in the central district of *Xi Cheng* in Beijing. It was founded in 1956, hence celebrations for the 50th anniversary was in 2006. I paid my first visit to this center back in 1991 and was surprised as I found a mixture of high-volume cardiac surgery with special dedication to congenital heart disease and also traditional Chinese medicine, almost unknown in Europe.

Associated to the Chinese Academy of Medical Sciences, Fuwai has a long history of dedication to clinical medicine and to research in cardiovascular diseases. It also serves as the base to a number of organizations like the National Center for Cardiovascular Disease of the Ministry of Health, the World Health Organization Beijing Center for Cardiac Surgery, the *Chinese Circulation Journal*, the *Chinese Journal of Pacing and Electrophysiology* and the *Chinese Journal of Molecular Cardiology*. It serves also as the National Training Center for Cardiac Surgery, Interventional Cardiology, Pacing and Electrophysiology of the Chinese Medical Association (Fig. 12).

This is a remarkable institution and I have seen its progression over the past twenty years becoming a modern hospital covering all aspects of the specialty. When getting through the main gate, it is clear that the patient will be taken care from the first-aid station. Today, Fuwai is a huge complex incorporating up-to-date equipment that allows their specialists to perform around 16,000 cases in the catheterization laboratory and use 11 operating rooms for a number of surgical cases of 4,700 by the end of 2004. Figures are always big in China and Fuwai is no exception, with about 12,000 cardiovascular admissions a year and a staff of nearly 1,500.

The evolution of Fuwai is an example of how the country changed in recent years. Fuwai is obviously not the single institution in the country. Many others are growing also at a very fast pace. The needs of such a huge country are enormous and a number of programs are getting operational to cope with them. We will witness many more changes in the near future as a reflection of the incorporation of China into the international arena and these are not to be neglected. In fact, they are not neglected at all by all those who see the world from a wide perspective.

## The Future

What we, Europeans, do expect from Europe? What we also do expect from China? Europe is a conglomerate of old cultures. Europe struggles to become united through a long-term project like the European Union that incorporates today 27 members with some more lining up to join the club in these first years of the 21st century. Europe may not be small but it is congested. The core of Europe is nowadays old, suffering from the diseases related to ageing, is physically handicapped by the lack of room to grow, mentally blocked by an immense bureaucracy and unable to compete with Asia and the Americas in terms of production. The European Working Time Directive [62] will definitely represent a major burden in the years to come, especially in Western Europe. The recently incorporated members of the European Union will bring youth and an eventually powerful workforce. However, there are still many problems to fix like unemployment, distribution of wealth, administrative stiffness, undesirable migration patterns, transnational organized crime and the consolidation of the European Union itself.

Western Europe is the destination point for many people that come from all over the world. Medical care is a political problem in most of the countries with socialized healthcare systems like Spain. The main issue is how big the bill is and who has to pay it. We see again in Western Europe diseases that were supposed to be eradicated like rheumatic fever among the youngsters. Coronary artery disease is still prevalent but interventional cardiology is taking over a significant proportion of patients that need less aggressive forms of treatment. There is too much politics in Europe and this is totally unpractical for the community and especially the medical community.

China, on the other hand, has already emerged. It is booming. Its main gates to the world, Beijing, Hong Kong and Shanghai are constantly busy regulating the inflow of visitors and traders. With this 1.3 billion people population is today seen by all as the major competitor for today and the future. The changes seen in recent years, its admission into the World Trade Organization, the coming Beijing 2008 Olympic Games, a heavily government-regulated economic growth leaning on double-digit figures have to be seen as the credentials for an immediate future. China has also a very old culture. Mandarin will be a must for future generations. Up to now we could say that by being fluent in English and Spanish you could easily tour around the world on an unrestricted basis and this is probably true. However, on practical grounds, young people will eventually need Mandarin as a third option for mobility and professional relations.

China is definitely at the crossroads [6]. We, Europeans, have to carefully watch future developments. Cardiothoracic and vascular surgery is no exception. This immense population will need and improvement in the healthcare system and current policies may become obsolete soon. The 10 top causes of death in China [63] with the expected mortality by 100,000 population include circulatory (235/100,000) being cerebrovascular (128/100,000) and heart disease (107/100,000), cancer (146/100,000), respiratory (79/100,000) injury and poison (36/100,000) and digestive (18/100,000). Mortality due to cardiovascular disease seems to be even for men and women according to regional data (33% men, 36% women) from the MUCA study [64]. The annual average coronary event rate per 100,000 in the region of Beijing is in the low range of the MONICA registry both for men and women but this may reflect different changes in the pattern of medical prevention and care but there are also interesting differences in mortality between the North, higher, and the South, lower [64]. In addition, the national statistics from the Ministry of Health show that there has been a slow but steady increase in mortality for ischemic heart disease both in urban and rural areas of China but with stronger impact of mortality in the urban conglomerates. The increasing obesity among schoolchildren in China in a decade has reached 8.5% at the end of 1995 according to regional statistics [65] and smoking now has an incidence of 60–63% of the population [66]. World estimates for overall deaths for the entire 21st century are in the range of 1 billion, which compared to 100 million for the total of the 20th century represent a significant 10-fold increase. China, then, may also suffer from this epidemic and our practice, affected [66].

The past history and current data on the healthcare in China and especially on cardiothoracic and vascular surgery are helpful to foresee the future. As more institutions are getting operational in the field, with a still growing population with a median age of 34 years, the activity will increase year by year. It is difficult to estimate when a plateau can be reached. However, based on some of the above-mentioned statistics, surgical activity will definitely increase. If European figures are to be extrapolated, it may not sound unrealistic to handle an average of 500,000 cardiac surgical cases per year in the future. The same can be estimated for general thoracic surgery, with or without video-assistance and especially endovascular surgery, provided costs are kept on the lower range. It is also a little unlikely that the private sector may start to develop soon although some political changes occurred that will eventually favor private activities in the near future. It is expected that one private hospital will start operations in Shanghai sometime in 2006.

China is a world in itself. But China is geographically and politically a part of another special world called Asia. Asia is an incredible conglomerate of geographies, cultures, societies, languages, ethnicities,… Putting all together, China, India, Indonesia, Pakistan and Bangladesh take into account for 48% of the world's population. Some of these cultures are even older than western cultures, back in the time more than 5,000 years. Asia as a whole has different values, this is well known and widely depicted by many different authors [67]. Our western perspective does not frequently allow us to realize about how deep the differences may be. Economics plays a role. This has been addressed by Amartya Sen, the 1998 Nobel Laureate for Economics [68]. Asian development is fascinating, is accelerated [69]. It is an emerging continent with China and India leading the pack. This applies to all activities, from demographics to politics and even surgery. Will then they play a stabilizing role in the world of the 21st century? Will Oriental Asia transform the entire world? Local, regional and transnational changes are underway. We see today a reverse colonial rule. It is true that oriental cultures tend to make the western world to behave in a different world [70]. The "Asian Tigers" may be responsible for this as they lead the economic regional development. The future of this region, of its individual components and the entire world sounds complex, but attractive.

## *Reflections*

This is a brief overview of some personal experiences in China over a span of almost twenty years. I have personally learnt a lot by getting exposed to a totally different environment than my hometown Barcelona, my country Spain and my region Europe. This is the value of traveling, especially when you are willing to learn from everybody. I believe I made the right decision when I decided to explore Asia in general and China and its area of influence in particular.

Cardiothoracic and vascular surgery is a fascinating part of medicine. Although I love Surgery—Surgery with capital letters—as a whole, I decided to embark in a cardiothoracic and vascular career when I realized about the consistency of such a school. From my very early days in Asia and in China I have been able to incorporate the following:

1. Do always open your eyes.
2. Do never underestimate anybody.
3. Be quiet, just listen.
4. Watch and see what the others do.
5. You will learn from good observation.

It has been impressive what you can get from traveling, observe and integrate. I am a graduate of the University of Barcelona School of Medicine and proud of it. However, there is no doubt that the best University you can attend is traveling and observation. China and its area of influence helped me a lot.

From my personal experiences I learnt that cardiothoracic and vascular surgery in China was more advanced as I expected when I first made this acquaintance. Lots of hands-on clinical experience was accumulated in certain areas in which we still were and probably are like schoolchildren, and the esophagus is a good example. I learnt that many people that I met have much more experience in almost everything but we were hardly able to presume this was true.

This has been the opinion of many others, European or not. Our British colleagues took advantage of the former British rule in many Asian countries but China and in continental Europe watched this from the distance. The American experiences like that of Leo Eloesser, one of the fathers of modern thoracic surgery [20], or the late Harry Windsor, one of the pioneers of Australian cardiothoracic surgery [71] were disputed by a handful of Europeans who had an early chance of incorporating some knowledge [72]. Today, China is seen by us as a mirror due to its incredible economics, complex politics, astonishing developments and the uncontrollable fast pace of growing. This will last for a long time. We have senior colleagues performing at the highest level like Yu-Guo Weng, a senior Shanghai-born surgeon, at the Deutsches Herzzentrum Berlin in Germany. We have European colleagues that have settled some links with China like Wolfgang Konertz from La Charité Hospital also in Berlin through an active institute in Shenyang. Through a senior colleague like Norbert Franz, links were also established at the Deutsches Herzzentrum Berlin, that has trained 58 people from China for more than two years since 1986. Fourteen of them received a German degree. This represents a way to cooperate and interlink two different worlds. There are other examples that follow the same path.

Recent major events like SARS have also shown how tough our Asian colleagues could be. Our editors Drs. Song Wan and Anthony Yim gave us a very detailed and dramatic description of the impact of such an event on the medical community as a whole and on individuals that suffered from this serious epidemic [73]. Things are not totally clear today and there are still risks now for large populations. What is the most important to me are the wise words from Dr. Wan, essential afterthoughts coming directly from the heart of a professional who dealt directly with the disease and death. No doubt these are remarkable words: "Small things can really add up" [73].

China and Asia are growing and will continue to do so for time. In our specialty, Asians can develop themselves very easily. Today there are a number of tools like meetings, conferences, journals, printed materials, the Internet, to communicate. As I personally stressed in the past [74], Asians have a good tool to use for communication and a regional journal like *The Asian Cardiovascular & Thoracic Annals* is an example of what can be done. The entrepreneurial work of an insider like the American Frank L. Tamru [75, 76], mentioned in association with the Pacific Biomedical heart valve project previously was crucial in making Asians aware that a regional journal could be a phenomenal tool for their own use. Frank took it upon himself to try and unify and uplift Asian surgeons by having their own scientific journal thereby increasing credibility in the eyes of Western colleagues. It was also a way to contribute something of significance to such a region. I am absolutely proud of having been closely associated with Frank and this project since its inception back in 1993. Its current managers, Executive Editor David Lik-Ching Cheung and Managing Editor Lindy Shuk-Kam Chan have gotten the relay and operating from Hong Kong offer a regional instrument that may have impact on China. China has used its own Chinese-published organs for national communication but any form of more comprehensible communication allowing expansion will include English as the language for understanding.

I can simply foresee the growth and expansion of my cardiothoracic and vascular surgery in China. I am confident on this.

## *Conclusions*

I guess the questions I was asking to myself on behalf of many others at the beginning of this chapter have been addressed by this quick trip through recent past times. I have learnt geography, history, and history of cardiothoracic and vascular Surgery in China. I got the chance to realize about how much we do need to watch, listen and share. China is in the right track. The famous Singaporean Chinese ophthalmologist Arthur Lim referred to the coming age of Asian surgery [77]. He was right as the years ahead of us were about to bring a number of developments. The 21st century will be that of the Oriental booming in medicine and surgery and China, with his cultural, ethnical, geographic and linguistic diversity but also with its negative aspects and problems still to be solved, will be an important part of this move forward. I am pleased and honored by having had the chance to witness on the spot many of these changes over the past twenty years.

## Acknowledgements

The author is deeply indebted to Ms. Lindy Shuk-Kam Chan from Hong Kong; Mr. Frank L. Tamru from Camden (NJ-USA) for his lifetime friendship and introducing me to Asia; Prof. Chuen-Neng Lee from Singapore for his teachings, friendship and guidance; Dr. David Lik-Ching Cheung from Hong Kong for having trusted me over the years for his hospitality and friendship; Dr. Song Wan from Hong Kong, the one who started as a guide and ended up as a true friend; Prof. Qing-Yu Wu from Beijing who introduced to me the Beijing world; Prof. Sheng-Shou Hu from Beijing for his willingness in cooperating and offering his personal help; and Prof. Anthony Yim for the honor of participating in this magnificient book. These people are just a representation of many others that I have met in the past and who were able to teach me about Asia in general and the Chinese culture in particular. The order in which their names appear may be considered arbitrary with the exception of Ms. Chan as she has been the most dedicated teacher in Chinese matters I ever came across.

## References

1.  Cressey GB (1934) China's geographic foundations. A survey of its land and its people. Chap 1: The geographical landscape. New York: McGraw-Hill, pp 1–34.
2.  Brunet R (1995) Géographie Universelle. Asie du Sud-Est-Océanie. Paris: Belin-Reclus.
3.  Weigtman B (2002) Dragons and tigers: geography of South, East and Southeast Asia. New York: Wiley & Sons.
4.  Burgos JA, Busquets A, Martinez D (2020) L'espai geogràfic de l'Asia Oriental. Open University of Catalunya. www.uoc.edu
5.  Lam WWL (1999) The era of Jiang Zemin. Singapore: Prentice Hall.
6.  Nolan P (2004) China at the crossroads. UK, Cambridge: Polity Press.
7.  (2005) US and EU turn up the heat on China. International Herald Tribune, May 18, p 4.
8.  (2005) China Central Bank & inflation. Dow Jones Newswires. Wall Street Journal Europe, May 24.
9.  (2005) Pakistan growth. International Herald Tribune, May 24.
10. (2005) Why the des res in catching on. Financial Times, February 16, p 8.
11. Greenlees D (2005) Last frontier of banking. International Herald Tribune, May 24, p 17.
12. Bradsher K (2005) Signs of cooling China economy. International Herald Tribune, May 19, p 19.
13. International Heart Forum Beijing 2005. www.ihfbeijing.org

14. Sloan H, Tashian J, Luis AHF (1982) The Beijing Cardiothoracic Symposium. Ann Thorac Surg 34:111–114.

15. Wan S, Yim APC (2003) The evolution of cardiovascular surgery in China. Ann Thorac Surg 76:2147–2155.

16. Zhu XD (1991) The evolution of cardiovascular surgical techniques at Fu-Wai Hospital. In: Xue GX (ed.) Proceedings of the 35th anniversary scientific symposium on cardiovascular surgery (Chinese). Beijing: Cardiovascular Institute of Academy of Medical Sciences, pp 1–7.

17. Shao LF, Li ZC, Wang MF (1986) Results of surgical treatment in 6123 cases of carcinoma of the esophagus and gastric cardia. Proceedings of the International Conference in Thoracic and Cardiovascular Surgery, 9–10.

18. Qian ZX (1986) Thirty years' experience of treatment if thoracic hydatid cyst. A report of 842 cases. Proceedings of the International Conference in Thoracic and Cardiovascular Surgery, 27.

19. Lan XC, GU KS, Wu YK (1985) History and present status of thoracic and cardiovascular in China. In Wu YK, Peters RM (eds.) International practice of thoracic and cardiovascular surgery in China. Beijing: Science Press, 23–27.

20. Wang YS, Cheng TO (2001) Leo Eloesser: an American cardiothoracic surgeon in China. Ann Thorac Surg 71:1387–1388.

21. Zhang MJ, Liu DD, Wan S, Chen MC, Lee CN, DeSmet JM, Mestres CA (1996) Coronary artery bypass graft in China. Asian Cardiovasc Thorac Ann 4:63.

22. Wan S, Marchant A, DeSmet JM, Antoine M, Zhang HB, Vincent JL, Vachiery JL, Goldman M, Vincent JL, LeClerc JL (1996) Human cytokine responses to cardiac transplantation and coronary artery bypass grafting. J Thorac Cardiovasc Surg 111:469–477

23. Wan S, DeSmet JM, Barvais L, Goldstein M, Vincent JL, LeClerc JL (1996) Myocardium is a major source of proinflammatory cytokines in patients undergoing cardiopulmonary bypass. J Thorac Cardiovasc Surg 112:806–811.

24. Wan S, DeSmet JM, Antoine M, Goldman M, Vincent JL, LeClerc JL (1996) Steroid administration in heart and heart-lung transplantation: is the timing adequate? *Ann Thorac Surg* 61:674–678.

25. Kissinger H (1999) Years of renewal. New York: Simon & Schuster, pp 136–142.

26. Saura E (2005) Cirugía Cardiaca en España 2003. El "otro" Registro. Cir Cardiovasc 12:67–68.

27. Igual A, Saura E (2005) Cirugía Cardiovascular en el año 2003. Registro de intervenciones de la Sociedad Española de Cirugía Cardiovascular. Cir Cardiovasc 12:55–66.

28. Wu YK (1947) Ligation of patent ductus arteriousus. Chin Med J 65:71–76.

29. Li XX, Wang SM, Chen W, Zhuang WQ, Chang GQ, Li SQ, Yang JY, Lin YJ

(2004) Endovascular stent-graft repair of aortic dissection. Asian Cardiovasc Thorac Ann 12:99–102.

30. Leung SY, Ng THK, Yuen ST (1993) Pattern of cerebral atherosclerosis in Hong Kong Chinese: severity in intracranial and extracranial vessels. Stroke 24:779–786.

31. Ting ACW, Cheng SWK, Cheung J, Ho P, Wu LLH, Cheung GCY (2002) Early and late outcomes in Hong Kong Chinese patients undergoing carotid endarterectomy. Chin Med J 115:536–539.

32. AhChong AK, Chou KM, Wong M, Yip AWC (2002) The influence of gender difference on the outcomes of infrainguinal bypass for critical limb ischemia in Chinese patients. Eur J Vasc Endovasc Surg 23:134–139.

33. Hultgren R, Olofsson P, Wahlberg E (2001) Gender differences in vascular interventions for lower limb ischemia. Eur J Vasc Endovasc Surg 21:2–27.

34. Yim APC (1996) Cost-containing strategies in video-assisted thoracoscopic surgery. Surg Endosc 10:1198–1200.

35. Ren H (1999) Thoracoscopic procedures for intrathoracic disease: current status in mainland China. Respirology 4:111–116.

36. He JX, Yang YY, Wei B (1996) VATS in 230 cases. Chin J Surg 34:73–75.

37. He JX, Yang YY, Chen MY (1996) Lobectomy using VATS. Chin J Surg 34:76–78.

38. Chen HY (1996) Video assisted thoracoscopic surgery should be enthusiastically and safely developed. Chin J Surg 34:67.

39. Zhan RL, Xiao H, Lin JX (1996) Thoracoscopic closure of PDA: A report of 22 cases. Chin J Thorac Cardiovasc Surg 12:7–8.

40. Lewis I (1946) The surgical treatment of carcinoma of the esophagus—with special reference to a new operation for growths of the middle third. Brit J Surg 34:18.

41. Fekete F, Lortat-Jacob JL, Richard CA, Maillard JN (1962) Present day treatment of cancer of the esophagus. Ann Chir 16:977–983.

42. Ellis FH, Jackson RC, Krieger JT, Moersch HJ, Clagett OT (1959) Carcinoma of the esophagus and cardia. New Engl J Med 260:351.

43. Le Roux BT (1961) Analysis of 700 cases of carcinoma of the hypopharynx, oesophagus and proximal stomach. Thorax 16:226.

44. Orringer MB (1984) Transhiatal esophagectomy without thoracotomy for carcinoma of the thoracic esophagus. Ann Surg 200:282–288.

45. Orringer MB (1981) Surgical treatment of esophageal strictures resulting from gastroesophegeal reflux. In: Dyde JA, Smith RE (eds.) The present state of Thoracic Surgery. Pitman Medical, London, pp 83–94.

46. Xu PQ, Ma XX, Ye XX, Feng LS, Dang XW, Zhao YF, Zhang SJ, Zhao LS, Tang Z, Lu XB (2004) Surgical treatment of 1360 cases of Budd-Chiari syndrome: 20-year experience. Hepatobiliary Pancreat Dis Int 3:391–394.

47. Victor S, Jayanthi V, Madanagopalan N (1996) Coarctation of the inferior vena cava. The Heart Institute, Madras, pp 5–13.

48. Wang ZG, Yu Z, Wang S, Pu L, Du Y, Zhang H, Yuan C, Chen Z, Wei M, Pu LQ, Du W. Liu M, Liu X, Johnson G (1989) Recognition and management of Budd-Chiari syndrome: report of one hundred cases. J Vasc Surg 10:149–156.

49. Wang ZG (1989) Recognition and management of Budd-Chiari syndrome. Exeprience with 143 patients. Chinese Med J 102:338–346.

50. Dong C, Wu QY, Tang Y (2002) Ruptured aneurysms of the Sinus of Valsalva: A Beijing experience. Ann Thorac Surg 74: 1621–1624.

51. Luo XJ, Yan J, Wu QY, Yang KM, Xu JP, Liu YL (2004) Clinical application of bidirectional Glenn shunt with off-pump technique. Asian Cardiovasc Thorac Ann 12:103–106.

52. Xiong YZ (1998) Swine production in China. Proceedings of the International Conference on Pig Production, Beijing, pp 109–112. www.paper.edu.cn.

53. Cheng TO (1004) The current state of cardiology in China. Int J Cardiol 96:425–439.

54. El Rouby S, Chan L, Chinese Cooperative Anticoagulation Group, La Duca FM, Zucker ML (2001) Warfarin requirements and frequent INR monitoring in Chinese patients with prosthetic heart valve replacement. A multicenter prospective trial demonstrates clinical efficacy of low dose therapy. Presented at the American Society of Hematology. Philadelphia.

55. El Rouby S, Mestres CA, La Duca FM, Zucker ML (2004) Racial and ethnic differences in warfarin response. J Heart Val Dis 13:15–21.

56. The Chinese Coordinating Center of OASIS Registry (2002) Clinical characteristics of acute ischemic syndrome in China. Chin Med J 115:1123–1126.

57. Sung JJY, Wong LKS, Li PKT, Sanderson J, Kwok TCY (2002) Principles and practice of clinical medicine in Asia. Treating the Asian patient. Philadelphia: Lippincot, Williams and Wilkins.

58. Spanish Society for the Study of Obesity (SEEDO) National Congress 2002; www.seedo.es.

59. Pan C (1989) Clinical analysis of 15,089 operations on the heart and great vessels. Results from the People's Republic of China. Texas Heart Inst J 16:37–43

60. Ghosh PK, Unger F (2004) Coronary revascularization in DACH: 1991?2002. Thorac Cardiovasc Surgeon 52:362–364.

61. Ng JYY, Tam SF, Man DKW, Cheng LC, Chiu SW (2003) Gender differences in self-esteem of Hong Kong Chinese with cardiac diseases. Int J Rehab Res 26:67–70.

62. European Working Time Directive.

63. Ministry of Health Centre for Statistics, 2000

64. Zhou BF (1998) CVD Prevention 1:207–216.

65. 1985 and 1995 national surveys of physical development in school children.
66. Yang G (1997) Smoking and health in China: 1996 national prevalence survey of smoking pattern. Beijing, China Science and Technology Press.
67. Sheridan G (1999) Asian values, Western dreams. Allen & Unwin. St. Leonards, NSW; Australia, pp 1–15.
68. Sen AK (1999) Beyond the crisis. Development strategies in Asia. Institute of Southeast Asian Studies. Singapore, pp 3–20.
69. Batalla X. Editorial (2005) La Vanguardia Dossier 16, p 3.
70. Weisbrode K (2005) The transformation of Asia. La Vanguardia Dossier 16, pp 6–15.
71. Windsor HM (1984) Cardiac surgery in China. Med J Aust 140:590–602.
72. Rodewald G (1979) A cardiac surgeon's impressions of China. Thorac Cardiovasc Surg 27:137–144.
73. Wan S, Yim APC (2004) At the epicenter of severe acute respiratory syndrome. J Thorac Cardiovasc Surg 17:1553–1557.
74. Mestres CA (2000) The growing role of the Asian Annals in cardiothoracic education. Asian Cardiovasc Thorac Ann 8:1–2
75. Tamru FL (1998) Memories, milestones and the millenium ahead. Asian Cardiovasc Thorac Ann 6:83–84.
76. Cho BK, Tamru FL (2001) CTSNet and Asia: A new horizon. Asian Cardiovasc Thorac Ann 9:157–158.
77. Lim ASM (1993) The coming age of Asian surgery. Asian Cardiovasc Thorac Ann 1:13A–14A.

# English for Chinese Cardiothoracic Surgeons

*John R. Benfield*

**M**andarin Chinese is the most commonly used language in the world and English is currently the second most common tongue. English is expected to drop to a four way tie with Spanish, Arabic, and Hindi/Urdu in second place by the year 2050. Among 6.5 billion people in the world, only about 8 percent speak English as their first language. Nevertheless, English is the language of science and international commerce. The Chinese, those who use the world's most common language work hard to master English, the second most common language (Fig. 1).

In cardiothoracic surgery about 60 percent of manuscripts in the *Annals of Thoracic Surgery* and in the *Journal of Thoracic and Cardiovascular Surgery* are from authors who do not speak English as their native tongue. Such authors were for many years referred to as non-native speaker (NNS). However, the term NNS as contrasted to native speaker (NS) has been challenged [1]. We prefer to use the term English as an International Language (EIL) and to refer to EIL authors and to identify those who previously were called NNS authors. In addition, we believe that with our privilege to use English on a daily basis, comes a responsibility to help EIL colleagues who must struggle with an "English Language Burden" [2].

The purpose of this chapter is briefly to review the history of English becoming the language of science and to describe some of the work we have done to help our EIL colleagues with the use of English. This chapter will limit itself to discussing the Introduction Section of manuscripts, leaving discussion of important topics like conference abstracts and correspondence with editors for later discussion. We also shall suggest ways in which Chinese surgeons might help themselves with English.

The earliest known written communications about surgery are the Edwin Smith Papyri, which came from Egypt in about the 17th century BC. These relics can now be found at the Royal College of Surgeons of England. In China, as I learned during a recent visit to Beijing, there were earlier (2698–2589 BC) medical writings—*The Yellow Emperor's Canon of Medicine*—ascribed to the ancient emperor [3]. Hippocrates (460–370 BC) is remembered for his medical

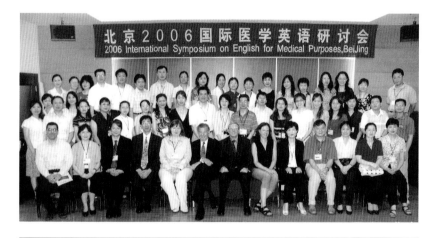

Fig. 1. *The second annual International Symposium on English for Medical Purposes in Beijing, July 2006. Professor Yong-Qan Bai (first row, fourth from the left), Dean of the School of International Studies of Xi'an Jiaotong University was the president. Wen-Xin Nie (second row, far right), Director of the school, was the organizer. Professor J. Patrick Barron (front row center), founder and head of Tokyo Medical University's International Communications Center gave the keynote address. Language professionals from throughout China were keen to advance the use of medical English in China. Medical professionals were represented by Professor John R. Benfield (front row, next to Barron) and Associate Professor of Neurological Surgery Wen-Bin Li of Capital University (second row, directly behind Benfield). Capital University currently teaches half of its medical school courses in English.*

leadership in Greece. Arabic was for a time the language of science. The relatively modern transition of the language of science from Latin to French to German and English is sufficiently well known so as not to require further details in this chapter. Suffice it to say that English became the dominant language of science after the end of World War II in 1945.

I am fortunate to speak German, Dutch and French as well as English. This has given me the opportunity during my visiting professorships to compare my communication where I speak the language against my communication with my hosts where I do not speak their tongue. My conclusion is that speaking is not the same as truly communicating. Communication occurs at various skill levels, somewhat independent of what might be one's native language. It was therefore that I responded to the question of how one defines a native speaker of English by urging that the term "native speaker" be abandoned in favor of the development of improved methods for assessing written and oral communication proficiency [4].

The difference between speaking a language and being able to communicate fully in that language is perhaps best illustrated in the Netherlands, one of the most multilingual nations in the world. Few people speak Dutch and almost every Dutchman speaks English. Virtually every Dutch physician is quite proficient in English, and so American and British physicians who have visited the Netherlands for professional purposes universally tend to say that the use of the English language is no problem in the Netherlands. However, medicine is an art as well as a science, and the science of medicine is imperfect. Therefore, the ability to communicate subtleties and to explain and to consider imperfections is an important part of medicine. In the Netherlands, physicians at all levels of experience were generally quite able to communicate fundamentally in English. However, they often expressed important (sometimes crucial) subtleties better in Dutch than in English. Since clarity is crucial in medicine, even in Holland, where essentially everyone speaks English, there is a need for improvement in English communication skills. If that is the case in the Netherlands, how is it in Latin America or China where relatively few people have a good command of

English? Another illustration of different levels of proficiency in English came from my 22 years' experience on the editorial board of the *Annals of Thoracic Surgery* and my service on seven other editorial boards and as an editorial consultant to 11 other journals. This experience made it readily apparent that most EIL authors express themselves easier and more clearly in their own languages as compared to English—the language of science.

In 1999, as the Honored Guest of the European Association for Cardiothoracic Surgery, I was asked to speak about the language of science [5], a topic that interested me although I had given it no formal attention. The requests that I deliver a major address about this issue made me somewhat anxious because I am neither a Linguist nor an Applied Linguist. At UCLA, my university, I was pleased to find Kathryn M. Howard, PhD, a superb young applied linguist who wanted to work with me. Together we studied five years of experience with EIL manuscripts that dealt with lung cancer, a subject in which I am expert. Howard was the language professional, expert in Applied Linguistics, and I was the peer expert in the surgical subject. The terms **subject expert** and **language professional** and **peer** are central to my message today.

While preparing for my address about the language of science, I was fortunate to develop a network of language professionals, including Professor Charles Bazerman at the University of California in Santa Barbara. He introduced me to Professor John Swales at the University of Michigan's English Language Institute (ELI) and his close colleague, Christine Feak—a master teacher of ELI students. Meanwhile, peer colleagues in Japan, all professors, and some former fellows of mine, introduced me to Professor J. Patrick Barron of Tokyo Medical University—the dean of medical applied linguistics in Japan. It was Barron who provided me with much of the information I needed to comply with a request to address the special problems of Japanese authors writing in English. In short, my learning continued while I was teaching.

At the request of the Society of Thoracic Surgeons, Christine Feak (language professional) and I (subject expert) designed and taught six unique annual programs based on reviewer comments about language. We conducted 18 interactive workshops for groups of 30–35 EIL authors. I'd like to stress the interactive nature of these workshops because I think it is very important. The curricula included areas of special challenge for EIL authors: Introductions, Discussions, Abstracts, and responses to reviewers and editors. Written evaluations and a follow-up survey showed that our programs were well received, always with requests for more.

Three other specialties in the US and in Asia have launched programs based on the Society of Thoracic Surgeons model. In addition, in 2005 and 2006, Elsevier Science Publishers invited us to Tokyo to address the 70 leading young gastroenterologists of Japan about how to improve their medical English. Most recently, I was pleased to learn more about China during an International Symposium of English for Medical Purposes in Beijing (Fig. 1).

What have we learned about teaching English to EIL in medicine? We recognized that there are at least seven categories of students (Table 1). We learned what portions of manuscripts and the business pertaining thereto are the most challenging for EIL authors: The Introduction Sections, the Discussion Sections and correspondence with the editors when the reviewers and editors have asked for revisions. We also learned that interactive workshops, whereby there is repeated contact between the EIL authors and the teachers work well. Such workshops should include some homework assignments.

**Table 1    International Students of English for Medical Purposes**

- Medical students
- Practicing physicians
- Faculty (Teachers and research workers)
- Industry (Pharmaceutical and device)
- Language professionals
- Editors
- Journalists

I shall illustrate our teaching method by stating some basic principles of composing an introduction, including the most fundamental one that introductions must capture the interest of readers. After reading an introduction, readers should be left with curiosity and a desire to study the remainder of the article. To accomplish this, there are two basic patterns for composing introductions. The first pattern is the so-called CARS Model—Create a Research Space—wherein there are three basic moves: Establish the research territory, create a place for the work to be described and then occupy the space. The second pattern is the so-called "Problem-Solution Model" wherein there are four moves: Describe the problem, highlight the problem, address the problem, and propose a solution for the problem. Table 2 summarizes the characteristics of a good introduction.

In his book entitled *In Search of Memory*, published in 2006, Eric Kandel, a Nobel Prize winner whose native tongue is German, quotes from one of his papers written in 1970. The following 143 word passage described what was to be his research strategy for the coming 30 years [6].

The **analysis of the neural mechanisms of learning and similar behavioral modifications** requires an animal whose behavior is modifiable **and whose nervous system is accessible for cellular analysis**. In this and the subsequent two papers, we have applied a combined behavioral and cellular neurophysiological approach to the marine mollusk Aplysia in order **to study a behavioral reflex**

### Table 2   Characteristics of a Good Introduction

- Organized according to an established model, e.g. CARS or Problem-Solution
- Brief and to the point (Not a literature review)
- Captures the interest of the reader
- Indicates the new knowledge the article will provide

**that undergoes habituation and dehabituation (sensitization)**. We have progressively simplified the neural circuit of this behavior so that the action individual neurons could be related to the total reflex. **As a result, it is now possible to analyze the locus of the mechanisms of the behavioral modifications.**

Does this introduction, about a research field other than our own, stimulate you to want to read more? Does it follow the CARS Model or the Problem-Solution Model is a question we might ask our students. We would then ask them to identify key phrases to support their answer. While there are elements of both models in this introduction, I think it fits the Problem-Solution Model best. For convenience, I have underlined and made bold the key phrases. First he addressed the problem, and then he highlighted and addressed it. Finally, by saying that—it is now possible to analyze the locus of the mechanisms of the behavior modification—he tells the reader that this paper will provide new information toward solving the problem. After reading this passage, I wanted to know more, and so it is an example of an excellent introduction that was capable of attracting my interest even though it was outside the purview of my specialty.

From the practical viewpoint, the next time you write an introduction, you might wish to assess it by asking yourself two questions: 1) Does it follow the CARS Model or the Problem-Solution Model? 2) Is it capable of capturing the interest of a reader whose field of practice and research is different from mine?

How do reviewers react to weak introductions? The following remarks of one reviewer are instructive: "(The introduction was) *difficult to follow and understand*. There were *multiple errors in language, syntax and grammar. I recommend considerable revision with an English translator for this paper to be considered for publication in an English-language journal.*"

What and who might an "English translator" be, and from whom might you obtain good editorial help the next time you write a paper or a chapter in English? We addressed this question in one of our recent papers [7], by saying:

In order for the revision process to move beyond the simple goal of "fixing" a text to a process in which EIL authors are developing their writing skills on the way toward becoming independent writers, input from both a language professional and an experienced peer is important. The language professional should ideally be a schooled and experienced applied linguist, and the peer a specialist in the subject matter of the manuscript. In reality, this ideal is difficult to achieve, in part because EIL authors may only have access to native English speaking "amateurs". Also, in addition, peers who are specialists in the discrete subject matter may be difficult to find.

Our answer to this question is not really original because it echoes the thoughts of applied linguist authors like Flowerdew and Parkhurst [8, 9]. These language professional authors, and we, are convinced that if one wants the highest possible quality of editing, one needs a language professional and a peer. Each alone is better than nothing, but each alone is insufficient. We further urge EIL authors to insist on knowing the credentials and experience of those who help them with manuscripts. Their manuscripts should be entrusted only to those who are properly educated.

My projection for the future (Table 3) includes that English will remain the language of science. However, let's not forget history wherein Greek, Arabic, Latin, French and German each had its period as the language of science. Therefore, I shall not predict what the language of science will be 100 years from now, and I shall remain humbled by the possibility that one day it may no longer be English. I am sufficiently optimistic to believe that the principles of scientific collegiality will override political considerations in governing how members of the international scientific relate to one another. Finally, I project that publishers, industry and government will eventually share with us the responsibility for taking the steps required to achieve universal excellence in the language of science. We are now very far from that goal.

My hope for the future (Table 4) is that English language medical education will start in medical school, and that it will be different from, and better than, the English education in our pre-medical

## Table 3    Projections for the Future of the Language of Science

- English will be the language of science for the foreseeable future, but not necessarily forever.
- The principles of scientific collegiality and not politics will, insofar as possible, govern how members of the international scientific community relate to one another.
- The responsibility for reporting science will be shared among scientists, publishers, industry and government.

## Table 4    Hopes for the Future of Medical English

- Linguists and subject specialists to work together
- Medical English education to start in medical school
- Education to be continuous—think in English
- EIL authors recognize that "native speaking" English does not make a linguist or an educator
- Funding sources will be generous

curricula. To make that happen, we are convinced that language professionals and medical subject experts should work together. Neither alone is sufficient. I also hope that education in the language of science will be continuous so that EIL professionals will learn to think in English. Continuity is fundamental and lack of it is devastating. I learned this when visiting some of my former international students when they had become professors 20–40 years after their time with us. A number of them had lost most of the English proficiency they had achieved while they were in the US. Therefore, I cannot stress too much the need for continuity. I also hope that EIL authors, who now pay for the help they get, will recognize that being a "native speaking" English person does not qualify one as an applied linguist or as an educator. Finally, I hope that there will be generous funding for EIL education.

My proposals (Table 5) are that medical English instruction programs would be subject oriented, starting in medical school and continuous, and extending into postgraduate and full career periods. I want again to stress that medical specialists and language professionals should work together. Fig. 2 is a reproduction of one of the world's great paintings that illustrates the merits of cooperation as compared to working alone.

I now inject a note of practicality. Active practitioners and academicians are likely to decline language education responsibilities in addition to their already busy schedules. However, recently retired subject experts (peers) are likely to be pleased to have the option of "remaining connected." Medical language education activities would

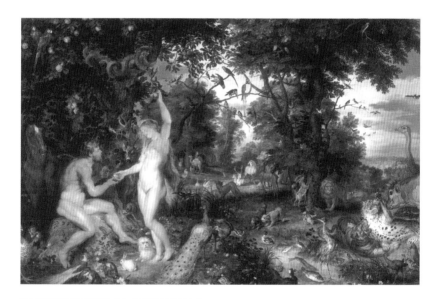

*Fig. 2. Working together. Adam and Eve in Paradise, painted by Peter Paul Rubens (1577–1640) and Jan Brueghel (1568–1625). Rubens excelled in painting people; Brueghel's special strength was in landscape painting. Each artist was powerful by himself, but together they were even better. Similarly, language professionals and subject experts (peers) working together are better editors than either alone. Original is displayed in the Royal Cabinet of Paintings Mauritshuis, The Hague, Netherlands. Reproduced with permission from the Mauritshuis.*

## Table 5    Proposals for Making Surgeons More Facile in English

- Medical English instruction programs should be subject oriented and continuous
- Medical specialists (recently retired) and language professionals should teach together
- Implementation should be via professional language and medical organizations
- Tests to evaluate medical subject oriented language proficiency should be improved
- Adequate funding sources should be pursued

provide them that opportunity. I believe that the services of recently retired medical professionals who work in language education should be rewarded with some appropriate payment just as language professionals need to be paid for their time and skill. I propose that the most efficient route to implementation of postgraduate medical English instruction is via professional organizations in medicine and in applied linguistics. All instruction programs merit monitoring with examinations. I question the practical validity of existing examinations in English insofar as medical English in the real world is concerned. Therefore, I propose that applied linguists and medical specialists work together to develop and to implement realistic and meaningful examinations of proficiency in writing, speaking, and understanding medical English in the forums of every day life.

Finally, I want to focus upon getting support for education programs in medical English. Under whichever political and economic system one works, money is needed if one wishes to start and to continue programs. Only 8 percent of the world population speaks English as its first language, but in cardiothoracic surgery about 50 percent (and sometimes more) of medical publications in the best peer reviewed journals now come from EIL authors. Thus, the need for funds to support EIL language education and assistance

# The Interaction between Chinese and Western Cardiac Surgery Communities—Reflections on the Personal Career of a Cardiac Surgeon

Guo-Wei He

U nlike the West, where the "Place of Birth" is key personal information, in China the "Origin of Family" is traditionally the column that must be filled in on all applications. In the Qing Dynasty this was determined by the birth-place of the grandfather. According to this regulation, my origin of family is Yuyao city, Zhejiang Province. Not only my grandfather but also my father were born there, and they immigrated to Shanghai, like many others from the region, in the 1930s. However when he was young my father left Shanghai and traveled to various places in China, despite the opposition of my grandfather who insisted that all family members (he had 5 children) should stay in Shanghai.

I was born in Wuhan, Hubei Province when my parents were there just before the revolution in 1949. After the revolution, my parents brought me and my siblings back to Shanghai. Rather dramatically, my father was given a job as Chief Manager in a petrol storage station, a government department in the capital city of Zhejiang Province, in 1950 and this made me a "real" Zhejiang person. Subsequently I grew up in Hangzhou, the city that was likened to Heaven in the Ming and Qing Dynasties.

Due to the fact that my father was considered an official of the previous Guomindang Government when he was in Wuhan, he soon lost his job in a political movement in 1955 and my family went to Hefei, Anhui Province because my aunt, who was supported by my father during her high school, found a job for my father there. My life was then changed and all my family had to fit into a new and uneasy life in this new place. Under such conditions my father soon passed away, due to heart failure that was caused by heavy physical work that he was not used to doing.

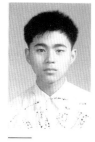

My parents and my big brother always told me that I was the most talented child in my family, although I am not sure. However, I did not waste their hopes in me and was a top student all the time. I graduated from high school in 1964 with full marks in all mathematical subjects and the highest marks for most other subjects in the class (Fig. 1). I dreamed of being a theoretical physicist, and was expecting and was expected to enter a top university in China.

*Fig. 1*

After the University entrance exam, I was even more confident about this because I believed that I had done very well. This was confirmed 2 years later. Back then, the results of the University entrance exam were top-secret and no students, parents, or teachers knew the exact results in order to avoid any questions about the admission, which was closely linked with the political background of the family of a student. This was just before the "Cultural Revolution" and political considerations were already the priority in choosing a student to enter a university, especially the good universities and those related to military or to what the government regarded as top science subjects. In the Cultural Revolution in 1966, the "Red Guards" broke into the Government buildings and took the files for the university entrance exams. Only then did I find out my exam results because one of my high-school classmates who was involved in this action found the report of my results and gave it to me. The report said that my score was the highest in the whole province, much higher than those who were accepted into Tsinghua or Peking University, which are regarded as the best universities in China.

Despite this, like many others who were from politically "unreliable families," I was assessed as "Not Suitable for University." This remark usually meant that the student would have to be refused by any university in China. In fact, in 1964, many top students were rejected by universities and had to go to the countryside to work as farmers. I was almost amongst them. I knew one who went insane because he could not take it psychologically.

However, I was relatively lucky. The story was explained to me 20 years later by the Communist Party Secretary of my class at the Anhui Medical College. He told me that I had been given the chance to get into the College only because I had the highest scores for the entrance exam in the province, a province with a population of about 60 million, and that the Chairman of the Education Committee, Mr. Fan-Fu Li who was also the highest officer of the Party for Education, Propaganda, and Health, was very sympathetic to me. He had ordered, against the usual regulations, that "this student must be accepted by a university." And so I was fortunate enough to be accepted by a "non-important, non-sensitive" university with regard to political or military subjects, a Medical College! This was why I, a top student who dreamed of being a theoretical physicist, became a medical student in China in 1964.

Twenty years later, when newspaper reporters interviewed me, they were all interested in this story and liked to write it in their report as evidence of that unusual period of history. But this is only the beginning of the story. The more interesting part comes after I was admitted into the medical college.

Not knowing the reason why I was only accepted by a local medical college, which destroyed my dream of becoming a theoretical physicist, and not knowing that I was really the luckiest one among thousands of students from "politically unreliable families," I was extremely angry about this fate and fell into deep contemplation of my life and my future. I was so anxious that despite the heavy political pressure during that period that I, a 17 year old young college student, took an unusual action that shocked all the political officers of the whole education system of the Anhui Province. I wrote a letter directly to Premier En-Lai Zhou to appeal against the "unfair" university entrance. The letter reached the Premier's Office and was sent back to the Committee of the Communist Party, Anhui Province. This later caused a new "movement" in the Medical College and I had to criticize myself in front of all the medical students and teachers of the College. However, owing to the fact that I was only 17, the youngest medical student, and the top student in the class, I was easily forgiven by the teachers and classmates for this action. But it made me "famous" in the College and became a focus of attention.

The reason I wrote the above paragraphs is to give the reader some idea of my academic background. Later, I gradually became deeply interested in medicine and determined to become a surgeon. However my interest in mathematics and physics never went away and I think this is why I have been so interested in research during my surgical practice.

Life as a medical student thereafter was smooth except for the Cultural Revolution that everyone was involved in. I actively participated in the "Great Revolutionary Link," meaning travels for revolutionary communications, and went to Beijing, Shanghai, Guangzhou and other cities. Unlike many others who often went to sightseeing, I spent most of the time in the famous universities. I am proud that I did not go to destroy any cultural treasures including books that were usually burned by the Red Guards, for membership of which I never did apply, partially because of my intrinsic love of ancient Chinese culture and partially because of my family background. In contrast, I collected some books during that period, particularly books on both Ancient Chinese and Western literature. I read a lot during that time. I had been fond of music since I was in kindergarten in Hangzhou (my music teacher was a professional violinist) and I had more time to practice violin and studied musical theory as a hobby. I remember that when I went to the most prestigious music school—"The Central Conservatory of Music, Beijing" (the equivalent to Julliard in China), I found that many textbooks had been thrown away. I collected some of them and started to study. I actually finished studying on my own the first-year textbooks for the Department of Musical Composition in the Central Conservatory, and even now I am still proud of my self-taught ability in music. In fact, I was a violinist in the College Band during the "Cultural Revolution" and my love to violin lasts till now although I had no time to practice due to busy daily schedule in the past 20 years.

My life in the next decade was rather usual for that period. I graduated from the College and was sent to a county hospital in a rural area to work as a general surgeon. I performed rather a large number of various operations, mainly in general surgery but also in orthopedic surgery; there was only an unspecialized department of surgery and a surgeon had to do everything. When the Cultural Revolution was almost over after the death of Ze-Dong Mao in 1976, the previous President of the Anhui Medical College Mr. Guang-Tao Li (who had accepted me into the Medical College in 1964), organized a new medical college. It was called the Wan Nan [South Anhui] Medical College and was based on a pre-Revolution USA-founded hospital, the Yi Ji Shan Hospital. Once again, I was given the opportunity by the President to work in this hospital. A remarkable thing during that period was that the President chose me among many applicants, all of whom were more senior than I was, to be trained in Cardiothoracic Surgery and to go to the National Training Class for Cardiac Surgery in the Shanghai Chest Hospital. Thus, I started my career in cardiothoracic surgery.

I settled in Wuhu and was married to my wife, Cheng-Qin Yang, who was my classmate in the Medical College. We had an only son. It was possible that I would have stayed in the Wan Nan Medical College all my life had there been no reform in China after Mao's death. Under the leadership of Xiao-Ping Deng, the famous "Reform" took place and soon involved the whole education system. Postgraduate studies were restored and gave an opportunity to a lot of young people who did not have a chance during the Cultural Revolution for further study and, perhaps more importantly, the opportunity to change one's place of work. During the Cultural Revolution, many excellent students were sent to do what they did not like. I was one of the lucky ones who continued with their profession. However I did desire to go to the national heart hospital in China, the Beijing Fuwai Hospital.

It was a great opportunity for me when I passed the tough exam to get into the Chinese Academy of Medical Science (CAMS) to which Fuwai Hospital is affiliated. I was the only graduate student admitted in the year of 1980 for the entire Fuwai Hospital. It sounds strange because there were more than 10 in the previous year, but it was due to the fact that in 1980, CAMS requested all applicants to take a more complete entrance exam that included mathematics and chemistry. For applicants to surgical disciplines there was also a requirement of at least 3 years experience in surgical practice. The problem for clinicians is that it is quite difficult to take high-level mathematics and chemistry exams. The result was that the most successful candidates were young university graduates who were still familiar with basic mathematics (calculus particularly) and chemistry. Those students were admitted into basic science institutions, but not clinical departments. My talent in mathematics and the physical sciences for the first time demonstrated its usefulness. I not only passed the exam but also obtained almost full scores for mathematics and had the highest total scores amongst all the CAMS applicants (there were hundreds of them!), according to the lady who was in charge of the Fuwai entrance exam and admissions.

I then left Wuhu and started my new life in Beijing alone. Although married and with a son it was difficult for my family to move to Beijing as residency permits for the capital city were difficult to obtain at that time. However, life was smooth in the environment in China in the early 1980s. My supervisor Professor Jia-Qiang Guo was the most active and successful cardiac surgeon and a real pioneer of cardiac surgery in China. He performed the first coronary bypass grafting and many other operations for as many as 18 complex congenital heart diseases. Professor Guo's influence on me was profound, not only in cardiac surgery but also in attitude to life, to people, particularly to the young people, as well as to professional success. Professor Guo was so kind to me that after a short period, he let me take charge of a cardiac surgery ward. This was the first time ever after the Cultural Revolution that a new generation had taken charge of a ward; those who were in charge of other wards were about 10 to 15 years older than I was (Fig. 2). In addition, with full trust, Professor Guo sent me to an Inner-Mongolian hospital to

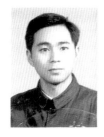

*Fig. 2*

help them start a cardiac surgery program. There I did 35 open-heart operations with great success. Again, this was an incredible trust as it was again the first time a young surgeon in China was given such an opportunity.

Professor Guo later told me that it was his personal experience which promoted this attitude of helping and trusting young surgeons. He was not given opportunity to go to Russia when he was a young surgeon due to the complicated personal relationships in Fuwai Hospital. During the 1950s, studying in Russia was an honor and meant a lot. I always remembered his words and later this also inspired me to do my best to help young people in their training and in finding a job, in both the clinical and basic science areas.

After a wonderful and enriching 4 years of experience in Fuwai Hospital, Professor Guo decided to send me abroad to gain more experience in complex congenital heart diseases, in the treatment of which he believed there was a significant gap between China and Western countries. I went to the Royal Children's Hospital, Melbourne, Australia to study under Mr. Roger Mee who was a pioneer in surgery for many complex congenital heart diseases (Fig. 3). Roger told me when I arrived that the RCH, Melbourne was among

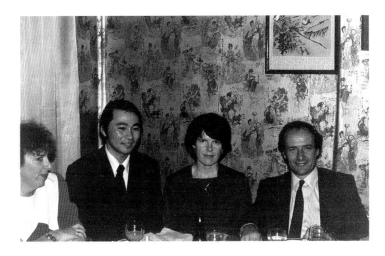

*Fig. 3*

the three best cardiac surgery units for congenital heart diseases in the world, together with Boston Children's Hospital and the Hospital for Sick Children, London.

I was thus exposed to a surgical practice very different from China's. I was very excited to be at the frontier of the new insights into open-heart surgery. Arterial switch operations, for which Roger gained world fame for being the first who had the operative mortality rate of less than 5%, as well as many other new operations such as MAPCAS (main aorta-pulmonary collateral arteries), were introduced to me. It was not only the operations but also the active thinking of the surgeon that excited and stimulated me. For example, for the first time I saw the right ventricular outflow tract (RVOT) patch being performed while the heart was still beating. In China we routinely did cardiopulmonary bypass (CPB) by snaring both vena cava, and stopping the heart. The variation in the CPB technique stimulated me to think a lot about the development of further techniques.

My life in the RCH was fruitful, although it was difficult sometimes because of Roger's famous bad temper during surgery. I was on call after a short period and was promoted to a formally employed position with full pay equal to the Australians (for the first time for a Chinese visiting scholar). Again, for the first time for a Chinese visiting surgeon according to Roger himself, he let me perform open-heart operations. I became a good friend of Bill Brawn (Fig. 4), the other surgeon with superior surgical skills. Bill later went back to UK and visited me when he came to Hong Kong 15 years later (Fig. 5). I think my work impressed both Roger and Bill a lot since after I left RCH for St. Vincent Hospital with Mr. John Clarabrough, Bill had discussions with Mr. Clarabrough and borrowed me back to RCH for another two weeks to be on call until a new fellow arrived.

After one year training in congenital heart diseases, coronary artery bypass surgery was another area in which I had to have experience, and Professor Guo again showed his foresight and support. I was approved to go to St. Vincent Hospital for experience in adult cardiac surgery. Surgeons were friendly there with better

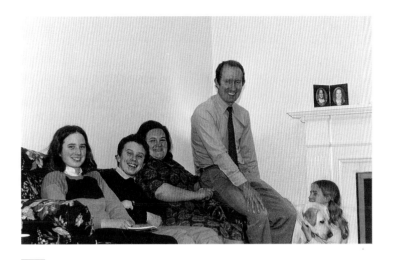

*Fig. 4*

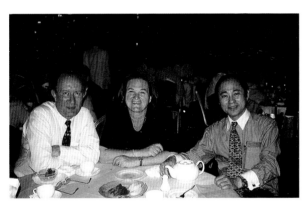

*Fig. 5*

tempers. Mr. Anthony Wilson even gave me a CABG case to do during the first month, which surprised Australian trainees. Some of them told me "this is incredible, he never gives us any cases to do!" Charles Mullany, who had just come back from the Mayo Clinic, and Antonia White, made a good team at St. Vincent Hospital. Miss White was very kind to children and she took my son to various events in Melbourne. Brian Buxton, who became world-famous in arterial grafting and with an enormous practice, was the main surgeon I assisted, both then at St. Vincent and afterwards at a private hospital, Epworth Hospital. The techniques of CABG I learned from him have helped me up until today (Fig. 6).

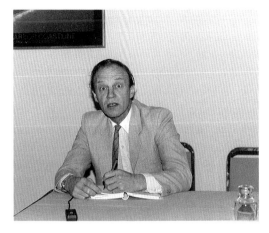

*Fig. 6*

It was interesting that my wife and son joined me in Australia when I was at RCH. This very "normal" and routine for Westerners, but it was a shock in the community of Chinese scholars and students in Melbourne, Australia. It was the first time that a Chinese scholar and students had been allowed to bring their family abroad and was a reflection of the Chinese "Reform." When Mr. Peng Li, the Commissioner of the State Education Committee who later became the Premier of China, came to Melbourne and met with delegates from the Chinese scholars and students (I was one of them), he announced that the Reform of China meant a "more relaxed environment" and that scholars were now allowed to bring their family abroad. I got my family to Australia so quickly because I wrote an application to the representative of the Chinese Embassy that same evening, immediately after the speech by Mr. Li, and it was immediately approved! It was soon proven that this was indeed a first in the history of the People's Republic of China when my family and I went to Canberra to attend a dinner party in the Chinese Embassy. Even the high-ranking diplomats were only allowed to bring their wife with them, but not the children, to prevent political defection. At the party my son, who was then 9, caused a great commotion. The diplomats happily yelled to each other "there is a child!" The Ambassador and his wife were so kind and came to us from crowd with smiles and talked to our son.

After my family arrived in Australia, I had to plan for my future. Whether I should go back to China after 6 months became the issue. I had gained experience in congenital heart and adult cardiac surgery, but it would be desirable to have a higher degree since at that time, a higher degree from Western countries was highly regarded in China. Quite a few scholars, after obtaining a PhD from the West and upon returning to China, were immediately promoted to professors, university chancellors, high-ranking administrators in the institutions of the National Academy of Science, or even ministers of education at different levels of the government.

I talked to Mr. Frank Rosenfeldt and he agreed to have me at the Baker Institute, which is affiliated to Monash University, to pursue a PhD degree. His decision was made after he talked to Roger and the St. Vincent surgeons who promised him continued surgical practice for me during the PhD period (Fig. 7). My only request was to carry on with surgery and to complete the PhD in the shortest period possible because I wanted to go back to Fuwai Hospital to practice surgery.

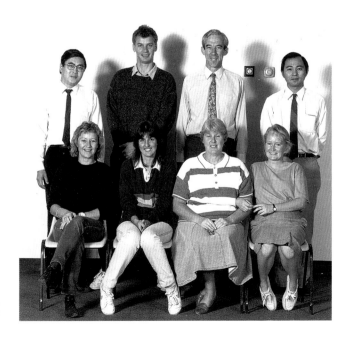

*Fig. 7*

My basic science talent played a great role in this period. I worked hard at Baker Institute under the dual supervision of Frank and a pharmacologist, Dr. Jim Angus, who gave me good guidance in pharmacological studies which were new to me. I was regarded as a "very determined person" by both Frank and Jim. Frank wanted me to do some work on the protection of saphenous vein graft, but I had more interest in arterial grafts. This was because my experiences in coronary bypass surgery with Mr. Brian Buxton made me believe that arterial grafts were more important to study, and use of arterial grafts was the new trend in coronary surgery. I found that the use of the internal mammary artery (IMA) gained a great surgical interest and therefore I wanted to study arterial grafts rather than vein grafts. The practice helped me maintain my surgical skill as well as supporting my family financially. Today, I must say that the Baker Institute provided me with a good opportunity, but on the other hand it did get a top student working for free. For the entire period of my PhD the Institute never supported me with one penny. I did not care; I was able to support my family by going to surgery regularly including at weekends with Mr. Brian Buxton, Mr. Jim Tatoulis, and the Alfred Hospital surgeons. Those surgeons were very kind to me during the whole period. However, years later, when I became supervisor to my own students, I felt badly about this because all my students are supported by either the university or my research funds. However I have to mention the support from the Head of the Department of Surgery, Professor O'Brian. Knowing of my excellent scientific progress, he strongly supported me as a candidate for PhD study when I was in difficulties. He even once paid the overseas student fee for me from the departmental funds when I could not afford it and there was no way to get any help from the Baker.

One thing I cannot forget at the Baker was that I submitted an abstract to the American Heart Association Annual Meeting on the pharmacology of the internal mammary artery, which was accepted. I was so keen to go to the USA to present the work, but the Institute did not want to pay for the travel or any expenses. Although I was presenting a paper for the Institute to one of the most important conferences on heart research, I had to pay for the travel and accommodation myself. This was too expensive for me, a research student who did not receive a penny from the Baker Institute. However, I went to Washington DC for the meeting (Fig. 8). Today I sometimes tell my PhD students how lucky they are because they all have full scholarships from the university or my research funds, which even pay them for trips to go to the USA to present their research work.

Nevertheless, with my work on arterial grafting based on the basic pharmacological method that I learned from Jim, I was able to finish my PhD thesis within the shortest period allowed by the university. I worked at weekends as well as sometimes at night. I often went home at 2 am and once, when I was so tired after the long day's work and I rode my bicycle home, I was hit by a car! Luckily, the accident was not serious. The only wish I had was to finish my work and leave the Baker as early as possible. During my PhD I published 5 papers in *Circulation*, *Journal of Thoracic and Cardiovascular Surgery*, the *Annals of Thoracic Surgery*, and the *Journal of Cardiovascular Pharmacology*. The editing by Frank and Jim of my papers helped me with my future research a lot. I shall never regret my experience at the Baker. I was able to go to many CABG operations with Brian,

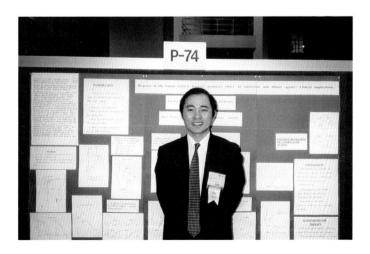

*Fig. 8*

Jim, and the Alfred Hospital cardiac surgeons: George Sterling, Bruce Davis, Jack Goldstein, and Gil Shardy, all of whom were very friendly to me. This gave me wonderful memories of the PhD study period and formed the basis for my surgical practice and scientific research later. Eleven years later, through my further research, I was awarded a Doctor of Science Degree by Monash University (Fig. 9).

I was back to full time clinical work when Mr. Clifford Hughes accepted me as senior registrar at the Royal Prince Alfred Hospital, Sydney. Mr. Douglas Baird was the Chief of the unit. The first year was the most unforgettable experience of surgery in my life. Most of the time there were 6 CABG cases per day and I went to two of those at least. Almost every other night, two or three registrars took turns to sleep in the ICU to look after the patients. Even meals were sent into the ICU. If the patients were stable, we slept on mattresses on the floor and went to surgery again the next day. When I was in Mr. Bruce Leckie's group he was so kind and gave me his cases to do. He kept saying to me "you have a very good pair of hands; you should do more surgery" (Fig. 10). With the support of Dr. Baird, I started a new laboratory in combination with the Department of Clinical Pharmacology, University of Sydney, to investigate arterial grafts. A lot of human tissues were available for study at the unit. My wife became my research assistant. With her background as a physician

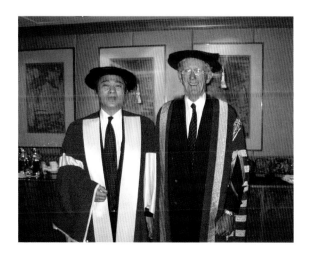

*Fig. 9*

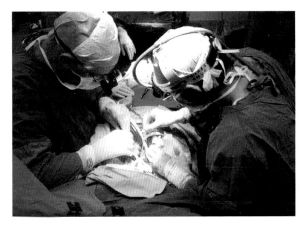

*Fig. 10*

for internal medicine, she mastered the technique of pharmacological study quickly. In addition to experimental studies, I found the surgical databases very useful. Again, my ability in mathematics and physics helped me do the statistical analysis and I quickly wrote a paper on the long-term survival of patients after combined CABG and mitral valve replacement that was published in the *Annals of Thoracic Surgery*.

Dr. Baird wanted to keep me in the unit but I had already decided to go to America, both for my own experience and for the education of our son. Another important reason was that for future work in China, it would be important to have American experience because the opening of China to the West meant that most Chinese scholars and students went to America for further experience and to have the opportunity to study in the most advanced country. Although I felt that Australian medicine was very advanced, and I did not see major differences in clinical medicine between Australia and America, the American experience was still particularly recognized in China. My plan was to go back to China but it should be at the optimal time. I appreciated the permission that Fuwai Hospital, through Professor Guo, gave me and I will never forget the support from Professor Guo. He once again granted me permission to gain experience in America. Such permission was not easy to get since I had been in Australia for a number of years already. In contrast with the attitude of some conservative Australians, the support of Professor Guo was extremely precious (Fig. 11)! However, I believe in human freedom and rights. This was echoed by Dr. Andrew Wechsler, who was another person from whom I felt I had much encouragement. He told me that "what you want to do is totally your own decision; it is illegal in the USA for others to interfere with your life and your rights" (Fig. 12). I thanked him and replied, "Give me liberty, or give me death!" These famous American words had long become a motto for me in my life.

I became a visiting scholar at the laboratory headed by Dr. Andrew Wechsler at the Medical College of Virginia. I knew that I would be welcome in a US unit. Although Mr. Buxton, who later became Professor of Cardiac Surgery at the University of Melbourne, very kindly arranged permanent residency for my family in Australia and provided a permanent position for me, for which I have always been appreciative and thankful, I went to North America. I immediately felt that there was tough competition as well as opportunities in America.

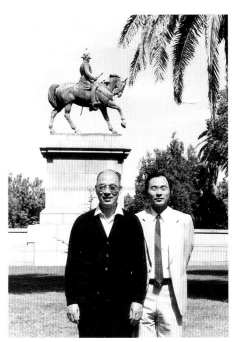

Entirely from the advertisements in the *Journal of Thoracic and Cardiovascular Surgery*, I applied for jobs in three places and was successful in two of them—Cardiothoracic Surgery Associates at North Texas (CSANT) and Dr. Albert Starr's institution, both as Director of Cardiac Surgery Research. I went to CSANT, Dallas, Texas first since the administrators at CSANT already got the H-1 visa for me.

*Fig. 11*

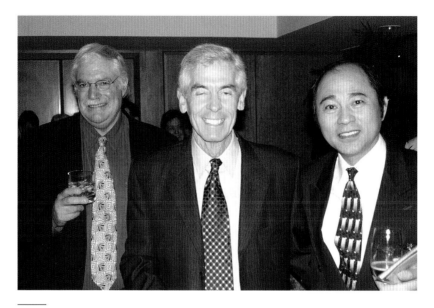

*Fig. 12*

Within 16 months, starting from scratch, I established a laboratory to study arterial grafts. Again, I found that there was a detailed database for cardiac surgery in CSANT that was at the moment used for administrative purposes. I looked into the database for risk factor analysis in CABG. Once again, my mathematical background played a major role in utilizing statistics. That was in early 1990s; the SAS program had no "Windows" version yet. The DOS version required a statistician to write a program for each calculation. I was fortunate to having an excellent computer analyst, Mr. David Roberts, who helped me with the programming. Within 16 months, I had written a large number of research papers and 7 of them were published in journals such as *JTCVS* and *Annals*. This certainly impressed Dr. Michael Mack (Fig. 13) who is the President of the organization. He wrote a recommendation letter to the American Association for Thoracic Surgery (AATS) a few years later saying that, "I found Professor He to be the most industrious and ambitious individual I have come in contact with in medicine." Mike, now one of the leading

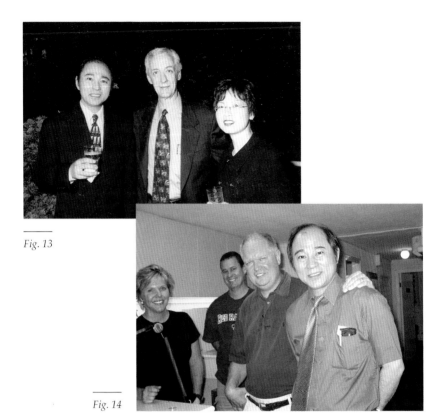

Fig. 13

Fig. 14

cardiac surgeons in CABG on the beating heart, became a very good friend of mine even though I left him for Dr. Albert Starr later. Mike supported me with my application to AATS and he was one of the major authors in the book I edited entitled "Arterial grafts in coronary artery bypass surgery." My friendship with another major surgeon in CSANT, Dr. Tea Acuff, who is also a leading cardiac surgeon in CABG on beating hearts, lasted for years. He helped me to get an institutional permit to be with him for his surgery in CABG as well as in congenital heart diseases, on which he had experience with Roger in RCH, Melbourne as well. The friendship has lasted until now and he was invited to operate at the heart institute I am now in charge of in Wuhan, China. A successful surgical ventricular restoration in Wuhan made us close colleagues (Fig. 14).

It was in this period that I started to think about arterial grafts as a whole. Why are they different? Can we find some intrinsic rules governing these mid-sized conduit arteries? I started to do a systemic investigation regarding the receptors in both endothelium and smooth muscle in a number of arteries used for CABG. Soon, I started to classify the arteries into three types that have now been widely accepted by the cardiac surgery community (Fig. 15). I also studied the segmental differences along the whole length of the artery in order to find out why some segments of the artery are more spastic than others. The experiments were performed by my wife who was now a skilled researcher (Fig. 16). I only needed to design the protocol and to look at the results, and to write papers. Even our son, who

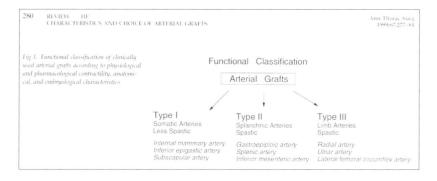

280   REVIEW   HE
        CHARACTERISTICS AND CHOICE OF ARTERIAL GRAFTS

Ann Thorac Surg
1999;67:277–84

Fig 1. *Functional classification of clinically used arterial grafts according to physiological and pharmacological contractility, anatomical, and embryological characteristics*

Functional Classification

Arterial Grafts

Type I
Somatic Arteries
Less Spastic

Internal mammary artery
Inferior epigastic artery
Subscapular artery

Type II
Splanchnic Arteries
Spastic

Gastroepiploic artery
Splenic artery
Inferior mesenteric artery

Type III
Limb Arteries
Spastic

Radial artery
Ulnar artery
Lateral femoral circumflex artery

Fig. 15

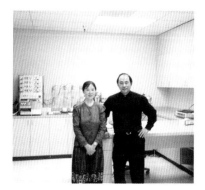

Fig. 16

was then an undergraduate student at the Department of Physics, Princeton University, contributed to my research by writing a very comprehensive computer program on the determination of the length-tension curve that is still currently used by my post-doctoral research fellows and students in my laboratories in the USA and Hong Kong.

The next phase of my life began when I left CSANT for Dr. Albert Starr in Portland, Oregon.

I once told Dr. Starr a story. During the Cultural Revolution when we had the "The Great Revolutionary Link," all transport for students was free. We could have free accommodation in a local school with free meals. I think this was the only good thing for us during the Cultural Revolution. When I visited the Shanghai Industrial Exhibition at the Shanghai Exhibition Hall, I saw a device that was placed in the middle of the exhibition room and which immediately attracted my attention. It was an artificial heart valve—"Starr-Edwards" prosthesis copied in China. Dr. Starr laughed and said "they did not ask me for permission!" when he later heard this from me. I was so amazed with this device and that was the moment, in 1966, that I became interested in cardiac surgery. I never thought that 25 years later I would become the Director of Cardiac Surgery Research at Albert Starr Academic Center for Cardiac Surgery. Dr. Starr was very interested in what I told him and he said to me once that we have a "natural connection" (Fig. 17).

As I am writing this, I have to say that the support Dr. Starr has given me cannot be over-stressed. As from Professor Jia-Qiang Guo, what I have learned from Dr. Starr is not only cardiac surgery, but also, perhaps even more importantly, an active attitude to life and the persistence to pursue science and technology. I also felt that the attitude to people from overseas in America is very different from that I had experienced at the Baker Institute: Dr. Starr at the interview told me that "since you are so good, you should work and live in America!"

Knowing my accomplishments Dr. Starr often introduced me to guests saying such things as, "I would like you to meet a young surgeon, Dr. He, a genius!" I am not sure that I am a genius, but I felt so warm when he praised me like this. In fact, Dr. Starr treated me

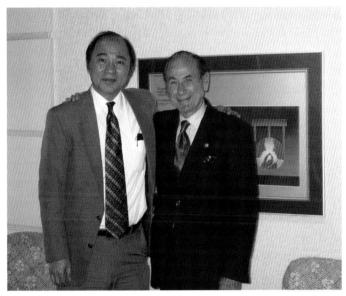

Fig. 17

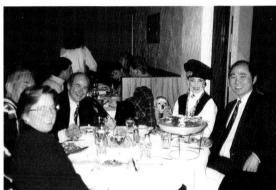

Fig. 18

not like a surgeon much junior to him but like a friend. Almost every Christmas, when I was in Portland, he would invite my wife and me for a Christmas dinner with him and his wife, Victoria, Dr. Peter Block, his Chief Cardiologist and his wife (Fig. 18). This made me feel important in his Heart Institute. The St. Vincent Foundation has since then, through Dr. Starr's efforts, raised funds for my research and the support continues.

The support from St. Vincent Medical Foundation for my research is enormous. It provides the money to rent a space, to buy equipment, and to pay for personal salaries. In return we have produced excellent research papers, have presented a large number of papers at international conferences, and have trained many young researchers. Dr. Starr and I have discussed in many meetings our desire to establish a "Cross-Pacific" Heart Research Center, and we want to make our research unit in Portland into such a center.

The St. Vincent Medical Foundation set up a scholarship named "Albert Starr—Guo-Wei He International Postdoctoral Research Fellowship," one for each period, to support young researchers. Since I am Chinese, I usually get such fellows from China, although this is not obligatory. Intrinsically though, I would like to have strong relationship with China. My fellows are from Beijing, Nanjing, Wuhan, Hefei, Shandong etc. The fellows have worked hard to obtain good publications and this has been successful. Everyone has published, as first author, 3-6 excellent research papers during the two year maximum period, derived from work done using such equipment as organ baths. Some of them may have realized that it is not the equipment that plays the major role in research. It is the researcher's brain which plays the major role, although some of them may not be aware of this even after the training. There have been 5 such fellows. One of them returned to China to work but all the rest have stayed in the US. I have never wanted to control them since I think this is their own decision, although I do make my views clear to them: it is in their own interests to go back to China to work.

During this period, I became particularly interested in research into endothelial cells. My work before was focused on arterial grafts, on physiology and on pharmacology. My research interest in blood vessels was deepened by coronary endothelium, which is an important issue in all kinds of open-heart operations. Similar interest was shown among basic researchers and cardiac surgeons world-wide; for the former, it was the nature of the endothelium-derived relaxing factor (EDRF); for the latter, it was the interaction between endothelium and cardioplegic solution during the ischemia-reperfusion period. This issue became my major interest thereafter and all my major research grants were written on this subject. It is this interest that made me gradually develop a surgical laboratory which can measure the single cell membrane potential; the single ion channel current by patch–clamp experiments; and the concentration of nitric oxide—which, of course, was after the discovery a few years later that nitric oxide is the EDRF. By researching this field we were able, for the first time, to discover the effect of high potassium in cardioplegic and organ preservation solutions on a particular endothelial factor—the endothelium-derived hyperpolarizing factor (EDHF)—and corrected the commonly believed theory that nitric oxide was affected by cardioplegic solutions. In these fields we had quite a large number of publications in international journals ranked highly in the cardiovascular category such as *Circulation, JTCVS, Cardiovascular Research.*

Endothelial research is important in medicine. This can be reflected by the fact that research on endothelial cells gave rise to two Nobel Prizes, first to John Vane for prostacyclin-related COX research in 1970s, and then to Robert Furchgott, Fred Murrad, and Louis Ignarro in 1998 for the discovery of nitric oxide as the EDRF. Dr. Ignarro later visited our research unit in Hong Kong, together with a renowned cardiac surgeon who was also one of the sponsors for my AATS membership and who gave me a lot of scientific support—Dr. Gerald Buckberg (Fig. 12 and Fig. 19). Dr. Ignarro was impressed by the electrochemical measurement of nitric oxide method and said "I don't have it!" (Fig. 19)

At the same time, Dr. Starr did his best to get an Oregon license for me to practice surgery. I was able to go to open-heart operations while I was full-time in Portland until I went to Hong Kong to take the position of Professor of Cardiothoracic Surgery at the University of Hong Kong in 1995. I call the period in Portland a "full-time" period because even now I am still the Director of Cardiac Surgery Research of the Albert Starr Academic Center for Cardiac Surgery at the Providence Heart Institute, the only difference being that I am "part-time" (I only go back to Portland 2–3 times a year but keep e-mail communication with my fellows on scientific guidance daily).

The generosity of Dr. Starr was not only shown in the aforementioned ways. When I felt that our research needed an

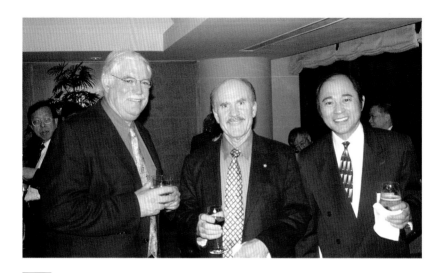

*Fig. 19*

academic affiliation, he supported me in exploring affiliation with Oregon Health & Science University (OHSU), the major medical school in Oregon State. Although it is generally thought that OHSU and Providence Health System are competitive organizations in Oregon State, the affiliation was also supported by the Officer in Charge of the Providence Heart Institute, Ms. Stacy Peterson. With their support I had an opportunity to meet the Chairman of the Department of Surgery, OHSU, Dr. John Hunter, who is a world expert and pioneer in minimally invasive surgery. I invited Dr. Hunter and his wife to China. After observing my two open-heart-operations, particularly after a total repair of Tetralogy of Fallot, Dr. Hunter was very impressed and he asked me, "Can I be trained as a cardiac surgeon now?" Although this was a joke this gave me encouragement in my work. Dr. Hunter quickly appointed me as "Clinical Professor of Surgery" and the appointment was endorsed by the Dean in 2001. I was then attached to the Division of Cardiothoracic Surgery headed by Dr. Ross Ungeleider, a renowned pediatric cardiac surgeon. The adult section headed by Dr. Matthew Slater, whom I later also invited to China to operate. Our publications were then affiliated to OHSU as well as to the Providence St. Vincent

Heart Institute and Albert Starr Academic Center for Cardiac Surgery.

It was during my stay in Portland that I felt that it might be the time for me to start working in China, although we felt even on arrival that Portland is an ideal place to live. It has probably everything other beautiful cities have: a wide river, beach, trees... but it has unique things: forest in the city, it is regarded as Rose City, or Bridge City, and it has 4 seasons! However I felt strongly that I had established myself in the West and my son's education was not a concern anymore. Despite my initial advice to choose medicine he, being interested in theoretical physics since his childhood, insisted on studying physics. What an irony it is, the lives of these two generations! The father wanted to become a theoretical physicist but went into medicine by fate, while the son went into theoretical physics despite the father wanting him to go into medicine!

Anyway, he was accepted by Princeton University in 1992 and studied theoretical physics in the Department of Physics, which had produced 15 Nobel Laureates. After his graduation as Summa Cum Laude, he received a scholarship from the US National Science Foundation and went to Cambridge University, UK, for an advanced mathematical certificate, followed by a PhD at Massachusetts Institute of Technology. I was much relieved as far as the duty of the father for the child's education is concerned.

Had I not seen an advertisement in the *Journal of Thoracic and Cardiovascular Surgery* for the position of Professor of Cardiothoracic Surgery at the University of Hong Kong, I would not have made the decision to go back to China. I applied and I was successful. The following 5 years in the University of Hong Kong was the most complicated sort of life for me. I was full-time university chair in a British-system university. I experienced the "hand-over" period of Hong Kong from British to Chinese rule. In order to describe how hard I worked for the University of Hong Kong, the best way is to state that I was a "full-time" cardiac surgeon and a "full-time" researcher" in Hong Kong with a "part-time" honorary research position in Portland, USA. I used to operate on at least 4 open-heart cases per week with a maximum of 10 cases when the Hospital Chief of Service (COS) was on leave. The type of operations I performed involved all kinds of cardiac operations. I was on second call for the service, even on the Chinese New Year almost every year, because others wanted to take a holiday during this period. I still remember that I did an emergency aortic surgery for a young man during the Chinese New Year who had had a car accident. His descending thoracic aorta was traumatically interrupted. I interpositioned an artificial aortic graft on his aorta. I did emergency repairs for more than 13 patients with acute type-A aortic dissection, with success in almost everyone of them. I reported my experiences at a conference in Beijing and I think the Fuwai surgeons who were my juniors when I was there were impressed. I was invited to give a lecture at Fuwai Hospital on radial artery grafting, of which I performed almost 30 cases in Hong Kong (I did the first radial artery grafting in Hong Kong in 1995). I also did the first one at the National Heart Center, Singapore in 1997 when I was appointed as a "National Expert" and "Visiting Expert" for a short visit there by the Ministry of Health through the Director of the Center, Professor Yean Leng Lim. The use of the radial artery in addition to the IMA became my routine practice for arterial grafting and this was extended to my later operations in China.

I was the first medical graduate from a medical school in mainland China to be appointed as Chair Professor at a clinical department in the Faculty of Medicine, University of Hong Kong, for at least 50 years. English was the only language I used to communicate with others, including colleagues and patients. When I talked to my patient, a nurse used to go with me and translate what I said in English (Fig. 20). This created a strange feeling but it worked.

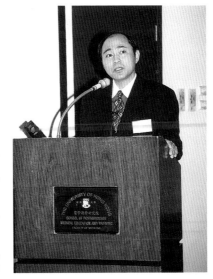

*Fig. 20*

I had excellent working relationships with all the nurses, particularly the nurses working in the Intensive Care Unit who looked after the patients I operated on. Some of them took the overseas courses of Monash University School of Nursing in Hong Kong for a bachelor degree. As a Monash alumni in Hong Kong and a Chair Professor in HKU, I was invited to be on the stage for their graduation ceremony and this left a wonderful memory (Fig. 21). I also have a good relationship with most doctors there. My experience has taught me that a system is the most important thing for success and I tried thereafter to establish a workable system when I came back to China.

The laboratory I established with the "Earmarked Grants" from the Research Grants Council, Hong Kong Government, was the only cardiac surgery research laboratory in the world able to do research on both large and microvessels, and with the ability to measure the membrane potential in a single cell and directly measure the concentration of nitric oxide derived from the endothelial cell.

After 5 years at the University of Hong Kong I came to The Chinese University of Hong Kong and quickly established a cardiovascular surgical research laboratory, with great help from Professor Anthony Yim. I was able to transfer my research grants to CUHK from the University of Hong Kong, as well as the equipment,

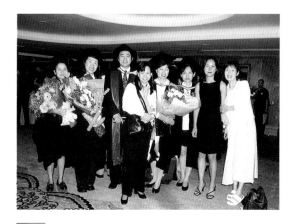

*Fig. 21*

with the support of RGC. We successfully held an international conference that invited distinguished speakers including Nobel Laureate Louis Ignarro and Sir Magdi Yacoub. We kept this laboratory at the highest level of research for cardiac surgery. The lab facilities and production have impressed many visitors including Dr. Denton Cooley (Fig. 22). We became even more capable with the facility to do single ion channel recording.

I must mention here that during the 10 year period in Hong Kong we supervised and trained a number of excellent research graduate students. They obtained their degrees because of their excellent research work, which made them active members of the research team. This point must be absorbed by mainland China: a supervisor trains a graduate student not simply for a degree. More important is to let them become an active part of the research projects supported by prestigious research grants.

However, my life became more complicated with my simultaneous surgical activities in China. In 1999 a surgeon from Anhui, China visited Hong Kong and watched my operations. He then reported to the president of his hospital, Dr. Xiao-Yin Yuan who immediately invited me to Anhui to be the Cardiac Surgeon-in-Chief

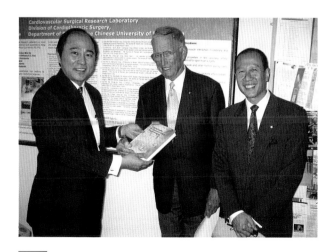

*Fig. 22*

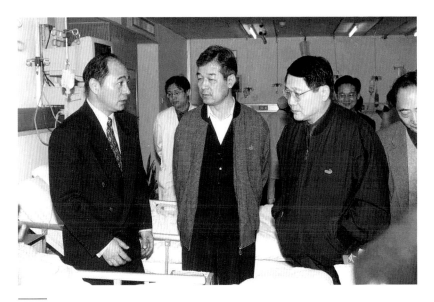

*Fig. 23*

and to establish a new Heart Institute. This activity in this province with a population of 70 million was greatly supported by the Minister of Health, Dr. Guang-Qiang Dai and was praised by the Vice Minister of the National Ministry of Health, Dr. Long-De Wang (Fig. 23). I spent some time each month there operating and 490 open-heart cases were performed under my supervision. I did the first successful Bentall operation, the first successful total repair of the totally anomalous pulmonary venous connection (TAPVC) etc. in that province and achieved zero mortality for the 130 valve replacements I did there. The success of the operations resulted in a series of newspaper reports in the National Health News in China. I was thinking of continuing the work there, but things changed unexpectedly.

An old friend who was my roommate when I was at Fuwai Hospital, Dr. Dao-De Cao, found me by reading the National Health News. We had not seen each other for nearly 20 years. He is now the President of the Central Hospital of Wuhan. As a previous cardiac surgeon, he was eager to establish a cardiac surgery service in his hospital. However the competition in Wuhan was enormous owing to the fact that this city has the first private heart hospital in the nation. After I had successfully performed 10 open-heart operations in Wuhan, I decided to work with him. Partly because I had already established a good unit in Anhui and it was time for me to leave.

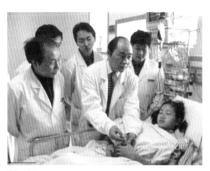

*Fig. 24*

It was rather difficult in Wuhan in the beginning because this was a totally new unit and I had to sleep in my office frequently after my operations. After two years an excellent unit was established with the full support of the hospital (Fig. 24). We are now able to perform more than 200 open-heart operations per year. We held our first international meeting and I invited my friend Dr. Tea Acuff and another friend Dr. Matthew Slater from Portland.

After 20 years of hard work in the West I have often been asked, by myself and by others, have I made contributions to cardiac surgery? Have I made contributions to the Chinese people as a whole? My return to China, although part-time, has made me very happy by developing a number of things. I was able to do what I really want to do: operating on both children and adults, developing new operative techniques, teaching young people, as well as melding myself into the Chinese community.

When I look back on my career, I sometimes still wonder whether I should have gone back to China earlier. On the one hand, that would mean that I knew more about the new system in China (the last 20 years have been the period of the most rapid changes in the entire history of China). On the other hand, I stayed in the West though with a conjunction of Eastern and Western cultures. The 10 years in Hong Kong have given me a clear vision of and insight into what we need to change and reform in China. Our work in cardiac surgery, including cardiac surgical research, has at least meant that Chinese names frequently appear in the most important cardiac surgery journals—*JTCVS* and *ATS*, and at meetings. I was invited to be the Chair of Symposium of endothelium in the Experimental Biology, San Francisco. I was invited to Japan three times to deliver a plenary lecture to the Japanese National Conferences in Cardiothoracic Surgery (Fig. 25). I was invited by many American surgeons from Harvard, Mayo Clinic, Cleveland Clinic etc., to present my work, although most of these have not been arranged due to my too busy schedule. I was invited to the Hungarian National Cardiac Surgery Conference to give talks about arterial grafting and endothelial function during cardioplegic arrest. The voice of Chinese in cardiac surgery is now frequently heard at important conferences around the world. *JTCVS* and *Annals* were among the very few journals that barred Chinese names in 1986 but today, if one opens these journals, there are plenty of Chinese names. I am very pleased to see the change.

Right from the beginning I insisted on keeping my name purely in Chinese style with no English names and spellings in order to make it known in my field that I am a native Chinese. The use of hyphenation in my name makes this even clearer. When I was accepted as an active member of the AATS, I was so proud since I

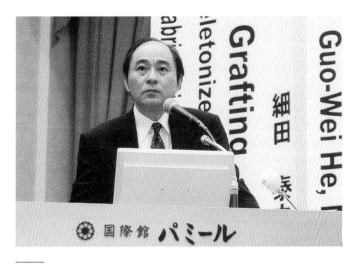

*Fig. 25*

was the first active member of this prestigious association ever elected from the so-called Greater Chinese Community. Professor Ying-Kai Wu (the former president of Fuwai Hospital) was an honorary member elected after the Cultural Revolution. In 2000, at the AATS Annual Meeting in Toronto, the first event of the Meeting was calling the new members to the stage. When my name was called, I stood up and walked to the stage with great excitement. Among the new members there was my old friend and mentor in cardiac surgery, Dr. Roger Mee. After working for years, I had been elected with him, my first Western mentor in cardiac surgery, and we stood together in the most prestigious Association for cardiothoracic surgery. I felt that I had done something for the Chinese people!

Even today, when Anthony Yim has also been elected to the AATS, we are the only two Chinese members in the association. Interestingly, we were both independently nominated to be a member of the Editorial Board of the *Annals of Thoracic Surgery*, another of the most-read cardiothoracic surgical journals. Tony and I see this as a good start for the involvement of Chinese in the high-level international community of cardiothoracic surgeons, and we wish to see more and more young Chinese surgeons getting to this level in the future.

Life is hard as a cardiac surgeon, particularly when starting a new unit. However the return for the hard work comes when my patients are discharged in good condition and grateful thanks. A patient on whom I performed a double valve replacement in Hong Kong sends a Christmas card every year that even follows my address changes. I am always excited when the children who have congenital heart diseases, particularly those with cyanotic ones, are discharged from my hands (Fig. 26). In fact, over the last 3 years I have performed 74 cases of complete repair of Tetralogy of Fallot. I feel that the time and the effort I have put in to establish new heart centers have not been wasted and I really receive more return than I deserve!

Another achievement in my life is the award of a Doctor of Science (DSc) Degree. This is probably not known to most people in China, even academics, because this is a degree within the British Education System. This higher doctoral degree is only awarded to those who

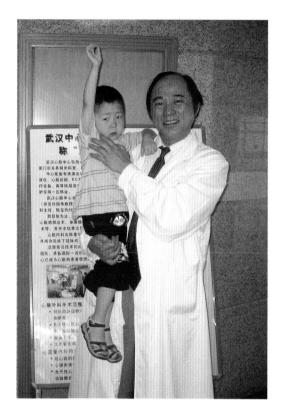

*Fig. 26*

are recognized as a world-authority in certain scientific research areas. The award is extremely rigorous. The minimal requirement is submission of a DSc thesis, that is a collection of published original work in renowned journals, a certain number of years after obtaining a PhD. Only if the Faculty of Science thinks the submission is worthy of examination can it then be sent to world experts for assessment. The final approval for the degree is given by the University Council and therefore very few of DSc are awarded. I went through all of this at Monash University and was the only DSc awarded by the University in 2003.

When I heard from Dr. Zheng-Xiang Luo (Fig. 27), one of the most senior cardiac surgeons in China, that in the cardiac surgery community in China some surgeons say that "you publish research papers and abstracts almost every week in international journals and

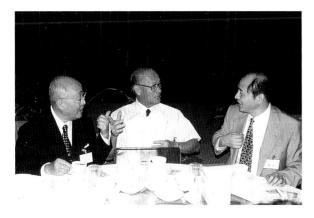

Fig. 27

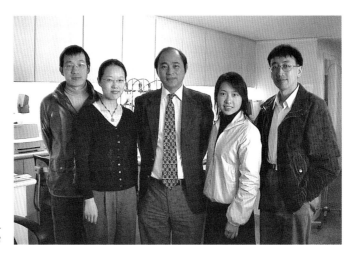

Fig. 28

meetings," I was very emotional and flattered. I felt that my work is worthwhile because there are people in China who know my work, although I have not done enough for the Chinese. More and more work will be done by my students in the future (Fig. 28). I must acknowledge the research work done by my long-time research assistant, my wife Dr. Cheng-Qin Yang and, also by my PhD students in Hong Kong after 1995 and the Starr-He International Postdoctoral Fellows in Portland, USA. They are: Drs. Zhi-Dong Ge, Zhi-Gang

Liu, Yue-Chun Liu, Zhen Ren, Ming-Hui Liu, Wei Zou, Qin Yang, Rong-Zhen Zhang, Zhi-Wu Chen and the current students Ying-Ying Dong, Min Wu and Post-doctoral fellow Li Fan. Most of them are still in America but some of them are back to China and Hong Kong and have taken up faculty positions. They have worked extremely hard to make our research active and, simultaneously, they have grown in science in this way.

Having worked in both Western countries and in China, I have a few observations that may help to promote cardiac surgery in China. In particular, I now know China better since I worked there before the "Reform" as well as under the present situation.

First, the health insurance needs to be improved. Many of my patients, particularly the patients with congenital heart diseases and from rural areas, have no insurance at all. Many of them saw a doctor for the first time just before the operation. With the great improvements in the transportation system, the only reason for this is financial problems. It is desirable to have the support from the government, both central and local, to establish basic health insurance.

Second, the relationship between the physician and the patient has reached abnormally levels of tension in China. The patient has high expectations of the physician even in the case of those diseases that are currently not curable. Any complications that are regarded as "normal complications" may cause complaints from the patient or relatives, and even lawsuits. In fact, a lawsuit is not so bad because worse things may happen. I have seen relatives put up big banners and posters criticizing the hospital and the physician in front of the hospital, as was done in the "Cultural Revolution." Some people say that this situation is mainly due to the irresponsibility of doctors. I agree that as medical professionals we should do our best to improve the quality of our service and to make patients feel warm and comfortable. However I do not agree with the opinion that the high-tension relationship between the physician and the patient is mainly due to the attitude of the former. In my observation, the intrinsic reason for this is related to the rapid progress of the new economic system and the improper propaganda on the relationship. The goal of this kind of action against the hospital and the physician is mainly financial compensation, although this is generally not admitted by the protesters. The media should make a fair assessment of this kind of relationship, and so should the government officials. The medical profession is highly respected in the West, but I do not see this happening in China at the moment.

Third, to properly restore the status of the medical profession, reform of the system is important. For example, the income of a physician should be judged by a normal and transparent salary system, not by the so-called "grey income." The latter causes a lot of problems. Due to the long education and training, the high responsibility and risk, as well as the nature of the work and long working hours, this profession should be highly respected and well paid. The formal income for a physician in China is less than that of a low-level salesman; this reflects the community's attitude to this great profession. I have seen surgeons resigning from hospitals to become salesmen. What a waste!

Further, China needs a formal "Residency Training Program," the enormous advantages of which are obvious. The matured "Residency System" in the West is a good example to follow. As I conclude this writing, I sincerely wish to the young Chinese surgeons training themselves in three aspects: professional, scientific, and ethical. The concord between these three aspects, the concord between the physician and the patient, the concord among surgical colleagues, and the concord between Chinese and Western surgical communities, will impact on the future of cardiothoracic surgery in China.

# Research Perspectives in Chinese Cardiothoracic Surgery: Towards the International Standard

Y. John Gu

C ardiothoracic surgery in China has experienced substantial achievements during the last century, especially after the birth of the heart-lung machine in 1950s that marked the new era of open-heart surgery. During these early years, surgical innovation and technological breakthroughs were the main stream on research and development undertaken by the pioneering Chinese cardiothoracic surgeons. However, these achievements were left much behind in comparison with the international society during the period of Cultural Revolution. After that period, cardiothoracic surgeons in China started to grasp the advanced technologies from the foreign countries through various scientific exchange programs and joint research projects. Meanwhile, younger generation of Chinese cardiothoracic surgeons started to study abroad and brought in advanced techniques from the world outstanding cardiothoracic surgical centers. Currently, molecular biology and gene technology have enabled the cardiothoracic surgeons to do research on different pathophysiological mechanisms in association with the surgical outcome. Advanced network and patient information systems have given more opportunities to design and coordinate multicenter studies for quality clinical research. Overall, a steady growth of scientific research, both in quantity and quality, is evident by scientific publications linked to cardiothoracic surgery in China in recent years.

In the future, there is a need to develop a large scale database for the Chinese population of cardiothoracic surgical patients. Such an achievement may further facilitate and strengthen the meaningful scientific research for cardiothoracic surgery in China.

## Research in Cardiothoracic Surgery in China: Past

The scientific and technological achievements of the cardiac surgery have been well recognized during the past century [1–3]. Among various achievements, the innovation and development of the heart-lung machine had marked a new era of the so called "open-heart" surgery in the early 1950s. The first successful open-heart operation was performed in 1953 in the United States by John Gibbon [4]. Since then, vigorous activities in research and development were stimulated and launched in the United States and Europe. During these early years, surgical innovation and technical breakthroughs were reported frequently in the field of repairing congenital cardiac abnormalities, later on in the treatment of valvular heart diseases, and currently in various procedures of treating coronary artery disease and heart failure.

In a close follow-up of the advance of cardiothoracic surgery of the international society, pioneering Chinese cardiothoracic surgeons wasted no time in catching up the international levels and made many impressive progress and national breakthroughs [5]. The first open-heart operation in China was performed in Xi'an in 1958 (5 years later than the world record) by Dr. Hong-Xi Su, who was returning from the United States after his surgical training and his witness of the early innovation of cardiothoracic surgery in the States. In the same year, Dr. Kai-Shi Gu in Shanghai performed the first open-heart case using the Chinese made heart-lung machine. In 1965, Dr. Yong-Zhi Cai in Shanghai performed the first successful mitral valve replacement with a Chinese made mechanical valve (also 5 years later than the world record). Since 1966, there was a period of stagnation of cardiac surgery in China because of the influence of the Cultural Revolution. In 1974, Dr. Jia-Qiang Guo in Beijing performed the first coronary bypass operation in China [6]. Since then, the number of coronary artery bypass grafting operations in China has increased year by year as the incidence of coronary heart disease has been increasing explosively [7].

In contrast to the fast development of the Chinese cardiothoracic surgery in the clinic, research and development of the cardiothoracic surgery in China were left much behind in comparison with the international society. During the period of the Cultural Revolution between 1966 and 1976, there were only a few publications linked to China about cardiothoracic surgery that can be traced from the Medline database (Table 1). Shortly after the Cultural Revolution in the period between 1977 and 1983, the amount of publications started to grow (Fig. 1). Since the early 1990s, a steady increase of scientific

### Table 1    Research Output on Cardiothoracic Surgery

| Years | (1) China | (2) Hong Kong | (3) Taiwan | (4) Hong Kong | (5) Taiwan |
|---|---|---|---|---|---|
| 1966–1976 | 3 | 0 | 0 | 2 | 1 |
| 1977–1983 | 38 | 0 | 2 | 0 | 2 |
| 1984–1988 | 28 | 0 | 2 | 2 | 6 |
| 1989–1992 | 67 | 1 | 24 | 6 | 27 |
| 1993–1995 | 90 | 7 | 22 | 14 | 41 |
| 1996–1998 | 126 | 17 | 22 | 43 | 48 |
| 1999–2000 | 86 | 24 | 8 | 31 | 51 |
| 2001–2002 | 130 | 21 | 16 | 26 | 60 |
| 2003–2005* | 177 | 28 | 23 | 32 | 95 |

Data are obtained from Medline using the commercial search engine SilverPlatter. Search key words are derived from the medical subject headings (MeSH) thesaurus. Column (1): obtained from the combination of key words "Thoracic Surgery" and "China or Chinese." Column (2): combination of (1) and key words "Hong Kong." Column (3): combination of (1) and key words "Taiwan." Column (4): combination of key words "Thoracic Surgery" and "Hong Kong." Column (5): combination of key words "Thoracic Surgery" and "Taiwan."

* Search results include the first four months of 2005.

publications appeared in the Medline database in the field of cardiothoracic surgery with a label of "China" or "Chinese." (Fig. 1) Among these publications, a considerable amount of papers were contributed by colleagues from Hong Kong or Taiwan (Table 1), as these two areas have had much more advanced infrastructure for research and development than those in the mainland China.

Next to the steady increase of the amount of scientific publications during the past years, the quality of publications representing the research of cardiothoracic surgery in China has increased as well (Fig. 2). During the period between 1984 and 1988, only 5 papers published in the journals with an impact factor higher than 2.0. The amount of publications in this category increased to 29 during the years 1993 to 1995. In the most recent period from 2003 to April 2005, the number of papers published in these relatively high-ranking journals climbed to 41. This improvement in impact factor linked to the publications

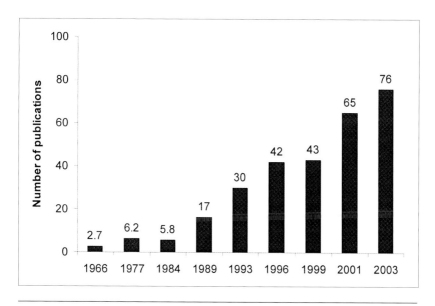

Fig. 1. *Amount of scientific publications in the field of cardiothoracic surgery retreived from the Medline database using the thesaurus keywords "Thoracic Surgery" and "China" or "Chinese." Note a remarkable increase during the recent 15 years. Data are the average amount of papers published each year from its respective period of time listed in Table 1.*

of cardiothoracic surgery in China, along with the growing number of published papers, indicates a growth of both the quality and quantity of research by the Chinese cardiothoracic surgeons during the previous years.

## Research in Cardiothoracic Surgery in China: Present

The current communication technology as well as the personal ability of the Chinese cardiothoracic surgeons has made the gap between the Chinese and the international cardiac surgical society shorter and

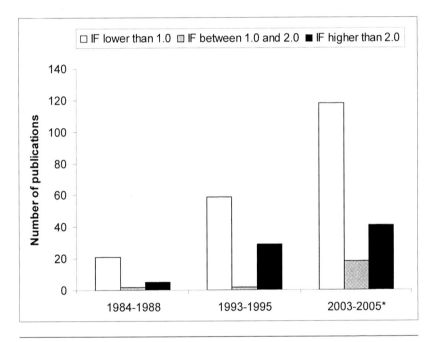

Fig. 2. *Quality as well as quantity of scientific publications related to the specialty of Chinese Cardiothoracic Surgery during different period of time. The impact factor (IF) is a criteria in assessing the ranking of a scientific journal, which is calculated by dividing the number of current year citations to the source items published in that journal during a certain period of past years. It is widely accepted that the higher the IF the better the quality of that journal. The above score of IF is obtained from the* Journal Citation Reports 2003 *by the Institution of Scientific Information Wed of Science Database.*
*\* Available until April 2005.*

shorter with regard to scientific research. After the Cultural Revolution, as more and more scientific exchange programs as well as joint research projects were initiated between the Chinese and international institutions, cardiothoracic surgeons in China started to acknowledge the advanced technologies from foreign countries. By the end of the last century, a majority of cardiothoracic surgical centers in China had implemented new methodologies on intraoperative management and the postoperative intensive care, which had lead to enormous improvement in the outcome of cardiothoracic surgery. These achievement in the clinic have also promoted scientific research. In the meantime, younger generation of Chinese cardiothoracic surgeons have involved various opportunities to study and learn advanced techniques in the world-leading institutions or centers of cardiothoracic surgery. Their achievements, both in gaining practical clinical experiences and the level in scientific research, contribute a great deal to the current development of cardiothoracic surgery in China.

Despite the fact that the research achievements in Chinese cardiothoracic surgery look quite encouraging, especially during the recent years, it covers only a very small portion of contribution to the world literature of cardiothoracic surgery. The international community of cardiothoracic surgery have published 69,119 articles in total since 1966. Within this amount of papers that can be retrieved from the Medline journals, only 741 were contributed by the Chinese authors. This is in line with the trend of global production of cardiovascular disease research published recently [8], from which the published articles from the Asia region are much less than the regions such as the United States and West Europe. Furthermore, regarding research quality, Chinese cardiothoracic surgeons have been publishing little in the world top-ranking clinical journals with high impact factors, such as the *New England Journal of Medicine* and the *Lancet*. In the current era, as a growing number of patients suffering from severe cardiovascular diseases are being treated surgically in China, it is no doubt that the research output in cardiothoracic surgery, either in its quantity or quality, should have a further increase.

## Research in Cardiothoracic Surgery in China: Future

The future is filled with potentiality for the research on cardiothoracic surgery in China. Different from the earlier era during which the Chinese pioneers of cardiothoracic surgery made their achievements with research, the modern era with advanced information and computer technology has given more opportunities to design and coordinate national or international multicenter studies with a relatively larger scale. In most of the developed countries or regions in the world, hospitals in which cardiothoracic surgery is presented usually have the centralized patient information systems. These networks facilitate the daily acquisition of the basic elements for research, such as data retrieval and collection systems from the laboratories, anesthesia and surgical procedures in the operating room, postoperative patient outcome in the intensive care unit, and even long-term follow up of patients discharged from the hospital. Large scale multicenter studies are the key elements in forming the so-called "evidence-based medicine" that collects various high-quality research evidence with different individual clinical expertise to help making appropriate health care decisions [9].

In this perspective, development of a national or at least regional database of cardiothoracic surgery in the Greater China area is of crucial importance as the Society of Thoracic Surgeons of the United States has benefited a great deal from its early initiative in building up a national adult cardiac surgery database [10–13]. Currently, this Database is the largest cardiothoracic surgery database in the world, having more than 500 participating sites and over 2.2 million patient records [14]. In China, developing such a large database for cardiothoracic surgical patients will help to identify a unique pattern of risk factors and prognostic models in predicting surgical outcome on different intervention procedures for congenital heart disease, valvular disease, as well as coronary artery disease. Eventually, Chinese cardiothoracic surgeons can rely on publications out of this/ these database(s) to keep a golden standard of surgical outcome for the Chinese population.

"In the scientific world, general laws are usually in the form of equations, and the world of cardiac surgery should be no exception. When outcomes are expressed in equations, the equations become extremely flexible and useful tools for predicting and comparing, the basic processes which should be the bases for most patient care and indeed even governmental decisions."[1]

## *References*

1. Kirklin J W (1990) The science of cardiac surgery. Eur J Cardiothorac Surg 4:63–71.
2. Cohn LH (2003) Fifty years of open-heart surgery. Circulation 107:2168–2170.
3. Edmunds LH Jr. (2004) Cardiopulmonary bypass after 50 years. N Engl J Med (14) 351:1603–1606.
4. Gibbon JH Jr. (1978) The development of the heart-lung apparatus. Am J Surg 135:608–619.
5. Wan S, Yim APC (2003) The evolution of cardiovascular surgery in China. Ann Thorac Surg 76:2147–2155.
6. Cheng TO (2004) The current state of cardiology in China. Int J Cardiol 96:425–439.
7. Wu Z, Yao C, Zhao D, Wu G, Wang W, Liu J, Zeng Z, Wu Y (2001) Sino-MONICA project: a collaborative study on trends and determinants in cardiovascular diseases in China, Part I: morbidity and mortality monitoring. Circulation 103: 462–468.
8. Rosmarakis ES, Vergidis PI, Soteriades ES, Paraschakis K, Papastamataki PA, Falagas ME (2005) Estimates of global production in cardiovascular diseases research. Int J Cardiol 100:443–449.
9. Evidence-Based Medicine Working Group (1992) Evidence-based medicine: a new approach to teaching the practice of medicine. JAMA 268:2420–2425.
10. Clark RE (1989) It is time for a national cardiothoracic surgical data base. Ann Thorac Surg 48:755–766.
11. Edwards FH, Clark RE, Schwartz M (1994) Coronary artery bypass grafting: the Society of Thoracic Surgeons National Database experience. Ann Thorac Surg 57:12–19.
12. Ferguson TB Jr, Dziuban SW Jr; Edwards FH, Eiken MC, Shroyer AL, Pairolero PC, Anderson RP, Grover FL (2000) The STS National Database: current changes and challenges for the new millennium. Committee to Establish a National Database in Cardiothoracic Surgery, The Society of Thoracic Surgeons. Ann Thorac Surg 69:680–691.
13. Shroyer AL, Coombs LP, Peterson ED, Eiken MC, DeLong ER, Chen A, Ferguson

TB Jr, Grover FL, Edwards FH (2003) The Society of Thoracic Surgeons: 30-day operative mortality and morbidity risk models. Ann Thorac Surg 75:1856–1864.

14. STS National Database. www.sts.org/sections/stsnationaldatabase. Assessed May 26, 2005.

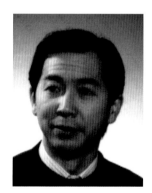

Y. John Gu

# The Development of Cardiothoracic Surgery in China: A Historical Perspective

*Ray Chu-Jeng Chiu*

"It is not his *possession* of knowledge, of irrefutable truth, that makes the man of science, but his persistent and *recklessly* critical *quest* for truth."

Karl R. Popper

## From Hua Tuo to Ying-Kai Wu

China inherited the great oldest continuing civilization in the world and is undergoing a spectacular revival in the 21st century. We may thus ponder how the past, present and future of cardiothoracic surgery in China, extensively and superbly covered in this book, fits into the big picture of Chinese history. Perhaps one can start with two great surgeons of China, Hua Tuo and Ying-Kai Wu, as prominent contributors to this story. Hua Tuo, the legendary father of surgery in traditional Chinese medicine, has been revered for his surgical skills and for introducing the use of general anesthesia with an effervescent powder, *Ma Fei San,* two millennia before anesthesia was practiced in the West. His great achievement and the lack of similarly prominent surgical figures in Chinese medicine in the following centuries symbolizes both the historical achievement and subsequent decline of traditional Chinese medicine. We will look at this more below.

Professor Ying-Kai Wu's contributions have been well described in this book by the editors who personally knew Dr. Wu. Although many other outstanding surgeons in China also played important roles in introducing modern cardiothoracic surgery into China in the early to mid 20th century, Dr. Wu was perhaps the best known domestically and certainly globally. His recognition as a pioneering modern Chinese surgeon was illustrated by the obituary published in the *Transactions of the American Surgical Association* when he passed away in 2003 (Fig. 1). The American Surgical Association is one of the oldest and certainly most prestigious surgical associations in the world, and very few foreign surgeons have been honored with membership in its nearly one and a quarter century history. Dr. Wu thus was recognized as a world-class surgical statesman, playing a key role in the birth and advancement of cardiothoracic surgery in China. Many younger leaders of cardiothoracic surgery in China deserve credit for the continuing progress being made today. Some of the contributors to this book, chosen by the well informed editors, are among those leaders.

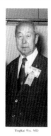

YINGKAI WU, MD
1910–2003

Professor YingKai Wu, Honorary Director of the Beijing Institute of Heart, Lung and Blood Vessel Diseases and former President of Beijing Anzhen Hospital, died of cancer on November 13, 2003, in Beijing at the age of 93, after failing to respond to meticulous medical treatment. He was born in 1910 in Manchuria, presently a Northeastern prov-

ince of China, the son of a teacher. He was 1 of 5 children, 4 of whom are doctors. His elder brother practiced occupational medicine, the middle brother is a chemist, the youngest brother a surgeon, and his sister an ophthalmologist.

Professor Wu received his medical degree from Liao-ning Medical College in 1933 and took his internship and surgical residency at the Peking Union Medical College from 1933 to 1939. The Peking Union Medical College was founded in 1915 by contributions from the Rockefeller Foundation and often has been referred to as the Johns Hopkins of the East.

After completion of his residency, he became an instructor in surgery at Peking Union Medical College and in 1941 was selected for a coveted fellowship in chest surgery under Dr. Evarts Graham at Barnes Hospital in St. Louis, Missouri. I am told that the famous Doctor Graham, a Past President of this Association, proudly performed his first successful esoph-

ageal resection while Dr. Wu was under his tutelage. During the discussion of the case, Dr. Wu modestly mentioned that he had already performed 6 such cases in China. Fortunately, he was not immediately dispatched on a slow boat back home!

Upon Professor Wu's return to China in 1943, he became head of the department of surgery at Chung-King Central Hospital in Tientsin for 2 years. In 1948, Professor Wu returned to Peking Union Medical College as associate professor of surgery under the direction of an American surgeon.

367

*Fig. 1. Ying-Kai Wu, Senior Fellow, American Association of Surgery, 2004; 122:367–368.*

## From Abroad and the Diaspora

Introducing modern cardiothoracic surgery to China in the 20th century and catapulting it on a trajectory of future success was accomplished not only by the pioneering Chinese surgeons mentioned above, but also by a number of dedicated foreign surgeons—some of whom contributing to this book—who forged global links with cardiothoracic surgery in China. Thus, another important figure in the birth of modern thoracic surgery in China is Dr. Norman Bethune, whose extraordinary career is documented elsewhere in this book. Prior to his legendary work in China, Dr. Bethune practiced thoracic surgery at the Royal Victoria Hospital of McGill University in Montreal, Canada, where many of the surgical devices he invented are still on display. In 1992 I found myself succeeding this extraordinary surgeon as the Head of Cardiothoracic Surgery in that institution where other founders of cardiothoracic surgery, such as Drs. Edward Archibald and Arthur Vineberg, also served (Fig. 2). The courage and compassion Dr. Bethune showed in caring for patients during the war illustrates the contributions of international leaders to cardiothoracic surgery for the well being of the people in China.

Among the huge Chinese diaspora residing abroad are cardiothoracic surgeons of Chinese origin serving their communities, some of them also contributing directly or indirectly to the advancement of cardiothoracic surgery in China. A number of such foreign cardiothoracic surgeons of Chinese ancestry are also represented in this book. For example, I was impressed by the high respect Australian cardiologists and cardiac surgeons held for Dr. Victor Chang of Sidney, Australia, whose parents emigrated from Shanghai, when I was invited to deliver the "Victor Chang Memorial Lecture" in 2003 at the annual convention of the Cardiac Society of

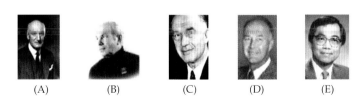

(A)    (B)    (C)    (D)    (E)

*Fig. 2. Professor Edward Archibald [A] was Chief of Thoracic Surgery at McGill University in Canada. He was succeeded by Dr. Norman Bethune [B], who later served and died in China. His followers as Chief of Cardiothoracic Surgery at McGill University included Drs. Arthur Vineberg [C], Anthony Dobell [D] and Ray C. J. Chiu [E].*

Australia and New Zealand. Dr. Chang was a leading cardiac transplant surgeon in Australia, and one of his major contributions was to train many young cardiac surgeons from Southeast Asia. My own participation in 1995 in the "National Conference to Improve Medical Residencies" in Wuxi, sponsored by the Ministry of Health of the People's Republic of China, allowed me to understand the urgent need to establish better residency training programs in China which is critically important to improve the quality of care for the patients. I am a believer of the proverb: *"Give a man a fish, and you feed him for a day; teach a man how to fish, and you feed him for a lifetime."* Although an expert surgeon donating his time to operate in a foreign country can benefit a few patients, providing assistance and advice to improve training of native surgeons will bring about wider and lasting benefits to patient care of that country in the long run. That was the main goal of the Workforce on International Relationships I chaired for the Society of Thoracic Surgeons in the United States during the last several years. It is my belief that those of us with experience in medical training programs of other developed countries could be helpful to our colleagues in China today for their similar endeavors.

Having said that, I, like many others often wonder why a great civilization which produced surgical giants like Hua Tuo thousands of years earlier had to import modern medicine such as cardiothoracic surgery from the West. Even today, the international exchange between China and the West for the knowledge and techniques of cardiothoracic surgery—perhaps with the conspicuous exception of esophageal surgery—has largely been an one way affair. It may be of interest to look into this question, since as it has been said often, learning the lessons of history might shed light for the future.

## The Parallelism of the History of Classic Empirical Medicines: East versus West

Traditional Chinese medicine of the "East" and the old "Western" medicine were the products of two great civilizations in the history of mankind, and they contributed to the health of huge proportions of the world's population. Both traditional medicines were empirical in nature, based on experience and tradition, with philosophical under-pinnings of earlier cultural beliefs. Today, Western medicine is seen widely as the orthodox modern medicine, while Chinese traditional medicine is often regarded as an "alternative" medicine (Table 1a). In 2002, to better comprehend their uneasy and sometimes competitive relationship, I attempted to examine their comparative time history, motivated in part by an invitation for a scientific award lecture which was delivered at the meeting of the Chinese American Medical Association in New York. It soon became apparent to me that most treaties on the medical history of the East and the West tended to look at each of them longitudinally, i.e. chronologically from the prehistoric to the present for the West, and then separately for the East, particularly for the era when global communication was limited. However, if one looks at them horizontally, comparing their progress at various time points in history, it is amazing to note that although these two civilizations were virtually isolated from each other for much of the known history, perhaps until the famed visit of Marco Polo to the imperial court of Yuan Dynasty in China in the 13th century, there were nearly parallel advances in some landmark developments of their medical histories.

In ancient Egypt and China, striking similarities in the ideographic depictions of elements and their relationships, which were thought to constitute the nature of the universe and effects on human health, can be noted (Fig. 3). By around 2000 BC, Egyptian papyrus recorded ancient medical practice in the West including the use of herbs such as willow bark, later known to contain aspirin;

**Table 1a    The "Parallel" View of Traditional Medicine**

Orthodox Medicine                 Alternate Medicine

(Western Medicine)                (Chinese Traditional Medicine)

Cardiothoracic Surgery

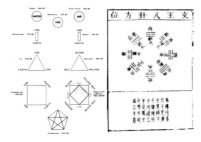

*Fig. 3. Ancient ideogram of nature and health. West (left) and East (right).*

while in the East the classic *Yellow Emperor's Pharmacopiae* appeared, describing cumulative knowledge available in that era. Some anatomical depictions of the heart and circulation appeared almost like a variation of the same sketch, with the blood leaving the heart and disappearing in the periphery (Fig. 4). Considering how these two solitudes existed without communication between them in ancient times, one wonders whether these similarities reflected certain commonality in mankind's pursuit of knowledge.

Other striking parallels include two great historic figures, Confucius (551 to 479 BC) in China and Hippocrates (460 to 367 BC) in Greece, living during almost the same historical life time. A more amazing parallel is the contemporary appearance of two great surgeons, Hua Tuo (110 to 207 AD) and Galen (130 to 218 AD) (Fig. 5). Galen of course was a titan in Western medicine whose ideas and teaching influenced European medicine for more than a millennium. Imagine while Hua Tuo in China was draining an abscess from the arm of the famous army general Guan Yu as he drank wine and played chess, Galen was amputating the mauled leg of a gladiator in the Roman theatre. If only they could have met in Rome or China at an international surgical conference to exchange their techniques!

Around this time during the second and the third century, a number of major treaties in Chinese medicine were written. Chung-Ching Chang (150 to 219 AD), who was known as the Hippocrates of China, wrote a 16-volume classic *Shang Han Za Bing Lun* (*Treaties on febrile Diseases*), which was credited for combining theory with clinical practice in medicine. Shu-He Wang composed the 12-volume

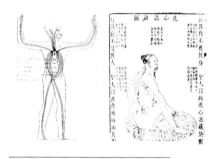

Fig. 4. Early concepts of "circulation."
West—Egypt (left) and East—China (right).

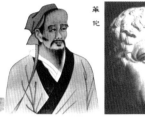
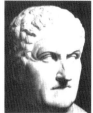

Fig. 5. Father of surgery. Hua Tuo, China—
East (left) and Galen, Rome—West.

*Mei Ching* (*Book of Pulse*), which still is consulted by its practitioners today.

## The Advent of Scientific Medicine in the West: The Renaissance

These theories and practices in the East, and Galenic teachings in the West dominated their respective medical practices for many centuries. Although some minor empirical advances were made in both sides of the world, it was not until the 16th century when a major turning point was reached in the West to verifying the classic teachings with testable facts. One of the most prominent efforts was to document the human anatomy with actual cadaveric dissection, which produced a number of anatomical masters such as Vesalius, Da Vinci and Fallopius. Accurate anatomical knowledge allowed the development of scientific physiology, such as William Harvey's work on circulation in *De Motu Cordis*, which described the modern concept of blood circulation in 1628. This great epoch in the West is known as the "*Renaissance*." From then on, Western medicine took off, transforming the empirical Western old medicine into a scientific global medicine, such that by the 20th century, highly advanced disciplines such as cardiothoracic surgery were able to evolve. Without its own renaissance, the East continued with the empirical traditional medicine and remained largely stagnant. This rather sudden schism between Eastern and Western medicines after the *Renaissance* was not so much due to sudden changes in resources or talent, but rather it was because of the failure of Eastern medicine to adopt "scientific methods" in medicine (Table 1b).

There have been many speculations as to why the Chinese traditional medicine never underwent the transformation to adopt scientific observations of human body, like its Western counterpart did. One suggestion was that in Chinese Confucian culture of ancestor worship, anatomical dissection of the deceased had been, and continue to be, considered socially undesirable. In contrast, in the ancient Egyptian religion with belief of human re-incarnation, the practice of creating mummies mandated anatomical dissection of cadavers. The revival and advance of anatomical dissections during *Rennaisance* provided sound anatomical knowledge, upon which the science of physiology and pathology could be built upon, ushering in the dawn of scientific medicine. Another thesis posits that although in its earlier history Chinese culture contributed significantly to

**Table 1b    The "Evolutionary" View of Traditional Medicine**

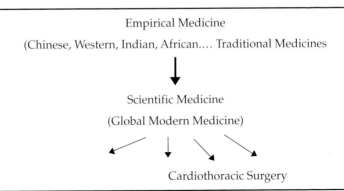

Empirical Medicine

(Chinese, Western, Indian, African.... Traditional Medicines

Scientific Medicine

(Global Modern Medicine)

Cardiothoracic Surgery

scientific discoveries, from astronomy to the inventions of paper, compass and gun powder etc., in the later years emphasis on literature, which provided key to Chinese bureaucratic advance, diverted the talents away from science and technology. Regardless of the reasons behind it, the fact was that prior to *Renaissance* in the West, the East had a dominant power in economy and culture, but after that point, the West rose, and the East declined. This bigger picture was reflected in the fates of Eastern versus Western medicines as well.

## Empirical versus Scientific Medicine

A famous quotation, which reflects Confucian wisdom, is: "Learning without thinking is useless, thinking without learning is dangerous." Perhaps to this one could add: "Unquestioned and unverified thinking and learning could be both dangerous and useless." As the philosopher of science Karl Popper succinctly postulated, in science, theories and hypotheses can be proven to be correct by observation or experimentation, but most importantly they can also be proven to be wrong. In other words, scientific theory is "falsifiable." In contrast a belief system such as a faith cannot be refuted. In science, a hypothesis thus can be used to predict phenomena, which can be tested to determine the validity of the original hypothesis. Such predictability could be either deterministic or statistical. In traditional medicine, the master's teaching, which has not undergone necessary validation, is accepted by his disciples in faith, from generation to generation.

## Scientific Medicine and the Development of Modern Cardiothoracic Surgery

Another major characteristic of science is the continuum of knowledge, which builds from basic sciences like mathematics, physics, chemistry and biology, to applied sciences like engineering and medicine. Such continuum of knowledge is crucial to developing highly sophisticated clinical specialties such as cardiothoracic surgery, where various branches of science must be integrated to create and advance the specialty. An example of interdisciplinary contributions in the advent of cardiac surgery is the crucial role of anticoagulants in cardiopulmonary bypass. Heparin was discovered by MacLean as a medical student in 1915 while searching for a pure pro-coagulant in dog liver. Without heparin, blood coming in contact with extracorporeal circuit tubing would clot, with disastrous consequences. Numerous other physiological and technological advances, now taken for granted, first had to be discovered to make first open heart surgery possible in 1953. In the early days of cardiac surgery, placing a patient on extracorporeal circulation was equivalent to performing a series of complex physiological experiments simultaneously. Without the scientific method, such a breakthrough could never have happened. Table 2 lists historical advances in surgery in general. Cardiac surgery required the cumulative advance of empirical, anatomical and physiological knowledge, plus major technological advances in the mid 20th century.

**Table 2    Evolution of Surgery**

|  |
|---|
| Empirical |
| + Anatomical |
| + Physiological |
| + Technological |
| + (Societal …) |

## A Renaissance for the East? … and a Vision for the Future

If the breakthrough in traditional Western medicine initiated by the *Renaissance* led to the advent of scientific medicine, which in turn culminated in the birth and advancement of modern cardiothoracic surgery, could a similar breakthrough occur in the East? I wish to submit that in fact this is in progress. Japan is now a highly developed country, which already contributed significantly to global scientific medicine during the last century. That became possible following the Japanese "Meiji Restoration" of 1868 to 1912, which achieved much of the same effect Europe gained through the *Renaissance*. The major difference was that in the original European *Renaissance, de novo* creation of scientific concept and methodology was needed, while in the Japanese "Meiji Restoration," rapid absorption of existing scientific knowledge from the West was required before native innovation was feasible.

In China, efforts to absorb Western technology started at the end of the 19th century during the late Qing Dynasty but was pursued on and off with limited success. However the reform movement initiated in 1979 by Xiao-Ping Deng has led to a full blown economic revival and may lead to a *de facto* "Renaissance" of Chinese culture and technology. This could provide the necessary foundation for advances in cardiothoracic surgery in China. One may then anticipate a short "catch up" phase followed by the creative application of scientific concepts and methodologies for a successful scientific "renaissance."

China has vast potential resources and talent to contribute to the further development of cardiothoracic surgery, which will serve the well being of the Chinese people. It has been predicted that the cutting edge of science in the 21st century will be biotechnology, and astounding advances in gene and stem cell therapies are already being made everyday. Nano-technology may revolutionize medical diagnosis and therapy. Continued advances in body imaging technologies and robotic minimally invasive surgery can be expected, such that ultimately image-guided computerized robotic surgery may become feasible. Cardiothoracic surgeons must keep up, integrating these scientific and technological advances to better serve our patients. Chinese cardiothoracic surgeons and investigators must participate actively in such future innovations, aiming for improving efficacy of therapy, minimizing invasiveness and complications of the procedures, and optimizing the cost effectiveness of the new approaches to make them affordable. The efficacy of new therapeutic modalities must be judged by properly designed clinical trials, which must be ethically sound and statistically valid. Clinical data bases must be established, and well organized training programs for future cardiothoracic surgeons and support professionals must be developed. Formal accreditation procedures for medical schools, residency programs and hospital services will ensure quality of education and clinical care in cardiothoracic surgery. This is an exciting time in the development of cardiothoracic surgery in China. The groundwork is being laid, but there is still much to accomplish. Professional support and exchange of knowledge within the country and internationally should be encouraged and expanded. The benefits of these efforts will contribute to the future well being of patients with cardiopulmonary diseases, not only in China but also worldwide.

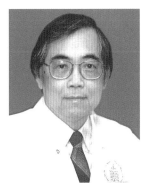

Ray Chu-Jeng Chiu

# A Selective Glossary

Anhui 安徽
Anzhen Hospital (Beijing) 北京安
    貞醫院

Ba-Da-Ling 八達嶺
Baiqiuen International Peace
    Hospital 白求恩國際和平醫院
Baoding (= Pao Ting) 保定
Beijing Heart Lung Blood Vessel
    Medical Center 北京市心肺血
    管中心
Beijing 北京

Cai, Yong-Zhi 蔡用之
Cao, Xian-Ting 曹獻庭
Cardiovascular Institute of
    Chinese Academy of Medical
    Science 中國醫學科學院心血管
    病研究所
Ceng, Xian-Jiu 曾憲九
Central Hospital, Chongching
    重慶中央醫院
Ch'i Po (= Qi Bo)
Chang Gung Memorial Hospital
    (Taiwan) 長庚紀念醫院
Chang, C. C. 張紀正
Chang, Chung-Ching 張仲景
Changhai Hospital (Shanghai)
    上海長海醫院
Changsha 長沙
Chaoyang Hospital 朝陽醫院
Chek Lap Kok 赤鱲角
Chen, Bao-Tian 陳寶田
Chen, Hai-Quan 陳海泉
Chen, Hao-Zhu 陳灝珠
Chen, Shu-Bao 陳樹寶
Chen, Wen-Hu 陳文虎
Chen, Yu-Ping 陳玉平
Chengdu 成都
China Red Cross Hospital 中國紅
    十字醫院
China Union Medical University
    中國協和醫科大學
Chinese Academy of Medical
    Sciences 中國醫學科學院
Chinese Surgical Association 中華
    外科協會
Chongqing (= Chungking) 重慶
Chu, Shu-Hsun 朱樹勛
Chung, S. C. Sydney 鍾尚志
Chungking (= Chongqing)

Ding, Jia-An 丁嘉安
Ding, Wen-Xiang 丁文祥

Eighth Route Army 八路軍

Fang, Zu-Xiang 方祖祥
Feng, Zhuo-Rong 馮卓榮
Fourth Military Medical
    University 第四軍醫大學
Fu, Pei-Bin 傅培彬
Fujian 福建
Fuwai Hospital 阜外醫院

Gansu 甘肅
Gao, Run-Lin 高潤霖
General Hospital of Shenyang
    Military Region 瀋陽軍區總
    醫院
Geng, Zhen-Jiang 耿振江
Gong, Lan-Sheng 龔蘭生
gou-kong 鈎孔
Gu, Fu-Sheng 顧復生
Gu, Kai-Shi 顧愷時
Guan Yu 關羽
Guangci Hospital (Shanghai) 上海
    廣慈醫院
Guangxi 廣西
Guangzhou 廣州
Guo, Ji-Hong 郭繼鴻
Guo, Jia-Qiang 郭加強
Guomindang (= Nationalist
    Party) 國民黨

Hainan 海南
Hakka 客家
Hangzhou 杭州
Hankou 漢口
Harbin 哈爾濱
Hatem, George (= Ma, Hai-De)
    馬海德
He, Bing-Xian 何秉賢

He, Guo-Wei 何國偉
Hebei (= Hopei) 河北
Hefei 合肥
Heilongjiang 黑龍江
Heishanhu Hospital 黑山滬醫院
Henan 河南
Hokkien 福建
Hongqiao 虹橋
Hongren Hospital 南洋醫院
Hopei (= Hebei)
Hou, You-Lin 侯幼臨
Hu, Jin-Tao 胡錦濤
Hu, Sheng-Shou 胡盛壽
Hua Tuo 華陀
*Huang Di Neijin* (The Yellow
    Emperor's Canon of Internal
    Medicine) 黃帝內經
Huang Di 黃帝
*Huang Jia-Si's Textbook of Surgery*
    黃家駟外科學
Huang, Chia-Ssu (= Huang, Jia-Si)
Huang, Guo-Jun 黃國俊
Huang, Jia-Si (= Huang, Chia-Ssu)
    黃家駟
Huang, Ou-Lin 黃偶麟
Huang, Wen-Kun 黃文昆
Huang, Wen-Mei 黃文美
Huang, Xiao-Mai 黃孝邁
Huangpu River 黃浦江
Hubei 湖北

Jiang, Wen-Ping 蔣文平
Jiang, Ze-Min 江澤民
Jiangsu 江蘇
Jiangxi 江西
Jilin 吉林

Jinan 濟南
Jin-Cha-Ji 晉察冀

Kai Tak 啟德
Kong, Ye 孔燁
Kunming 崑明

Lan, Hsi-Ch'un (= Lan, Xi-Chun)
Lan, Xi-Chun (= Lan, Hsi-Ch'un)
　蘭錫純
Lanzhou 蘭州
Li, Bing 李冰
Li, Peng 李鵬
Li, Ying-Ze 李穎則
Liang, Qi-Chen 梁其琛
Liaoning 遼寧
Lin, Chiao-Chih 林巧稚
Lin, Xun-Sheng 林訓生
Linxian 林縣
Linxian Esophageal Carcinoma
　Hospital 林縣食管癌醫院
Liu, Fang-Yuan 劉芳園
Liu, Hui-Ping 劉會平
Liu, Jin-Fen 劉錦紛
Liu, Wei-Yong 劉維永
Liu, Xiao-Cheng 劉曉程
Liu, Yu-Qing 劉玉清
Long Cun 龍村
Long, Guo-Cui 龍國粹
Lujiazui 陸家嘴
Luo, Zheng-Xiang 羅徵祥

Ma, Hai-De (= Hatem, George)
Mao, Tse-Tung (= Mao, Ze-Dong)
　毛澤東
Mao, Ze-Dong (= Mao, Tse-Tung)

Medical College of Nanjing
　Central University 南京中央大
　學醫學院
*Mei Ching* 脈經
Mei Fei San 麻沸散
mian bao 麵包
Military Thoracic Hospital 解放軍
　胸科醫院
Ming 明
Moukden Medical College 奉天
　(瀋陽) 醫學院
Mudanjiang Cardiovascular
　Institute 牡丹江心血管中心

Nanjing Gulou Hospital 南京鼓樓
　醫院
Nanjing 南京
National Shanghai Medical
　College 國立上海醫學院
Nationalist Party (= Guomin-
　dang)
New Fourth Army 新四軍
New Life Movement 新生活運動
Nie, Rong-Zhen 聶榮臻

Pan, Shao-Chuan 潘少川
Pan, Zhi 潘治
Pao Ting (= Baoding)
Peking Union Medical College
　(PUMC) 北京協和醫學院
Pudong 浦東

Qi Bo (= Ch'i Po) 歧伯
Qian, Zhong-Xi 錢中希
Qing 清
Qinghai 青海

Qiu, Fa-Zu 裘法祖

Renji Hospital (Shanghai) 上海仁濟醫院

Ruijin Hospital of the Shanghai Second Medical College 上海第二醫學院附屬瑞金醫院

Shandong Provincial Hospital 山東省醫院

Shandong 山東

*Shang Han Za Bing Lun* 傷寒雜病論

Shanghai Chest Hospital 上海胸科醫院

Shanghai Children's Medical Center 上海兒童醫學中心

Shanghai Fudan University 上海復旦大學

Shanghai Zhongshan Hospital 上海中山醫院

Shansi 山西

Shao, Ling-Fang 邵令方

She, Ya-Xiong 佘亞雄

Shen, Qiong 沈瓊

Shenyang 瀋陽

Shih, Mei-Xin (= Shih, Mei-Hsin) 石美鑫

Shih, Mei-Hsin (= Shi, Mei-Xin)

Shi-Ma-Tai 司馬台

Sian Incident (= Xi'an Incident)

Songjiazhuang 宋家莊

Su, Hong-Xi 蘇鴻熙

Su, Ying-Heng 蘇應衡

Su, Zhao-Kang 蘇肇伉

Sun, Han-Song 孫寒松

Sun, Jui Lung (= Sun Rui-Long)

Sun, Rui-Long (= Sun Jui Lung) 孫瑞龍

Sun, Shao-Qian 孫紹謙

Sun, Yan-Qing 孫衍慶

Sung-yen K'ou 松岩口

Taihang 太行

Taihu 太湖

Taishan 泰山

Taiyuan 太原

Tao, Shou-Chi (= Tao, Shou-Qi) 陶壽淇

Tao, Shou-Qi (= Tao, Shou-Chi)

Teochew 潮州

*The Pulse Classic* 脈經

Tian-An-Men 天安門

Tianjian Medical College 天津醫學院

Tin, Ka-Ping 田家炳

Tongji 同濟

Tongren Hospital (Shanghai) 同仁醫院

Tseng, Hsien-Chiu 曾憲九

Tsinghua 清華

Tung, Chen-Lang 董承琅

Wan, De-Xing 萬德星

Wan, Feng 萬峰

Wang, Da-Tong (= Wang, T. T.) 王大同

Wang, Shu-He 王叔和

Wang, T. T. (= Wang, Da-Tong)

Wang, Xin-Fang 王新房

Wang, Zeng-Wei 汪曾煒

Weng, Yu-Guo 翁渝國

Wu, Jie-Ping 吳階平
Wu, Qing-Yu 吳清玉
Wu, Shan-Fang 吳善芳
Wu, Wei-Zhong 吳維中
Wu, Xia 吳遐
Wu, Xian-Zhong 吳咸中
Wu, Y. K. (= Wu, Ying-Kai)
Wu, Ying-Kai (= Wu, Y. K.) 吳英愷
Wu, Zhen-Zhong 吳振中
Wu, Zhi-Zhong (= Wu, Chi-
　　Chong) 吳執中
Wuhan 武漢
Wuhu 蕪湖
Wutaishan 五臺山
Wuxi 無錫

Xi Cheng 西城
Xi'an 西安
Xi'an Incident (= Sian Incident)
　　西安事變
Xi'an Jiaotong University 西安交
　　通大學
Xi'an Medical University 西安醫
　　科大學
Xia, Qiu-Ming 夏求明
Xiamen 廈門
Xiao, Ming-Di 肖明第
Xie, Tao-Ying 謝陶瀛
Xijing Hospital (Xi'an) 西京
　　醫院
*Xindianxue Zazhi* 新電學雜誌
Xinhua Hospital of the Shanghai
　　Second Medical College 上海
　　第二醫學院附屬新華醫院

Xinjiang 新疆
Xinmin 新民
Xinqiao Hospital (Chongqing)
　　新橋醫院 (重慶)
Xu, Chun-Li 徐春棣
Xu, Le-tian 徐樂天
Xu, Zhi-Wei 徐志偉
Xu, Zhi-Yun 徐志雲
Xue, Gan-Xing 薛淦興

Yan'an 延安
Yang, Bi-Bo 楊碧波
Yang, Gui 楊貴
Yang, Wen-Xian 楊文獻
Yeung, C. K. 楊重光
Yu Yi-Fei 余翼飛
Yushan 玉山
Yuyao 餘姚

Zhang, Bao-Ren 張寶仁
Zhang, Chao-Mei 張超昧
Zhang, Ji-Zheng 張紀正
Zhang, Shi-Ze 張世澤
Zhang, Yu-De 張毓德
Zhang, Zhi-Tai 張志泰
Zhang, Zhong 張忠
Zhao, Qiang 趙強
Zhejiang 浙江
Zhengzhou University 鄭州大學
Zhou, Guan-Han 周冠漢
Zhou, Yun-Zhong 周允中
Zhu, De 朱德
Zhu, Min 朱敏
Zhu, Xiao-Dong 朱曉東